James Wherton
10-1-88

REVOLUTION
AT THE TABLE

HARVEY A. LEVENSTEIN

REVOLUTION AT THE TABLE

*The Transformation
of the American Diet*

New York ∗ *Oxford*
Oxford University Press
1988

Oxford University Press

Oxford   New York   Toronto
Delhi   Bombay   Calcutta   Madras   Karachi
Petaling Jaya   Singapore   Hong Kong   Tokyo
Nairobi   Dar es Salaam   Cape Town
Melbourne   Auckland
and associated companies in
Beirut   Berlin   Ibadan   Nicosia

Copyright © 1988 by Harvey A. Levenstein

Published by Oxford University Press, Inc.,
200 Madison Avenue, New York, New York 10016

Oxford is a registered trademark of Oxford University Press

Library of Congress Cataloging-in-Publication Data
Levenstein, Harvey A., 1938–
Revolution at the table.
Bibliography: p.   Includes index.
1. Food habits—United States—History.
2. Diet—United States—History. I. Title.
GT2853.U5L48   1988   394.1'2'0973   87-22006
ISBN 0-19-504365-0

2 4 6 8 10 9 7 5 3 1

Printed in the United States of America
on acid-free paper

To my sister, Esther

Preface

It is difficult to pinpoint how my interest in this topic evolved. My friends all assume that the book is related to my love of cooking and eating; indeed it has been difficult to disabuse some of them of the notion that it is some kind of weird cookbook. However, as a glance at its contents will show, it has virtually nothing to do with how to cook and only little more with how to eat. Moreover, although it does deal with the history of eating in America, it offers little in the way of vicarious gastronomic satisfaction by re-creating the delights (or horrors) of eating in the past. Rather than emerging from my own interest in eating, it derives much more from my interest in the question of why other people eat and in particular why and how they change or do not change their food habits. Perhaps the first thing that piqued this curiosity occurred in the late 1950s, when a study of G.I.s taken prisoner during the Korean War received widespread publicity. Among its disturbing conclusions was that many American P.O.W.s died of malnutrition-related diseases, not as a result of a deliberate policy on the part of their Chinese and Korean captors, but mainly because they refused to change their diets. The food in most P.O.W. camps approximated the military rations of their captors in quantity and nature. Those who died of nutrition-related ailments were often those who refused to eat much of it because they found it repellent. The Turkish and other American prisoners who ate all they were served survived at much greater rates.

This idea that although they certainly were not consciously willing their own deaths, some people would die rather than eat certain kinds of food has stuck in my mind thereafter, and it made me curious about how food habits do and do not change. Raising two children, one of whom was a "difficult" eater, further impressed upon me the essential conservatism of many people with regard to food. Yet, on the other hand, human food habits have changed over the eons, and it is likely that never have they changed so markedly and rapidly as during the past one hundred years, when industrialization and urbanization have transformed much of the world.

It is easy to ascribe most changes in food habits merely to different material conditions of life and to increased availability (or unavailability) of certain foodstuffs, but to do this is to forget those Korean P.O.W.s, or my daughter Lisa. Clearly, there is and always has been much more involved—considerations of class, status, religion, and, let us not forget, the physiology of taste. However, the modern world has also brought us another dimension, something which I find particularly fascinating: deliberate attempts to change the food habits of large numbers of people for secular purposes. Whether because of a desire to improve the lot of the poor, the health of the middle class, or the state of their own balance sheets, the past one hundred-odd years has seen an increasing number of people and forces trying to change popular eating habits. Some have succeeded and others have not. In combination with the forces changing the food supply, those who have succeeded have managed to change radically not just the food habits of the United States but of most of the modern industrialized world. To me it seems this transformation was substantially accomplished in a relatively short time: in the case of the United States in the fifty or so years between about 1880 and 1930. As we shall see, most of us would find it quite difficult to adjust to the eating habits of Americans of any class in 1880. We would find it even more difficult to stomach their ideas about food. However, transported back to 1930, we would find the essence of the ideas which still guide our food choices well established. I have tried to analyze the economic, social, and ideological forces, the complex interplay among networks of reformers, scientists, industrialists, faddists, and hucksters which brought about this change.

Today, when we see large numbers of people in the Third World go hungry while anthropologists and agronomists struggle to persuade them to change their food preferences and introduce crops deemed ecologically and nutritionally superior, this foray into the stories of those who tried to change the food habits of Americans cannot be completely irrelevant. Nor can reading about the large doses of misinformation which the scientists and other experts of the past passed off as nutritional science fail to temper our attitudes towards the advice of their contemporary successors. It might also do no harm for people such as the director of advertising for Pepsi-Cola, who recently boasted to *Adweek* that his firm had "made cola into a necktie product" by persuading people that "what you drank said something about who you were" (*The Times Literary Supplement,* Dec. 26, 1986), to realize that their apparent successes have historical roots. I also hope that the book adds to our understanding of other aspects of social history: women's history, labor history, history of medicine, history of social work, immigration history, even history of science. Most of all, however, I hope that it is "a good read."

This book represents a rather marked shift from my previous work, which dealt mainly with labor unions in the United States and Mexico, and a number of people deserve thanks for helping ease the transition by reaffirming that I was not embarking on some kind of frivolous venture. Royden Harrison and Tony Mason at the Centre for the Study of Social History in the University of Warwick, England, where I spent two very pleasant and stimulating years, created an atmosphere which encouraged me to think of working-class and social history in very broad terms. Alice Kessler-Harris, who was there during one of those years, was very encouraging and pointed out the relevance of my work to various facets of women's history. Jay Winter, now of Pembroke College, Cambridge University, opened up a whole new (for me) dimension of the topic by introducing me to the demographic literature on the subject. John Davis, now director of the Centre, was supportive and introduced me to Maurice Aymard, of the Maison des Sciences de l'Homme in Paris, who opened me up to new approaches to food history and put me in touch with a network of French social scientists interested in food and its history. In particular, Claude Fischler of the Centre National de Recherche Scientifique has been a great help. He has read and commented intelligently on much of my *oeuvre* in this *genre,* including large parts of this manuscript, making excellent suggestions and saving me from some rather serious *gaffes.*

Joe Conlin, my erstwhile collaborator on other food projects, has helped me in many ways, including making particularly apt (if devastating) comments on the first part of the book. (Indeed, I might reverse the usual procedure and say that any of the failings of the first two chapters are completely his responsibility.) Peter Lawson took time off from tracking the fates of Tudor criminals to initiate me into some of the mysteries of SPSS, feed the computer-analyzable data into the monster mainframe computer, overcome numerous glitches whose nature was beyond my comprehension, and help me make some sense of what emerged. My wife Mona read the first rambling drafts of the entire manuscript with an appropriately critical yet sympathetic eye, making excellent suggestions for excision and improvement. My daughters, Lisa and Monica, helped by being sensitive to the travail of writing and giving me a wide berth while I was upstairs staring blankly at the word processor. Lisa also helped me check footnotes and choose photographs during two very enjoyable days at the

Library of Congress. Monica (the "good eater") provided incisive analyses of late adolescent and teenage food habits and fads which kept me abreast of that topic.

Much of the research for this book was done in libraries such as the Library of Congress, the National Archives, the New York Public Library, the various Harvard University Libraries, Columbia University Libraries, Stanford University Libraries, the British Library, and the Boston Public Library whose size and nature hardly breed chuminess between readers and staff. Nevertheless, I cannot think of an occasion in which the staff I encountered in these institutions were not courteous and as helpful as they could be to me, even though I was unknown to them (and a foreign non-taxpayer to boot!) The staff at one of the smaller institutions, the Schlesinger Library at Radcliffe, were especially helpful. So have been the staff at the Hamilton Public Library and the McMaster University libraries. My particular thanks to the embattled women in the Interlibrary Loan department of Mills Library at McMaster, who have put up with my torrents of often-zany-sounding requests, as well as the occasional delay in returning material, with remarkable good humor.

The enthusiasm of Sheldon Meyer of Oxford University Press for this project was most encouraging, and Rachel Toor has been a fine editor: skilled, understanding, and supportive. I am also grateful to Sondra Beame, of Hamilton, who did such a fine job in preparing the index for my previous book, for taking on this one as well.

Much of the research for this book was funded by the Social Sciences and Humanities Research Foundation of Canada, supplemented by grants from the Nuffield Foundation of Great Britain and the McMaster University Arts Research Board. I would like to express my gratitude to all of them.

Some sections of this book have appeared elsewhere in articles I have published, and I would like to thank the following for permission to reprint portions of them: The American Studies Association, for "The New England Kitchen and the Origins of Modern American Eating Habits," *American Quarterly*, Vol. 32, No. 4 (Fall 1980); the Organization of American Historians, for " 'Best for Babies' or 'Preventable Infanticide'? The Controversy over Artificial Feeding of Infants in America, 1880–1920," *Journal of American History*, Vol. 70 (June 1983); and Presses Universitaires de Nancy, 25 rue Baron Luis, 54000 Nancy, France, for "The Servant Crisis and American Cookery," *La Revue Français d'Etudes Américaines*, Vol. 11, No. 27/28 (*fevrier* 1986).

Hamilton, Ontario, Canada   H.A.L.
January, 1987

Contents

REVOLUTION
AT THE TABLE

INTRODUCTION

The British-American Culinary Heritage

The United States may have won its political independence from Great Britain in 1783, but during the hundred-odd years that followed, Americans never liberated themselves from the British culinary heritage. Americans tended to eat more corn, pork, molasses, and indeed (according to nineteenth-century travelers from Britain) much more of everything than did the British. They drank more whiskey and cider but less ale and tea. In the grand scheme of things gastronomical, however, the American table remained what Louis Hartz claimed its polity to be: the product of a fragment of British culture.

Much about the edible flora and fauna of the Northern and Middle colonies was distinctive, and the semi-tropical South provided an abundance of foods that temperate Britain could not produce. And yet, as Waverley Root pointed out, the colonists "turned their backs on most of the new foods, often refusing to eat them until after Europe had accepted them and re-imported them to the land of their origin."[1] The potato and tomato, which originated in native American Indian civilizations just to the south of them some millennia before, reached Anglo-America late in the eighteenth century, only after gaining grudging approval in Britain. Colonials accepted the pumpkins of the New World because they resembled European squash. Indian corn was integrated into the colonial diet mainly out of necessity: strains of European wheat did not begin to adapt to and thrive in America until the later eighteenth century, and wheat

3

remained expensive until the 1820s and 1830s. On the other hand, the colonials imported as many plants and seeds from Britain as they could, including their beloved apple trees, which flourished in the New World.[2]

British-American culinary conservatism can hardly be ascribed to the universally high regard with which British cuisine has been held, even by the British. (As Alistair Cooke has remarked, "A Briton telling an American about cooking is like the blind leading the one-eyed.") And yet, Americans manifested a remarkable degree of resistance to the culinary influence of other cultures. Even before independence, waves of immigrants from Europe and Africa washed onto America's shores, but left few traces of their cuisines on the American table. This continued to be the case after 1783, even though the proportion of immigrants of non-British origin rose. Then, only the Germans could be said to have substantially influenced American cooking, and they were Northern Europeans whose cuisine resembled that of the British.[3]

Vegetarian crusades of the 1830s and 1840s, inspired by Romantic and Puritanical notions, faced an enormous challenge, for people on both sides of the British North Atlantic were carnivores of the first order. Jean-Jacques Rousseau, a romantic with profound vegetarian leanings, found evidence for his contention that meat was the brutish food *par excellence* in the fact that the British loved it so.[4] Before the 1860s, pork was consumed in such large quantities in America that wags often suggested that the United States be rechristened "The Republic of Porkdom." Yet beef reigned supreme in status. "We are essentially a hungry *beef-eating* people, who live by eating," proclaimed a proud mid-nineteenth-century American frontier newspaper.[5] Poultry and lamb were also held in high esteem in both nations, and raised breads, made of wheat, rye, oats and other grains, constituted, if not quite the traditional "staff of life," at least the staple filler. Porridges made from a variety of grains also provided sustenance, and puddings and pies containing a wide variety of meats and other foods were popular favorites.

On the other hand, consumption of vegetables and fruits was limited, relative to present-day standards. Like their counterparts in Britain, early New Englanders thought of vegetables as sauces to accompany meats, much in the way applesauce accompanies pork today, and they commonly referred to them as "garden sass." By the middle of the nineteenth century the potato and the cabbage were the predominant vegetables. Peas, beans, turnips, and onions joined them on the table with some regularity, but were served in relatively small portions. While lettuce was much appreciated among a small segment of the social elite attuned to the popularity of green salads dressed with oil and vinegar in France (it was called "French salad" in America),[6] green and leafy vegetables were generally disdained. Other vegetables, such as tomatoes, were used mainly as condiments and were served in even smaller quantities. Root vegetables were as often grown for fodder as for human consumption. An 1879 cookbook admonished Americans "to realize the wealth of green food abounding in their gardens and fields, which they have too long abandoned to their beasts of burden."[7]

Apples remained the most common fruit. The belief that they had medicinal properties was well-established by the nineteenth century. *Hall's Journal of Health* advised families to maintain a supply of at least two to ten barrels of apples, for they had "an admirable effect on the general system, often removing constipation, correcting acidities, and cooling off febrile conditions, more effectually than the most approved medicines." If Americans substituted them for pies, cakes, candies, and other sweets, "there would be a diminution in the sum total of doctors' bills in a single year."[8]

The narrow range of foods consumed by most British-Americans before the mid-nineteenth century has led many modern observers to remark on the monotony of their gastronomic lives.[9] Contemporary critics, however, rarely remarked on this. Rather, many deplored its binding nature. The enormous amounts of meat and starch and the short shrift given to fresh fruits and vegetables made constipation the national curse of the first four or five decades of the nineteenth century in America.

As for the ways in which these foods were prepared, the major characteristic was an overwhelming heaviness. The favored method for preparing meat was to roast large fatty joints. Big chunks of meat or whole fowls were also boiled, but boiling was particularly popular for preparing vegetables, which were often subjected to this treatment for hours before being mashed into paste. It was commonly thought that the only way to rid potatoes of their supposed poisonous qualities was to boil them for extended periods of time. Foods fried in large quantities of lard or butter were also well appreciated, particularly in America.

Stewing, which elsewhere called for smaller pieces of meat, more seasonings, and the addition of a variety of vegetables, was not well regarded, particularly if the outcome was highly seasoned. The British upper classes spiced their food and beverages formidably until the mid-1660s, but by the late seventeenth and eighteenth century a modicum of restraint had gained the upper hand. Salt and small amounts of pepper, cloves, cinnamon, mace, ginger, nutmeg, and a few herbs were the main British/American seasonings.

A relatively light hand with spices continued to characterize cooking in both countries during the nineteenth century. Not only were spicy foods blamed for inducing a craving for alcohol, many people shared the notion of antebellum American food reformer Sylvester Graham that they stimulated inordinate appetites for sex. Thus, although intrepid sailors, businessmen, and soldiers of both countries now roamed the world, only occasionally were the exotic spices and herbs of the non-Northern European world adopted in sufficient quantities to add more than, say, the minor titillation which a touch of "curry powder" gave to a bland white sauce.

Although today's reconstructed herb gardens of any number of ersatz "pioneer villages" demonstrate that many herbs were grown, they were used mainly for medicinal rather than culinary purposes. An 1873 article on "potherbs," that is, those used for imparting taste in cooking, in *Godey's Lady's Book and Magazine* discussed only parsley, sage, thyme, marjoram, mint, and savory, remarking that the last was seldom used.[10] Herbs "should be used in small quantities and only by those who require a stimulant," warned *The Ladies' Magazine* in 1833.[11] Needless to say, the glorious garlic bulb was little known and regarded with a mixture of horror and awe. "Gar-licks," said one of America's first cookbooks in the early nineteenth century, "though used by the French, are better adapted to medicine than cooking."[12]

Spices were more common in desserts, for when sweetness was involved Anglo-American taste buds lost their delicate sensitivity. Particularly after 1750, the two nations seem to have shared the Atlantic world's greatest sweet tooth, with America running second only to Britain in per capita consumption of sugar.[13] By the mid-nineteenth century, falling prices for cane and beet sugars encouraged soaring consumption of these sweeteners among all classes. British "puddings," originally main course fare, now became progressively sweeter and more diverse, mutating into an incredible variety of hot, cold, baked and steamed puddings, pies, tarts, creams, molds, charlottes, bettys, fools, syllabubs, junkets, and ices.[14] These recipes were avidly imitated in the United States. In 1879, when 175 genteel women of Virginia pooled their favorite recipes into a cookbook, over one-third of the book consisted of recipes for desserts, including separate chapters not only for cakes and pies but also for icing, gingerbread, pudding sauces, fritters and pancakes, ice cream and frozen custard, jellies, fruit desserts, preserves and fruit jellies, as well as thirty-six pages of pudding recipes, and another long chapter devoted to jelly, blanc-mange, Charlotte russe, baked custard, creams, and various other desserts.[15]

Many of these concoctions used heavy doses of cinnamon, cloves, ginger, and mace to complement a level of sweetness which would set many a modern amalgam filling to screaming. The Beecher sisters, Catharine and Harriet Beecher Stowe, condemned the American taste for over-spiced "heavy sweets," and put the blame squarely on their "phlegmatic ancestors," the English. "Witness the national recipe for plum pudding," they wrote. "Take a pound of every indigestible substance you can think of, boil into a cannon-ball, and serve in flaming brandy."[16]

Sweetness also served to counter the blandness or excessive saltiness of many so-called savory dishes. Sweet or sweet and sour condiments were particularly popular as accompaniments for meats, and as sugar prices declined in the nineteenth century they soared in popularity. Cucumbers, onions, and other vegetables were preserved in sugar, salt, and vinegar. Tomatoes and mushrooms were boiled down with sugar, salt, pepper, and vinegar to produce "catsup." The result was a cuisine which, even excluding desserts, relied more on sweetness than did any other major cuisine in the world.[17]

To nineteenth-century observers, the major differences between the American and British diets could usually be summed up in one word: abundance. Virtually every foreign visitor who wrote about American eating habits expressed amazement, shock, and even disgust at the quantity of food consumed. In his description of mid-century America the English novelist Anthony Trollope warned English readers to bear in mind "that 10,000 or 40,000 inhabitants in an American town . . . is a number which means much more than would be implied by any similar number as to an old town in Europe. Such a population in America would consume double the amount of beef which it would in England . . . ."[18] Long before Americans' overflowing self-serve "salad bars," "all-you-can-eat buffets," and "smorgs" came to symbolize to overseas visitors an obsession with quantity, the groaning boards of America's hotels struck Europeans the same way. Unlike most of their European counterparts, the hotels which spread out across the country in the 1840s and 1850s included meals in their prices, the so-called "American Plan," and they vied with each other to make the "boards" upon which their food was served literally groan. The enormous breakfasts aroused particular comment. The Englishman Thomas Hamilton's first encounter with an American breakfast, in a New York City hotel, was a table "loaded with solid viands of all descriptions . . . while, in the occasional intervals, were distributed dishes of rolls, toast and cakes of buckwheat and Indian corn." Had it not been early morning, he would easily have mistaken it for a dinner table.[19]

Even later in the century, when dishes came to be ordered from menus, the apparent indifference of American hotel patrons to wasting food struck Europeans as a product of its abundance in America. "The thing which strikes me most disagreeably . . . is the sight of the tremendous waste of food that goes on at every meal," wrote a European recalling his sojourns in nineteenth-century American hotels. "There are rarely fewer than fifty different dishes on the *menu* at dinner time. Every day at every meal you see people order three or four times as much of this food as they could under any circumstance eat, and picking at and spoiling one dish after another, send the bulk away uneaten."[20] Actually, his estimate of fifty choices on the *menus* was rather low. Two authors in a subsequent issue of the same magazine refer to dinner menus of one hundred and ten items and breakfast menus with at least seventy-five, while the dinner menu of the New York City Brevoort House hotel for an ordinary Thursday some years earlier, in November 1867, listed a choice of 145 items.[21]

Critics of American cooking often blamed abundance for encouraging poor preparation. The Englishwoman Frances Trollope, a caustic critic of American manners during the Jacksonian era, was impressed by the "excellence, abundance, and cheapness" of the food in the market in Cincinnati, where she lived. However, she thought that this abundance contributed to sloppy preparation and that "the ordinary mode of living was abundant but not delicate."[22] The Beecher sisters declared the American table to be inferior to that of France and England because "it presents a fine abundance of material, carelessly and poorly treated. The management of food is nowhere in the world, perhaps, more slovenly and wasteful. Everything betokens that want of care that waits on abundance."[23] "In no other land," wrote Juliet Corson, the genteel head of the New York Cooking School in 1879, "is there such a profusion of food, and certainly in none is so much wasted from sheer ignorance, and spoiled by bad cooking."[24]

Many were struck by the American attachment to the frying pan and the consequent greasiness of American foods. "To a gentleman with a keen appetite, the *coup d'oeil* of the dinner table was far from unpleasing," wrote Hamilton of a typical American hotel dinner. "The number of dishes was very great. The style of cooking neither French nor English, though certainly approaching nearer to the latter than to the former." However, "the dressed dishes were decidedly bad, the sauces being composed of little else than liquid grease." Only the sheer multitude of dishes enabled him to discover "some unobjectionable viands," proving again the wisdom of the old adage, "in the multitude of counsellors there is wisdom."[25]

Abundance also seemed to breed a vague indifference to food, manifested in a tendency to eat and run, rather than to dine and savor. For the American man, said Chevalier, "meal time is not . . . a period of relaxation, in which his mind seeks repose in the bosom of his friends; it is only a disagreeable interruption of business, an interruption to which he yields because it cannot be avoided, but which he abridges as much as possible."[26] The national motto, according to one European, was "Gobble, gulp, and go."[27] Foreigners often remarked on the eerie silence that reigned at American dinner tables, as diners seemed to concentrate on getting the tiresome burden of stuffing themselves out of the way in as short a time as possible. Charles Dickens found American banquets funereal and stupefyingly boring. Judging from the silence, he said, one would think the diners were assembled to lament the passing of a dear friend, rather than to joyfully contribute to their own survival.[28] "In my neighborhood there was no conversation," recalled the genial Hamilton of a typical hotel dining room. "Each individual seemed to *pitchfork* his food down his gullet, without the smallest attention to the wants of his neighbor."[29]

But generalizations about national food habits can go just so far before they run aground on the rocks of class as well as regional differences. Not all Americans were stuck in the British culinary rut, neither were all the British. Moreover, by 1880, in both Britain and America, the old ways were being challenged by new ideas regarding how and what people should eat.

CHAPTER 1

The American Table in 1880: The Tastes of the Upper Crust

By 1880, upper-class Americans had discovered, as had their British counterparts, the delights of fare more sophisticated than their national cuisine. In the years since the outbreak of the Civil War, the ranks and fortunes of the very wealthy in America had grown enormously. Fueled by Civil War bonanzas and the rapidly accruing profits of industrial and commercial expansion, businessmen in post-Civil War America had amassed fortunes unheard of among the wealthiest of the antebellum elite. Awash in wealth, the new upper class steamrolled through the older elite of more modest resources, marrying its daughters, buying its properties, and casting aside the simpler, more "republican" tastes and manners of previous generations. In their view, a new "Age of Elegance" was being inaugurated.[1]

Their own culinary heritage may have been abundant, but it had little in the way of elegance to offer, so they turned to Europe, in particular to the cuisine and dining manners of France. The French tradition was by no means a mystery to the American elite. French food had been synonymous with elegance and sophistication in America long before the Civil War. Many Americans, among them Thomas Jefferson, had returned from travels in Europe with a reverence for French food. French chefs had migrated to New Orleans in the early 1800s, exerting a lasting influence on that city's cuisine, and some of New York City's finer hotels hired French chefs shortly thereafter.[2] Since its founding in 1832, Delmonico's restaurant in New York City functioned as a major beachhead of French food, stimulating an appreciation among the Northeastern elite. The rush of gold-seekers to San Francisco after 1849 also sparked a rush of French chefs to the Bay Area as newly rich miners bought a taste of the elegant life symbolized by French cuisine.[3]

However, the taste for French food never entered the mainstream. Jefferson enjoyed his fine French foods and wines in private, but avoided proselytizing it as he did so many other of his whims. New Orleans developed a wonderful variation on French cooking but it remained a regional cuisine, affecting the national diet hardly at all. Delmonico's spawned a number of antebellum imitators, but together they influenced only a small number of the elite, mainly New Yorkers.

There was not merely an indifference to French food. As Whig politico Thurlow Weed wrote, there was a general prejudice against "fancy French cooking."[4] He and his party successfully exploited this in defeating the New York Jacksonian Martin Van Buren in his bid for re-election to the presidency in 1840. Van Buren's weakness for French food—denoted by his hiring a French chef for the White House—was used against him in a smear campaign labeling him an aristocrat intent on the restoration of monarchy. The Whig candidate, William Henry Harrison, was extolled as living on "raw beef and salt." Middle-class cookbook authors who tried to apply lessons learned from the French to American cooking were defensive about it. In their household manual, the Beecher sisters pleaded that they should be able to take some leaves from foreign books "without accusations of foreign foppery." Their suggestions that American housewives serve smaller, more attractive looking cuts of meat were met with "Oh! We can't give time here in America to go into niceties and French whim-whams."[5] In her 1877 cookbook, Juliet Corson felt compelled to defend herself against the charge that undue preference was being given to foreign ways of cooking by citing the thriftiness of French cooking.[6]

These defenses were of simple French *bourgeois* cuisine, with its economical *pot au feu* and scrap-ingesting stockpots, rather than the *haute cuisine* of Delmonico's and the *beau monde* of Paris. Yet it was the latter cuisine that now inspired the American upper classes, eagerly taking their cues from the French capital. Paris was the "headquarters of elegance," said America's best-selling etiquette book in 1884.[7] "We have imitated whatever we have considered wisest and pleasantest in the habits of the French, English, and other nations," said another handbook on etiquette, but particularly those of the French, whose ways were "less heavy and more graceful" than those of the English.[8]

The results, in terms of public dining habits, are well known: meals of not just the traditional enormous proportions but of great sophistication as well. A dinner for thirty given in 1880 at Delmonico's in honor of General Winfield Scott Hancock, soon to be the Democratic party's standard-bearer in that year's presidential election, was typical of this genre.

The meal began, as most did, with raw oysters, whose abundance and popularity at that time made them perhaps the closest thing to a classless food.[9] A choice of two soups was followed by an *hors d'oeuvre* and then a fish course. The preliminaries thus dispensed with, the *Relevés*, saddle of lamb and *filet* of beef, were then carved and served. These were followed by the *Entrées*, chicken wings with green peas and lamb chops garnished with beans and mushroom-stuffed artichokes. Then came Terrapin *en casserole à la Maryland*, some *sorbet* to clear the palate followed by the "Roast" course, canvas-back ducks and quail. For dessert, or rather desserts, there was *timbale Madison*, followed by an array of ice creams, whipped creams, jellied dishes, banana mousse, and the elaborate confectionery constructions so beloved by the French pastry chefs of the day, made to be a feast for the eye, rather than the palate. Fruit and *petits fours* were then placed on the table while coffee and liqueurs were served. With the exception of the canvas-back duck, all the foods were prepared in a distinctly French fashion and labeled in French.[10]

When unrestrained by the kind of political exigencies that may have dictated that this meal should have a relatively American flavor, Delmonico's meals were indistinguishable from the finest Paris had to offer. Two months after the Hancock dinner chef Charles Ranhofer prepared a dinner for 230 in honor of the great canal-builder Ferdinand DeLesseps. For this occasion, truffles went into the *timbales* and covered the *pâté de foie gras*, the number of *entreés*, all from French cuisine, multiplied, and exotic imported pineapples capped an imposing array of desserts.[11]

To the modern reader, the most striking aspect of these menus is, of course, the sheer volume of food. To the obvious question: Did people actually eat all the food placed before them?, the answer would seem to be that most of it was indeed consumed. There is no evidence, for example, of the thriving industry which arose in nineteenth-century Paris to dispose of the monumental amounts of leftovers from the tables of the very rich by selling them to the poor.[12] While one must give credence to foreigners' remarks on the amount of food left on American hotel and restaurant tables, the photographs of men attending these formal dinners provide ample evidence that they did not merely peck at their food. Row upon row of rotund white-clad bellies protrude from black jackets, crowned at the apex with eye-catching silver or gold watch chains, clear indications that girth and appetite were sources of pride.

Women were expected to be daintier eaters. The thought of women indulging in any kind of physical passion to excess alarmed Victorians, and a modicum of gastronomic restraint was therefore expected. Nevertheless, by our standards their appetites and figures were both large. Plumpness was widely regarded, by health experts and connoisseurs of female aesthetics alike, as a sign of good health. Rather than churning out starvation diets, health experts and faddists wrote books such as *How to Be*

Plump, which recommended eating starchy foods, fats, and sweets in order to achieve what the author (an M.D. as well as a homeopath) called "florid plumpness."[13]

Contemporary fashion complemented this with clothes that emphasized and distorted ample busts and bottoms. In the 1880s, the so-called "voluptuous woman" became the ideal.[14] Stage star Lillian Russell, "airy, fairy, Lillian, the American Beauty"—after whom America's favorite rose was named—whose hourglass (while corsetted) figure with its ample hips and very full bosom was the late nineteenth-century ideal, weighed about two hundred pounds.[15] Her enormous appetite was almost as legendary as her beauty, even challenging the rather latitudinarian Victorian ideas regarding female restraint at the table. Young Oscar Tschirky, who was later to exercise his own kind of mastery over the world of fashion as *maître d'hôtel* at the Waldorf, took a job at Delmonico's largely because Russell, whom he worshipped from afar, dined there three or four times a week. Finally placed in charge of the private dining rooms, he at last had his chance to serve her while she dined with "Diamond" Jim Brady, who also had an impressive appetite. Alas, Tschirky later told his biographer, "I had the surprise and disillusionment of my lifetime. Lillian Russell ate more than Diamond Jim."[16]

It has been suggested that corpulence is regarded as attractive in societies characterized by food scarcity.[17] But this makes the vogue of voluptuousness all the more puzzling, for nineteenth-century Americans were little concerned by food shortages. Indeed, quite the reverse was true. As David Potter pointed out some years ago, their self-image was that of "people of plenty."[18] More to the point would seem to be Thorstein Veblen's suggestion that the upper classes engaged in "conspicuous consumption" to distinguish themselves from those lower on the socioeconomic scale.[19] This emphasis on consumption patterns as the mark of status represented a distinct change from the past. Except, perhaps, in the South, with its fictionalized ideal of a chivalric landed gentry, the century's previous generations of well-off Americans were presumed to have gained their status through contributions to the productive process, and their tables were expected to reflect this straightforwardness of purpose and achievement. The two most influential domestic economy writers of the pre-Civil War era, Sarah Hale and Catharine Beecher, strongly disapproved of excessive displays of consumption and leisure even in upper-class households. "In giving dinners, avoid ostentation, which will not only be very expensive, but will make your guests uncomfortable," wrote Hale. "To ensure a well-dressed dinner, provide enough, and beware of the common practice of having too much. The table had better appear rather bare than crowded with dishes not wanted," she advised.[20] Beecher admonished American upper-class women against imitating the languorous attitude of the English aristocracy towards the home, warning that it led to melancholia and other forms of "mental distress."[21] Entreaties of this sort were ignored and rejected by the postbellum rich. By 1880, nowhere did Ray Ginger's label, the "Age of Excess," apply more aptly than to the consumption patterns of the rich, and nowhere was it more appropriate than as a label for the way they consumed food.

In a country characterized by relative abundance of food, conspicuous consumption would have to consist of much more than just eating large quantities. The food would have to be prepared and served in ways only those in the highest echelons could afford. The cuisine of the French upper class of the Second Empire, as adapted by the *haute bourgeoisie* of the Third Republic, fit this bill admirably. Here was a cuisine whose basic ingredients were not exotic to most Americans, but behind whose elaborate methods of preparation, foreign code-words, and complex dining rituals the wealthy could find refuge from those trying to scale the ramparts of their newly acquired status.

It is interesting that Tschirky was disillusioned by Lillian Russell's gluttony, for as maître d' at the Waldorf he went on to play an important role in helping the social elite develop a code of dining by which they would distinguish their eating habits from those of *parvenu* millionaires such as Jim Brady and *demi-monde* successes such as Russell. And an elaborate code was necessary, for by 1880 New York City had emerged as the nation's arbiter of elite tastes and manners. The wealthy upper class of the rapidly expanding metropolis was now involved in a vicious scramble for social status resulting in a veritable orgy of display and entertainment. Elaborate and expensive dinner parties featuring *haute cuisine* were major weapons in the social armory. Chefs imported from France struggled to outdo each other at the dinner tables of massive new mansions. Delmonico's and its competitors provided other venues for well-heeled forays in what could be called the Wars of Entertainment. One dinner party at Delmonico's in the early 1880s, for which a thirty-foot-long artificial lake—complete with live swans—was constructed as the centerpiece, cost its genial host $10,000. Remarking on the great post-Civil War strides in extravagant entertainment, Ward McAllister, a syncophant anointed by Mrs. William Astor as the social arbiter of the 1880s and 1890s, noted that in 1862 New York City was so backward that "there were not more than one or two men in New York who spent, in living and entertaining, over sixty thousand dollars a year. There were not more than half a dozen *chefs* in private families in this city."[22]

By *chefs,* of course, McAllister meant French *chefs,* and to demonstrate their superiority he once arranged a kind of cook-off between a renowned Southern black cook and a French *chef.* Together they cooked different dishes for a dinner of sixty in Newport. While acknowledging that "both were great artists in their way," McAllister declared that "the *chef* came off very much the victor" because of the superior refinement of French cooking. "The *chef*," he said, was "an educated, cultivated artist," while the black cook merely possessed "a wonderful natural taste, and the art of making things savory, i.e. taste good."[23]

The art of making things taste good was not enough for *chefs* because their clientele possessed the most cultivated of tastes. People like Jim Brady and Lillian Russell liked things that merely tasted good, and could polish off ten pounds of Southern fried chicken with the same gusto as they attacked a plate of *foie gras*. Only the truly elegant could appreciate the superior sophistication of French food. Francophilic attitudes also encouraged sneering at much of non-French European cooking, particularly that of central, eastern, and southern Europe. Germany was "a land . . . whose kitchen is an abomination to all other nations," wrote America's foremost etiquette authority of the 1880s. "Not that one does not get an excellent dinner at a German hotel in a great city. But all the cooks are French."[24]

The ascendancy of French cooking is evident in many of the menus that survive from the upper and upper-middle-class hotels of the postwar era. In the late 1860s and early 1870s they tended to be mainly English/American in their offerings and language, with only an occasional French touch. By the mid- and late 1870s, however, a wholesale invasion of French terms and French dishes was under way.[25] The change was evident even in boom towns on the gold and silver mining frontiers. Like their Bay Area predecessors, when miners struck it rich, or believed they were going to, they celebrated their entry into the upper class with French *haute cuisine*. Thus, by the mid-1870s, towns such as Tombstone, Arizona, Virginia City, Nevada, and Georgetown, Colorado, boasted fine French restaurants. The Hotel de Paris restaurant in Georgetown even attracted such customers as Denver-based financier and *gourmet* Jay Gould, who assembled parties of friends to take the narrow-gauge railroad up to the town just for a fine French meal.[26] This was despite the fact that Denver itself boasted at least six restaurants serving *haute cuisine*, including the famed Carpiot's, "the Delmonico's of the West."[27]

Imitation of the French could go just so far, however. The American upper class drew the line at the traditional American breakfast. Instead of accepting the French repast of breads and butter washed down with coffee or tea,[28] hotels at the elite's favorite watering places continued to offer breakfast menus of beefsteak, broiled chicken, broiled salmon and other fish, liver and bacon, kidneys, lamb chops, tripe, clams, omelettes, cold cuts, many kinds of potatoes, beans, breads, and so on.[29] Even in the Children and Nurses' dining room of the Grand Union Hotel in Saratoga an array of rolls, breads, and hot cereals followed by beefsteak, mutton chops, ham, fresh fish, liver and bacon, codfish cakes, boiled or scrambled eggs, kidneys, corned beef hash, tripe, clams, and various kinds of potatoes was served.[30]

There were attempts to make breakfast a more genteel event, at least in some upper-class homes. The habit of sleeping late often pushed breakfast into the late morning, turning it into something like our "brunch." Mary Sherwood's popular etiquette book gave a prescription for one of these "family breakfasts" in 1884:

> Flowers should be placed everywhere in summer. The napkins, silver and glass and china should be spotless; the butter should be golden, the honey fragrant and fine, and the fresh rolls delicious, the coffee clear and the tea strong. Fruit should be served when in season; berries and cream, peaches and cream, and all the hot cakes. Broiled chicken, fried eggs, beefsteaks, which our omnivorous people demand should be had for the asking. Finger bowls should be within reach, and the favorite beverage, ice water, should be particularly attended to. In our very prolific fruit seasons, to begin with a melon and end with a peach is a good "Alpha and Omega."[31]

For some years, in the early 1880s, it became fashionable to entertain guests at these relatively informal meals, particularly in the summer at places like Newport, where the men could be spared the affliction of evening dress and arrive in lawn tennis or hunting suits and the women could wear "morning dresses." Then, game, veal cutlets, sweetbreads, and *pâté de foie gras* were commonly served as well.[32]

If "conspicuous consumption" was the hallmark of upper-class life, nowhere was it more apparent than in the way they entertained each other at their own dinner tables. As the historian Samuel Eliot Morison, who was raised in the innermost of Boston's elite circles in the 1880s and 1890s, wrote: "the social flavor of that period was expressed largely in dining out. People were always giving dinner parties or going to friends' dinners; and these affairs, from our standpoint, were characterized by an excessive amount of food; eight courses seem to have been considered the proper thing."[33]

The new emphasis on dining was accompanied by a new method of serving. Serving *à la Russe* had swept the dining rooms of the British and French elites in the 1850s and 1860s and became fashionable in the United States in the 1870s. Instead of placing a goodly number of dishes on the table at once, with the host carving and serving them while guests helped themselves from other dishes placed around the table, a butler carved and served each course at a sideboard, arranging it attractively on individual plates or platters from which servants would then serve the guests. Menu cards (usually in French) faced each diner, informing them of what lay ahead (and in front) of them. Not only did this method allow the hosts to devote more time to charming conversation with their guests, it also drew attention to the quality and sophistication of the individual dishes. "Dish after dish comes round, as if by magic," enthused one fan of the new system, "and nothing remains but to eat and be happy."[34]

The new fascination with sophisticated food helped to move the hour at which dinner, the main meal, was served well into the evening. Before the 1870s, dinner time varied but was usually in the early or mid-afternoon. Tea and supper were generally taken in late afternoon and evening. However, once dinner parties became the centerpiece for entertaining guests, it made more sense to stage them in the evening, particularly in America, where upper-class males liked at least to appear to be engaging in productive activities during the day.[35]

Dinners were not the only occasions for impressive spreads of food and beverages. Upper-class women also hosted sumptuous lunches and elaborate teas. When Morison's grandmother's chapter of the Daughters of the American Revolution lunched at her house, the ladies were treated to, among other things, chartreuse of grouse, creamed oysters, lobster farci, turkey salad, fourteen dozen sandwiches, and three and a half gallons of ice cream and water ice.[36] Teas were served around 5:00 p.m. and ranged from relatively simple affairs, calling for an array of thin sandwiches and cakes, to "high teas." The latter were given on Sundays in cities or on any day in country "watering places," and included such items as scalloped oysters, fried chicken, partridge, mushrooms on toast, *pâté de foie gras,* and thin-sliced cold ham.[37]

By 1880, the prodigalities of the American upper class at their tables were regarded as remarkable even among French chefs, who were by no means easily impressed in those matters. One chef wrote of "the Americans, those robust gourmets who, newly arrived in the arena, have nevertheless made remarkable progress, in cooking as well as gastronomy. But the luxuries of the table in that country of voracious appetites have assumed such extraordinary proportions as to make one involuntarily think of the famous excesses of the feasts of Ancient Rome."[38]

Although they might wrinkle their noses behind their patrons' backs, the new prodigality proved to be a boon to French chefs, who found themselves in increasing demand in America. In 1883, the Hoffman House Hotel in New York City hired the head chef of the famous *Café des Anglais* in Paris, formerly chef to the Rothschilds, for the then astronomical salary of $300 a month.[39] It also meant a greater demand for servants. By removing the array of bowls and platters that had formerly cluttered dining tables, *service à la Russe* allowed tables to be decorated with elaborate centerpieces and an astonishing array of glassware, silver, and devilishly clever devices for extracting, seasoning, and eating the wide variety of foods served.[40] These were set and removed with great care by teams of servants and then cleaned, scrubbed, and polished. "Nowhere has the growth of luxury in this country been more apparent than in the pomp and circumstance which now accompanies modern dinners," wrote a proud contemporary commentator.[41] Morison, commenting on his family's dinner parties, wrote that "even with the abundant domestic staffs of that era, supplemented by 'accommodators' on dinner nights, there must have been an appalling amount of planning by the lady of the house, and cooking, serving, and dishwashing by the servants." His grandmother's notes for her D.A.R. lunch contained the notation "Had one extra cook. Two extra waitresses, two women to clean up, two men to move furniture, two carpenters to take off the doors."[42]

The lines separating the classes were no clearer in 1880 than they are today, and the imaginary dividing line between the upper class and the upper-middle class is impossible to plot with any precision. It is doubly difficult in the case of food, for in societies characterized by considerable social mobility, there is often a tendency for those lower on the social order to try to emulate the food habits of those above them by eating the same foods. However, a line of demarcation can be found in service; in the higher economic strata the number and quality of servants probably played a more important role than the cost of ingredients in determining what people could and could not serve.

The number of servants in an upper-middle- or middle-class household varied, of course, with family size, income, region, personal inclination, and other factors. However, while upper-class families generally had at least four or five servants, upper-middle-class families usually got along with three or four.[43] Middle-class families, particularly in larger cities, tended to have one or two servants, especially during the woman's child-bearing years. Relatively few middle-class families seem to have been able to operate on a servantless basis. By 1880, almost one-quarter of all urban and suburban households employed at least one servant.[44] One of the most popular middle-class housekeeping manuals of the 1880s, a fiction-alized account of a young couple setting out to economize, claimed that by adopting a variety of housekeeping economies a young couple could live on ten dollars a week for housekeeping. Yet even there, the housewife supervised a German immigrant maid ("a thick, short, strong but stupid-looking girl") hired for ten dollars a month.[45]

The fact that the middle class could afford fewer servants than the upper class, and that their servants normally had less training and skill, inevitably affected the preparation and serving of food in the household. Rare was the middle-class household that could afford a cook versed in French cuisine. Thus, for the most part, upper-middle- and middle-class house-hold cooking remained stolidly Anglo-Saxon American. Roast meats, scal-loped dishes, thick gravies—simple recipes that could be mastered by the succession of immigrant cooks under the watchful eye of the housewife remained the backbone of the cuisine.

Still, by 1880 technological change was enabling the middle-class kitch-en to widen its culinary horizons. Iron stoves and ranges replaced the open hearths which had been the mainstay of cooking until just before the Civil War. These new coal- and wood-burning monsters opened up vast new possibilities in the kitchen, making it possible to regulate heat more precisely and cook a number of sophisticated dishes simultaneously. An astounding outpouring of new utensils, mainly metal, also helped. In her 1880 cookbook for middle-class families Maria Parloa, generally an advocate of restraint in cooking and dining, listed ninety-three different utensils as "essential" for a kitchen. Along with a whip churn, melon mold, jagging iron, larding needle, apple corer, and squash strainer, among the essentials were no less than forty-four pots and pans to be used for cooking.[46]

Armed with new technology, the middle classes were able to use their kitchens and dining rooms in the never-ending struggle to secure or elevate their often shaky status. Dinner parties at home became the vogue. If one could not rival the Astors in elaborate cooking, one could still impress one's guests with expensive ingredients. Middle-class dinner parties were not places to cut corners on the family budget. The finest cuts of beef and game, exotic seafoods and fruits, served in large quantities, were expected to grace the dinner table when guests were present. When Maria Parloa suggested an "economical" meal in her popular 1881 cookbook for the middle class, it still featured fillet of beef—as expensive a cut then as now—as the *pièce de résistance.* Her assurances that a meal for twelve need not cost more than twenty-five dollars does not smack of penny pinching. Ten dollars a week was a good wage for a semi-skilled worker in 1881, and laborers in the iron and cotton mills of upstate New York earned about a dollar a day.[47]

Still, in 1880, middle-class food was only beginning to reflect the ascendancy of French food in the class above. While the straightforward simplicity of the likes of Catharine Beecher and Sarah Hale was beginning to seem outmoded to those in tune with the latest trends, the newer advocates of "fancy cooking" (normally meaning watered-down French *haute cuisine*) had not yet made a deep impression on the middle classes. "Talleyrand said England was a country with twenty-four religions and only one sauce," wrote one cookbook author in 1881. "He might have said two sauces, and he would have been literally right as regards both England and America. Everything is served with brown sauce or white sauce. And how often the white sauce is like bookbinder's paste, the brown a bitter, tasteless brown mess."[48]

Cooking schools aimed at middle-class housewives who wanted to learn how to cook (or rather to supervise cooks) and entertain in the new manner were becoming a feature of big city life, but the most successful generally concentrated on mainstream Anglo-American cookery, with only occasional forays into *haute cuisine.* Maria Parloa's suggested "bills of fare" for entertaining would seem to reflect the new middle-class aspirations quite well. A typical dinner for twelve began with two quarts of oysters on a block of ice, *consommé à la royale,* and then baked fish with hollandaise sauce. A cheese soufflé was the next course, followed by roast chicken with mashed potatoes, green peas, celery, and cranberry jelly. Then came fourteen oyster patties followed by lettuce salad with French dressing. The meal was to be rounded off by crackers and Neufchâtel cheese, orange sherbet, frozen cabinet pudding with apricot sauce, *Glacé Meringue* [*sic*], sponge cake, fruit and coffee.[49] We will never know if anyone ever served exactly that meal, although given the popularity of Parloa's books, it is likely that some did. However, what is interesting is that a mere fifteen years earlier it would have been inconceivable for anyone to even suggest that a dinner of this sophistication could or indeed *should* be cooked and served in a middle-class home.

While the middle class could not afford the number and quality of servants necessary to pull off formal *service à la Russe,* by 1880 "modified *service à la Russe*" was replacing the headlong cavalry charges on an array of heaping platters and overflowing bowls that often characterized ante-bellum American middle-class eating habits. Servants now served some dishes from the sideboard, while the host or hostess carved and served the *pièces de rèsistance* onto the diners' individual plates. As with the upper classes, this made for more courses, longer dinner parties, and allowed the guests to note the quality of the individual dishes.

Although the middle class could not match the upper class in sophistication of cooking and serving, it could try to match them in terms of etiquette. A new formality now surrounded middle-class dinners, as guests were invited to even modest homes by means of engraved invitations, sat down in front of the appropriate place card to read from little menus set on tables covered with fine damask tablecloths, linen napkins, silver, an array of crystal wine and water goblets, cruets and cut-glass containers of various kinds, and elaborate floral and other centerpieces. Elaborately carved sideboards became the second most expensive items in middle-class houses, (surpassed only by the ubiquitous carpeting), their Gothic style exuding a quasi-religious aura over the dining ritual.[50] By the mid-1880s, so formal had dinners become that some bemoaned the passing of the old-fashioned hospitality, which concentrated on making guests feel comfortable, and the rise of a new style of entertaining that seemed concerned mainly with impressing guests with the magnificence of homes and meals. So consumed were people with putting on a better show than their neighbors, said the *Ladies' Home Journal* in 1886, that both guests and hosts now were denied the old-time comfort.[51]

As with the upper class, the vogue for dinner parties helped bring a profound shift in previously flexible hours of eating. In 1865, a typical middle-class cookbook had no suggested mealtimes at all, merely recommending that "they must, to a certain degree, be conformed to family convenience, but ought to be quite independent of the caprices of fashion."[52] In the 1870s, *Godey's Lady's Book and Magazine* was equally hazy:

"Nature has fixed no particular hours for eating. When the mode of life is uniform, it is of great importance to adopt fixed hours; when it is irregular, we ought to be guided by the real wants of the system as dictated by appetite."[53] But by 1880, not only was the growing popularity of having guests for dinner pushing mealtime into the evening, so was the changing nature and geography of middle-class occupations in urban areas. In the colonial city middle-class men tended to work out of or very near to their residences. In the early nineteenth century, as the work force expanded and the nature of middle-class occupations changed, work and residence often became separated. Still, the distance between the two was often not so far as to preclude a walk or ride back home for a large mid-day meal. By 1880, middle- and upper-class residential areas in and around the larger cities were quite a distance from where most of their denizens worked, and many pursued occupations that did not have the old flexibility of hours which allowed for long mid-day dinners. Mid-day meals thus tended to become earlier and smaller: lunches were taken in the vicinity of the workplace, and evening meals with families or guests became larger and more leisurely.

As for the nature of those evening meals with the family, by 1880 middle-class home cooking seems not to have been much more sophisticated than that of 1860. One factor in keeping it simple was a decline in beef prices following the opening of new cattle lands in the West. Beefsteak thus played an even more important role than hitherto in their diets. It was even considered *de rigueur* for the big breakfasts of the day. "Beefsteak deserves the highest rank among breakfast fares," said an 1882 cookbook. "This Bible and chemically sanctioned food, purposely designed for man, is very satisfying to the stomach and possesses great strengthening powers. To replenish the animal spirits there is no food like beef . . . . It is iron which gives the red color to flesh. Beef is not wanting in this life-giving element."[54]

The supremacy of beef provided grist for the mills of those who complained that the middle-class American diet was too restricted. The common refrain of cookbooks advocating a more varied diet was that middle-class American cooking was mired in a rut of porterhouse steak, roast beef, and potatoes.[55] The beef and potatoes syndrome was reinforced by a disdain for pork, almost universally availabile in antebellum days. Here too, the middle class followed their social superiors, who shunned fresh and salted pork and deigned only to eat an occasional slice of smoked ham.[56] Although its low price induced them to consume much more pork than it did the rich, in middle-class eyes pork ranked far below not just beef, but lamb, poultry, and game as well. When *Godey's Lady's Book and Magazine* described the pros and cons of various meats in 1877, beef came off the best by far. Pork and ham, on the other hand, were called difficult to digest, often unwholesome, and unhealthy for people with certain disorders.[57] Not only do Maria Parloa's suggested menus for dinner guests contain absolutely no pork or ham, neither do her twenty-one suggested menus for family dinners.[58] This disdain for pork continued into the next decade. "As an article of food, pork, of late years, does not generally meet the approval of intelligent people and is almost entirely discarded by hygienists," sniffed *Good Housekeeping* magazine in 1890.[59]

Curiously, the traditional high status staple, white wheaten flour, consumed in the form of raised breads, rolls, muffins, pies, and pancakes, continued to be highly regarded among the middle class even though its price had been dropping quite steadily for well over a hundred years, particularly since the opening of the Erie Canal in 1817. New flour milling processes introduced in the 1840s and 1870s produced cheaper, whiter flour and made it affordable to most Americans. Yet a very high proportion of middle-class housewives (probably about 80 percent) continued to bake their own bread, taking great pride in its whiteness and lightness. "Nothing in the whole range of domestic life more affects the health and happiness of the family than the quality of its daily bread," said *Mrs. Lincoln's Boston Cook Book* in 1883.[60]

While the cookbook recipes for breads and pies might appear toothsome, the reality was not always so. "To cook indigestible lumps of pastry, to feed a nation on pies, on heavy bread," lamented an etiquette book in 1880: "Who can expect greatness, wisdom, or honesty from a nation of moody dyspeptics?"[61] When one takes into account the quantities of heavy, greasy, sweet, and generally difficult-to-digest foods (let alone the amount of alcohol) consumed by the average middle-class adult male, it is no wonder that "dyspepsia," a catch-all term for stomach pains, upsets, and disorders of all kinds, gradually replaced constipation as the bane of the mid- and late nineteenth-century middle-class male.[62] Like "neuresthenia," the psychological disorder which crippled so many of their wives and daughters, dyspepsia was part fact and part fiction. It was true that the middle-class diet seemed to lag in adjusting to the increasingly sedentary nature of urban life and that overeating, even by the standards of the day, was rampant.[63] But it is also likely that behind much bemoaning of the condition of stomachs was the fact that, like neuresthenia, dyspepsia was a rather trendy disorder. In the same way that neuresthenia signified that its female sufferers were card-carrying members of a leisured class, without the extra resources of nervous energy which the hurly-burly of the modern competitive world demanded, so dyspepsia signified that its male victims were surrounded by so much material abundance that it had become a kind of curse. The many cures, diets, and tonics to combat it were rarely promoted among the working class, even though their diets were much more coarse and burdensome, for to them full bellies were both too much a source of pleasure and much too serious a business to serve as a scapegoat for what ailed them.

CHAPTER 2

How the Other Half Ate

While industrialization and urbanization created a wealthy and expanding middle class in the first half of the nineteenth century, they also inaugurated an era of increasing inequality and poorer nutrition for American workers.[1] This was reflected in the decreasing physical stature of Americans. After almost reaching modern levels in the later eighteenth century, around 1830 their mean stature began a prolonged decline which lasted until at least the 1870s, mainly as a result of the poor condition of many of the expanding working class.[2]

Exactly what later nineteenth-century workers ate is by no means clear. Middle-class writers such as Catherine Owen called it "coarse" and "substantial," and warned that to the "cultivated appetites" of the middle class "it would not be eatable," but they never described it in any detail.[3] The first systematic survey of workers' standards of living, done in Massachusetts in 1874, tells us as much about their food habits by what it did not ask as by what it did: salted meats, potatoes, and cabbage were such ubiquitous features of the working-class diet that surveyors did not even inquire about the frequency with which they were consumed. The survey, whose 397 subjects were mainly the families of skilled and semi-skilled workers of American or British origin, portrays workers as committed carnivores who loved sweets but consumed few vegetables other than potatoes and cabbage. Over half of the families ate fresh meat two or three times a day. Twenty-six of them even managed to eat fresh meat three times a day, quite a feat when the supply of fresh beef and pork in towns and cities was still rather erratic. Over 42 percent, that is, 169 families, reported that sweets such as cakes and pies were an integral part of all three meals and an additional sixty-five families said that at least two meals included sweets. Vegetables were not nearly so popular. One hundred and seventy families reported that they ate vegetables other than potatoes and cabbage at less than one meal a day and 218 at only one meal a day. Only seven ate these vegetables at two meals a day and nine three times a day.[4]

A compilation of a number of studies done in the mid-1880s covering about 8,000 workers' families in twenty-four states reinforces these impressions, confirming that American workers not only loved meat but revered beef most of all.[5]

Of course this comes as no surprise. Senator James G. Blaine needed no survey to tell him the American workingman worshipped at the shrine of fresh beef. He played on this adroitly in appealing for working-class support in his campaign to restrict Asian immigration. "You can not work a man who must have beef and bread, and would prefer beef," he said, "alongside of a man who can live on rice. In all such conflicts, and in all such struggles, the result is not to bring up the man who lives on rice to the beef-and-bread standard, but it is to bring down the beef-and-bread man to the rice standard."[6]

Coffee was the non-alcoholic beverage of choice for most workers' families, regardless of income, and those in the lower income brackets managed to guzzle almost as much of it as those in the top bracket.[7] Regionalism was still an important factor in workers' diets in the 1880s. Workers in the New England, Midwest and mid-Atlantic ate much more beef and potatoes and less pork and corn meal than those in the Southern and border states, who were very much part of the "hog 'n hominy" culinary world.[8]

But means and averages camouflage individual idiosyncrasies in food tastes, and the great variations in the proportion of their income that different families are willing to devote to food. For example, one of the few commonly accepted universal laws of dietary budgets is that propounded by the German Ernst Engel, who in the late 1870s declared that as incomes rise the proportion of them spent on food tends to fall. Yet an 1884 survey of Illinois workers included two families, both of the same Scandinavian origin, whose expenditures ran completely counter to this pattern. One, a family of eight living on $420 a year, spent only $165, or 39 percent of its income on food. The other, a family of five, earned $632 that year and spent an astonishing $425, or 67 percent of it on food.[9]

Averages also obscure variations resulting from local or occupational circumstances. Many of the American-born coal miners and steel workers in smaller communities, for example, were recent migrants from farms who used their rural skills to grow food and raise livestock in their new surroundings. A study of 2,500 families living in the principal coal, iron, and steel regions in 1890 indicated that about half of them had livestock, poultry, vegetable gardens, or all three. Almost 30 percent purchased no vegetables aside from potatoes during the course of the year, but this does not mean they ate none.[10]

Most of all, though, means and averages obscure the fact that there was no homogeneous working class in America. Workers were divided by religion, ethnicity, skill, and occupation. The latter two were particularly important, for they involved great disparities in income. In the iron and cotton industries, for example, the wage rates of the top categories of skilled workers were commonly about five times those of the unskilled at the bottom.[11] As a result, by 1880, the pattern that was to reign even more strongly by the end of the century was already incipient: in terms of standard of living, there were two de facto working classes. One was composed primarily of skilled and semi-skilled workers whose incomes were more than sufficient to provide them with housing, clothing, and food of the quality they desired. One estimate is that in the 1880s this labor elite, earning from $800 to $1200 a year, comprised about 15 percent of the nation's work force.[12] The rest, comprising the vast majority of the unskilled, hovered around what came to be called the "subsistence level." Just over half of the workers' families in the two New York state industrial towns whose standard of living in the 1880s Daniel Walkowitz studied seemed to have lived at or slightly above this line, in what he calls "secondary poverty." They earned enough to provide the minimum, plus additional costs for medicine, education, transportation, drink, old debts, and so on, while about 20 percent lived below it.[13]

Most American workers lived in rented housing, generally cramped and shabby, in parts of towns and cities with only the most rudimentary sanitation services. The revolution in kitchen equipment that transformed middle-class cooking by 1880 had hardly touched them. The Gothic invasion of dining room decor passed them by because most did not have dining rooms. While middle-class people were able to bake white bread in ovens, most of the poorer workers' wives cooked over open fires or on small stoves and were dependent on commercial bakers for this, their filling staple.

Nevertheless, there is no indication that many of even the poorest workers suffered from insufficient quantities of food. Rather, the problem was in the quality and variety of what they ate. While even the poorly paid could afford some fresh fruits—particularly apples—and vegetables during the summer and fall, the winter and spring saw affordable supplies dry up, forcing them back on the monotonous routine of potatoes, cabbage, and perhaps some turnips. These would be punctuated and enlivened by powerful doses of pickled condiments, but not in large enough quantities to overcome the absence of fresh fruits and vegetables. Milk prices also fluctuated markedly, and the poorer areas of the cities relied on "swill milk," a yellow brew made from the milk of scrawny cows fed on brewers' and distillers' wastes, often surreptitiously whitened with chalk or other additives.

The tables of the labor elite, on the other hand, epitomized the "American Standard," hailed as the birthright of the American worker by Samuel Gompers and those skilled and semi-skilled workers who joined together in 1886 to create the American Federation of Labor. Some owned their own homes and most owned ovens, allowing their wives to take the pride in their home-baked bread. Although, like the poorer workers, they had summer and winter diets, well-off workers could afford some imported fruits and vegetables. Commercial canning had taken great strides during the 1870s, and made fish, fruit, vegetables, and milk available to them all year round in this high-status form. They did not have to buy swill milk from the street vendor's suspect cans, and by the mid-1880s could afford to buy farmers' milk in new glass bottles. While the mid-1880s surveys indicate that they did not consume these vitamin and mineral supplying products all that freely, they were never short of protein, for not only did consumption of steak and roast beef rise with higher income, so did that of eggs, butter, and, likely, poultry as well.[14]

Although they did not share in the riches of the elite's tables, the other 85-odd percent of workers generally shared the conviction that American workers ate better than those in any other country. Their points of reference were usually the places from whence they or their forebears hailed: the British Isles, Northern Europe, or crisis-ridden rural Quebec.[15] Yet many were also immigrants from rural America, and while they too must have harbored few doubts that their diets were superior to those of Europe and Asia, they may have been more dubious regarding their dietary advantages over those who remained behind to cultivate the American "Garden."

Despite a widespread belief that rural America constituted a verdant garden, many rural folk never saw the proverbial cornucopias and lived on diets even more nutritionally deficient than those of the poorest urban workers. In his extensive travels through the Southern slave states in the 1850s, Frederick Law Olmsted noted that the more modest Southern planters (by far the large majority of the slave-owning class) lived on little more than bacon, corn pone, and coffee sweetened with molasses. He thought that even their slaves seemed somewhat better off because they supplemented their salt pork and corn diet with some vegetables in the summer and fall and sweet potatoes in the winter.[16] The slave diet was by no means exemplary. Very high infant mortality rates, an indication of poor nutrition, were the norm for the black people of the rural South, slave and free, throughout the entire nineteenth century.[17] Emancipation, which saw slavery replaced by various forms of tenant farming, hardly improved the nutritional condition of the ex-slaves, for the "three M's," that is, meat (meaning salt pork), meal, and molasses, continued as the core diet. Sharecroppers usually moved too frequently to develop the vegetable gardens slaves had often cultivated and, beginning in the late 1870s, the white flour they bought from the landowner for biscuit and pancake-making was processed in new, high efficiency roller mills and deprived of many of its nutrients. Some years later, new methods for milling corn did the same to cornmeal.

Poor white farmers were hardly better off. Indeed, a belt of tragic poorly nourished "dirt-eaters" stretched across the sand barrens and pine woods from South Carolina to Mississippi. These yellow-skinned, pot-bellied, unfortunates derived their name from the clay and resin they chewed to relieve the pain of the hookworms which infested them.[18] Like the blacks and whites of the cotton belt, their diet of processed corn meal and bolted flour likely led to many cases of pellagra, although that dietary-deficiency affliction did not come to public attention until the early twen-tieth century.[19] Even those who were better off suffered nutritional defi-ciencies. Cattle raising—beef or dairy—was not common in a South trans-fixed by cotton, tobacco, and the traditional staple crops. Even where cattle were raised the lack of cold storage facilities meant that milk could not be marketed commercially and that fresh beef was normally available only in the few cool winter months.

Sharecropping and other forms of tenant farming were by no means confined to the Southeast. Along with infinite variations on the crop lien system, they dominated large parts of the Southwest and border states as well. The nature of these tenancy systems undermined farmers' diets. Landowners anxious to be paid in cash discouraged the production of non-cash crops such as fruit and vegetables. Because they profited from the sale of salt pork, flour, molasses, and sugar on credit to the tenants they strove to maintain the diet based on these, and sometimes forceably pre-vented tenants from raising their own livestock in order to preserve their monopoly over the supply of salted pork.[20] As a result, milk and fresh meat, even fresh pork, were usually rarities on croppers' tables. Only some scrawny chickens and the eggs they laid provided year-round alter-native sources of animal protein to the omnipresent salted pork, and egg-laying was by no means a consistent process.

In the summer time, greens and berries could be gathered and, if local conditions allowed, squirrels, racoons, or fish could be caught to supple-ment the diet, but the rigors of planting time in the spring, and harvest time from August to December, normally inhibited those endeavors, par-ticularly in the cotton belt. Indeed, the life of a sharecropper's wife, which often demanded twelve-hour days in the fields, normally allowed little time for food preparation at all. Typically, she would rise at 4 a.m. in a one- or two-room cabin to prepare breakfast: thinly sliced fat salt pork fried over an open fire and corn bread spread with fat and molasses. There would be no time to clean the kitchen before going to work in the fields until about 10 a.m., when she would gather firewood to cook the main meal of the day. This was served around 11 a.m., and usually consisted of leftovers from breakfast, supplemented, if the family was lucky and it happened to be summer or fall, by collard or other greens. Then, it was back to the fields, again leaving the dirty pan and dishes where they were. Supper, before and after which all the other household chores were performed, was usually a repeat of the mid-day meal.[21]

The only farmers whose diets may have rivaled those of the southeastern and southwestern tenants in monotony and meagerness were those still staking out new farms on the rapidly disappearing northwestern frontier. Living in sod huts or shanties for the first years, their diets also revolved around corn and pork. But they raised their own corn, ground their own meal, and ate their own hogs, both fresh and salted, lean meat as well as fat. When fortune began to smile upon them, said a historian of Minnesota's Norwegian-American farmers, they could "emancipate themselves from the benevolent tyranny of the pig" and branch out into raising other animals.[22] This in turn would pave the way for the more varied diets of the farmers in more settled areas to the East.

Aside from these relics of an earlier era, the large majority of farmers of the Northeast, Midwest, and West likely ate much better than the lower paid urban workers.[23] Free of the systems of farm tenancy and the devotion to cotton which impoverished and restricted the diets of the large majority of southern farmers, they could raise dairy cows, poultry, and cultivate vegetable gardens to provide some variety in their diets. By 1880 a number of processed foods became common on farms, particularly outside the South. Although corn meal, molasses, and sorghum continued to be consumed in considerable quantities, white wheaten flour and refined sugar became staples on most farms. Dried fish made frequent appearances and canned varieties were not unknown. Biscuits or crackers were purchased in bulk at village general stores, lessening the burden of baking. The invention of the Mason jar in mid-century and improvements in home canning processes in the 1870s allowed fruits and vegetables to be "put up" for the winter and spring in something approximating their natural form, instead of being highly sweetened or vinegared.

Still, in 1880, transportation difficulties and cash shortages meant relatively few farmers had easy access to much in the way of affordable processed or exotic foods. Local geography was therefore still the most important factor in shaping rural diets, helping to preserve the regional culinary traditions of the past. Harvest times might bring bountiful tables and considerable variety, but for much of the year farmers' diets were restricted to the staples of their region and to foods that could be preserved over winter and spring. The winter and spring diets of New England farmers still revolved around the region's "great trinity" of bread, bacon, and beans, supplemented by some root vegetables. In the Midwest, particularly after the 1870s, when corn cultivation replaced wheat cultivation in much of the region, the pig, salted, smoked, and pickled, was the farmer's great storehouse for corn over the winter and dominated that long season's diet. Yet by the 1880s dairy farming was expanding rapidly in both regions, providing fresh milk, butter, and cheese all year round, and growing stocks of poultry provided other sources of protein.

An ample variety of food on the tables did not come easily. For most farm families, food gathering and preparation was a terribly time-consuming process, and women were regarded as indispensable for these chores. The son of a Kansas farmer recalled that in the early 1880s his German-born mother grew and gathered her own vegetables, fruits, berries, and melons in spring and summer and preserved them in the fall for use over the winter. She churned her own butter and pressed the juice out of sorghum cane and boiled it down into a kind of molasses, which she used instead of sugar. Vinegar, essential for pickling, was made from molasses, rain water, and yeast, while "coffee" was made from browned rye grain.[24] The food still needed to be preserved and cooked, wood stoves had to be fed, stoked, and cleaned, and these and a multitude of other kitchen tasks kept farm wives virtually chained to their kitchens. Although "hired hands" commonly helped men in the fields, relatively few farm women (or men) employed help in the kitchen.[25] An Englishman who farmed in Iowa and Wyoming in the late 1870s and early 1880s wrote home that American farmers "can't understand a man paying a woman to cook for him when he might as just as well marry and get it done for nothing." Nine-tenths of them married "as a matter of business and economy . . . and half of them value their wives just in the same way one values a horse."[26]

While the food consumed may have reflected regional differences, rural food habits and methods of preparation retained their roots in the Anglo-Saxon culinary tradition. Although the opening of the West ultimately helped to change the American diet by expanding food choices and food supplies, it had remarkably little effect on the way Americans prepared and ate their food. The Native American influence was obliterated. The Spanish/Mexican tradition was shunted aside, its remnants lingering unappreciated in backwaters. The food habits of the Northern European settlers of the Upper Midwest and Northern Plains merged almost invisibly into those of the dominant culture.

CHAPTER 3

The Rise of the Giant
Food Processors

The westward expansion of the railroad opened up vast new lands for wheat cultivation. New varieties of hardy spring wheat and improvements in the technology of planting and harvesting allowed wheat to be cultivated on a massive scale in Minnesota, the Dakotas, and even in parts of what was still called "the Great American Desert," lowering the price of the farmer's wheat and the consumer's flour. The westward expansion of the wheat belt was accompanied by the expansion of the corn and hog belts into much of the Midwest previously devoted to wheat. In a number of states, particularly Wisconsin and Iowa, this was followed by the rise of a dairy cattle industry.

Many New England farmers, unable to compete with either the midwestern corn and hog economy or western wheat economy, moved to industrial towns. Others turned to dairy farming, or, if they were near railroads with direct access to the markets of industrial cities, to "truck" farming, growing vegetables and fruits for nearby urban markets. Although some farmers had used greenhouses to extend the growing and harvesting seasons of pricier produce since the 1840s, only in the 1870s, with the extension of the railroad networks, did cities begin to receive noteworthy supplies of hothouse produce.[1] By the later 1880s, railroad networks radiating from cities provided daily pick-ups of fresh milk, fruits, and vegetables in the exurban areas of the Middle Atlantic and Great Lakes states. Thanks mainly to these new networks the quantity of whole milk sold from American farms rose from 2 billion pounds in 1870 to over 18 billion pounds in 1900.[2]

Earlier, the railroads had opened up the grasslands of the Great Plains to giant herds of beef cattle. Most of the cattle were shipped eastward on the hoof, for slaughter close to their markets, but some midwestern pork packing houses had expanded into beef as well, turning out corned and canned beef for domestic and foreign markets. In 1879, Gustavus Swift, a dour, sharp-eyed easterner obsessed with gaining control of the meat trade, helped fulfill an important part of the American Dream by developing a system that allowed beef to be fattened and slaughtered in Chicago and shipped East in refrigerated railroad cars, fresh, dressed, and cheaper than beef on the hoof.

Meanwhile, the extension of the Illinois Central Railway down to New Orleans opened the booming market of Chicago and the north-central Midwest to fresh southern vegetables, shipped back on trains which carried midwestern wheat, corn, and salted pork to the South. The railways snaking their way down to the southeast through Maryland, Delaware, and Virginia encouraged fruit and vegetable growing for northeastern urban markets along their pathways, extending the season and lowering the prices of items such as fresh peas and strawberries. The Georgia peach industry, on the verge of extinction, was saved in the late 1870s by the expansion of the Northern railroad network into the state, allowing its new breed of longer-lasting peaches to reach northern cities before they rotted. Refrigerated cars were a boon to growers and shippers of perishable fruits and vegetables from these and other warm climes. They gave a major boost to fruit and vegetable production in California, which shipped its first box-car load of fresh fruit east in 1869, and later in Texas and Florida as well.

Lettuce, too tender and perishable for the new transportation to handle economically, remained an expensive, upper-class delicacy until the turn of the century. However, in 1903, agricultural science came to the rescue and almost single-handedly redirected the path of the modern American diet by developing a strain of lettuce called "iceberg," which seemed virtually indestructible.[3]

For farmers, these changes proved to be a two-edged sword. While some prospered, others were caught in a desperate race between mounting debts incurred to buy the new land and machinery to increase production and falling prices for the foodstuffs they produced. For the urban consumer, however, the benefits were visible on the table. Beef prices declined fairly steadily in the 1870s and 1880s[4] and while the price drop slowed in the ensuing years, the quality of beef in eastern markets improved. Before the refrigerator car, the grass-fed cattle that arrived in eastern cities had generally been scrawny and stringy. Those that were fattened before slaughter were often fed the residues from brewers' mash or other malodorous substances which imparted unpleasant tastes to the flesh. The new system, which allowed beef to be "finished" on corn before being slaughtered in Chicago or Kansas City produced beef Americans regarded as much better tasting. By the mid-1880s, easterners thought they were living in the "Golden Age of American Beef."

Other commodities experienced more striking falls in price. Whereas one dollar would buy fifteen pounds of flour in 1872, and close to twenty pounds in 1881, in 1897 it could buy thirty-four pounds. Indeed, in 1898 one dollar could buy 43 percent more rice than in 1872, 35 percent more beans, 49 percent more tea, 51 percent more roasted coffee, 114 percent more sugar, 62 percent more mutton, 25 percent more fresh pork, 60 percent more lard and butter, and 42 percent more milk.[5]

The boom in production and shipping took place in an America in the throes of industrial reorganization. In food, as in petroleum, iron, and steel, quests for technological innovations to reduce costs and eliminate dependence on skilled, artisanal labor went hand in hand with drives to merge and consolidate businesses in order to gain control of market forces. An example is the sugar industry. In the decades before the Civil War, new methods for refining sugar brought down the price of white sugar and greatly increased its consumption. From 1839 to 1849 the wholesale price of sugar dropped from about sixteen cents a pound to about eight cents, remaining at that level for the next decade.[6] New technological advances then brought even further reductions in refining costs so that by the 1870s newcomers could build a state-of-the-art refinery for only half a million dollars or so. As a result, much to the chagrin of most refiners, by the 1880s something close to pure competition reigned in the industry, bringing down the price of white granulated sugar to rock-bottom levels. Desperate to gain control of production and restrict price competition, the sugar refiners created what became a classic oligopoly. Led by a brace of New York and New Jersey scions of the Havermeyer family, who had been influential in the sugar industry since early in the century, the industry leaders employed a crafty banker to model a "trust" on that which John D. Rockefeller had recently used so creatively to gain control of the petroleum industry.[7]

Although the resulting creature, the American Sugar Refining Company came up with a brand name—"Domino"—for its sugar, the "Sugar Trust" concentrated mainly on beating down competition and spent relatively little on advertising or promotion. However, it did mount a successful campaign to denigrate brown sugar, whose refining it did not completely control, by cleverly reproducing blown-up photographs of horrible-looking but harmless little microbes, taken through newly invented microscopes, and warning the public of the supposed dangers of eating brown sugar. So successful was this effort that in 1900, the best-selling *Boston Cook Book* accepted this as scientific wisdom, warning readers that brown sugar was inferior in quality to white sugar and was prone to infestation by "a minute insect."[8]

But this was all quite unnecessary, for consumers did not really have to be told that brown sugar was of a lower order than the white variety. White sugar, like white bread, had been more highly regarded than brown long before anyone thought of forming a "Sugar Trust."[9] The combination of relatively low prices and historically high status proved to be unbeatable, and after 1880 white granulated sugar swept all competition aside. Farmers abandoned molasses and home-made sorghum, workers gave up molasses and brown sugar, and between 1880 and 1915 per capita consumption of white granulated sugar doubled.[10]

The campaign against brown sugar showed that, although they were not about to lead the food industry into the bright new world of modern advertising, sugar refiners were at least dimly aware of one of the keys to food advertising in advanced industrial countries: that once individuals ingest an adequate number of calories in their diets, most changes in food consumption will be the result of the substitution of one food for another.[11] Although it was an idea whose time would not really come until the 1920s, other food processors were already acting on that basis by the 1890s.

Those most successful in encouraging the substitution of one kind of food for another were also the zaniest: the entrepreneurs of the breakfast food industry who almost single-handedly destroyed the traditional American breakfast. Historically, industrial and economic development has been accompanied by the substitution of meat for grain in the diet.[12] Yet while that was indeed the overall trend from 1870 on in America, the breakfast food manufacturers managed to promote the opposite process at breakfast: the replacement of the traditional slabs of meat with various forms of highly processed grain.

The rise of Kellogg's "Corn Flakes" and Post's "Grape-Nuts" and "Toasties," which led the way, held important lessons for other food processors. First, there was the link to health, very effective among the middle classes who, by the turn of the century, were becoming very concerned about the link between food and good health. Corn Flakes had been invented as a vegetarian health food at the Seventh-Day Adventist "sanatorium" at Battle Creek, Michigan, by William R. Kellogg, the dogged if somewhat colorless brother of the institution's flamboyant director Dr. John Harvey Kellogg, whose mixture of vegetarianism and hokum had turned the modest little outpost into a thriving health resort attracting thousands of non-Adventists, including many of the era's rich and famous, to its cures. Initially, much of Corn Flakes' success in the wider market derived from this link with good health. So effective was the sanatorium tie thought to be that when an ex-patient, a peripatetic St. Louis real estate promoter named Charles W. Post who had already entered the health food market with a cereal-based beverage he modestly called "Postum," lifted Kellogg's idea and started producing "Grape-Nuts," a similar ready-to-eat breakfast food, he purchased property in Battle Creek to imply a sanatorium connection. So did about forty other imitators who soon emerged. Post, a master of the dubious health claim whose genius lay in slogans that implied everything but promised nothing, marketed his cereal as a "brain food" which was also likely to cure consumption, malaria, and loose teeth.[13] Second, of course, there was convenience. The appeal of breakfast foods which required no cooking was not to be denied in the majority of American homes, which did not have servant girls to arise early in the morning, light the wood stove, and begin frying bacon and stirring porridge pots. Third, there was hygiene. The existence of bacteria had been discovered in the 1880s, and even before the pure-food scare of the early 1900s, middle-class Americans were greatly concerned that "germs" infested everything. The neatly packaged cereals promised absolute cleanliness and, presumably, germ-free food.

Most important, though, Kellogg's and Post's success seemed to derive from successful promotion and advertising. The catchy "brand names" they thought up for their products were regarded in the industry as the key to their success. "Toasted Corn Flakes" and "Grape-Nuts" were easily read, easily remembered, and distinctive. Post met little success in marketing a second breakfast food under a label, "Elijah's Manna," which played mainly on the health food factor. He soon realized, however, that the main barrier to its success was not the outcry of those disturbed by the implication that the old prophet himself had originated its formula (although a court injunction prohibiting its sale in England was obtained on these grounds). Rather, it was the name itself, which was just not "catchy" enough. When he changed the name to "Toasties," sales took off. In 1906, William Kellogg, more attuned to new business methods than his tight-fisted brother—who imagined himself to be one of the giants of modern medical science—took the breakfast food operation out from under his brother's wing because the doctor, who continued to dither with unprofitable ideas for health foods, refused to spend money on the promotion and advertising necessary to keep Corn Flakes in the forefront of the burgeoning industry.[14]

Once armed with a promotional budget as potent as Post's, Kellogg's company regained the lead. To other food processors the success of Kellogg and Post thus provided striking evidence of the effectiveness of packaging, advertising, and promotion in selling food products. And for good reason: their clever use of the new promotional techniques had created a mass market for a food product that had not even existed before, one which replaced, not supplemented, competing foodstuffs.

Advertising and promotion also became crucial to more conventional sectors of the food industry. Improved transportation opened up possibilities of national markets for mass-produced food products, but it also exacerbated a marketing problem that resulted from the improved processing technology: the advances which allowed the production of items such as flour, biscuits, sugar, salt, and canned goods on a massive scale also produced foods that were absolutely uniform in appearance, quality, and taste. Since most manufacturers used essentially the same technology, there was little to choose from among the products. This put a premium on advertising, promotion, and the brand names they created and touted.

The accounts of the nation's largest advertising agency of the time, N. W. Ayer, reflect the growing importance of advertising in the changing food industry. In 1877 food advertisements accounted for less than 1 percent of the agency's business. By 1901, food accounted for almost 15 percent of its business and remained the single most advertised class of commodity until the 1930s, when it was overtaken by automobiles.[15] The advertising techniques of the time were, by contemporary standards, primitive and unsophisticated. Today, the National Biscuit Company's name for its soda crackers, "Uneeda," seems the ultimate in corniness, but in 1899, when it was invented, it smacked of genius. Indeed, the story of the rise of "Uneeda" crackers is significant, for National Biscuit was a typical product of many of the forces transforming the food industry.

Soda crackers and biscuits had long been an American staple, and the cracker barrel, with fresh crackers periodically added on top and leftovers gradually crumbling into a sodden mass to please the rodents nesting at the bottom, was the center of the traditional general store. Most crackers were supplied by wholesalers, who distributed the crackers and biscuits of biscuit bakers in their regions. The railroad, however, opened the regional and local markets to competition from biscuit bakers across the nation. In the resulting competitive scramble, a series of mergers by the large manufacturers attempting to limit competition ultimately led to the formation of one giant, the National Biscuit Company, which accounted for an astonishing 70 percent of the entire industry's sales.

In order to head off lowering prices or lose the market share to smaller, upstart bakers, Nabisco broke through the old bulk supply system by wrapping its crackers in colorful, sanitary-looking packages and giving them a memorable brand name. It then made an end run around the wholesalers by building its own sales team and selling them directly to grocers. These grocery shops had grown enormously in number since 1880, and in all but the most remote rural areas replaced the old general store. With its enormous resources, National Biscuit was then able to mount an advertising campaign large enough to render the cracker barrel a sodden bit of nostalgia and ensure "Uneeda" crackers domination of the market for many years.

The usual array of upstart imitators assumed, wrongly, that much of "Uneeda"'s success lay in the clever name itself, and turned out crackers with such names as "I Wanta Cracker," "Taka Cracker," and "Hava Cracker." Their failure demonstrated, however, that marketing genius was not enough. While their names and packaging might have been every bit as brilliant as Uneeda's, they fell far short of matching Nabisco's advertising budget, and it was the name's repeated exposure on billboards, in newspapers, magazines, and on the sides of streetcars that made it so effective.[16]

Typical of another new kind of food giant was the company built up by Henry J. Heinz, which rode the crest of that most-remarked-upon phenomenon of the time, the substitution of products and services manufactured outside the home for those traditionally produced at home. Through brilliant promotion, Heinz was able to capitalize on the taste for sweet and sour condiments and persuade American housewives that his pickles and other condiments were as tasty, yet healthier and more convenient, than home-made ones. Americans had always preserved vegetables and fruits in brine and vinegar and stored them in air-tight crocks or, since mid-century, in Mason jars. But in the late 1870s, a new method of packing under steam pressure greatly reduced the heating time and made large-scale production of glass-jarred pickles possible. Similarly, canning, a European invention, had been in America since 1819, and, although it derived considerable impetus from the Civil War, it was not until 1874, when a similar application of steam pressure resolved some of its problems, that a wide variety of canned goods could begin to be produced for a mass market. Heinz was one of the first to realize the size of the potential market for preserved and canned foods, and was soon claiming to produce "57 Varieties" of them.

Although few questioned the quality of his product, Heinz himself would have been among the first to admit that his company's phenomenal success was based largely on promotion and advertising. The Heinz display at the Chicago World's Fair of 1893 was one of the smash hits of the fair, attracting over one million people to visit it, to taste a free sample, and to pick up a tiny green metallic reproduction of a Heinz pickle, to be attached to key chains or charm bracelets. Heinz arranged demonstrations of his products at grocery stores, offered a money-back guarantee, opened his factories to public tours, gave away millions of samples, and invested heavily on the most expensive form of advertising of the time, the electrically illuminated sign. He personally designed and had erected the first large sign of this kind in New York, a six-story "HEINZ"-emblazoned green pickle which dominated the intersection of Fifth Avenue and Twenty-third Street until it was replaced by the Flatiron building in 1906. In 1899, he opened the Heinz Pier in Atlantic City. Stretching nine hundred feet into the sea behind immense neo-classical portals, for the next forty-five years it lured millions to view its sumptuous furnishings, paintings and sculpture, cooking demonstrations, and to munch on the inevitable free samples.[17]

Heinz also pioneered another feature of the booming food processing industry, vertical integration. As early as 1880 he helped develop improved seeds for his cucumber pickles and was contracting with farmers to plant and grow them for him at a pre-arranged price, a system picked up by other giants in the fruit and vegetable canning industry. By 1900, 20,000 people worked on 16,000 acres of farmland devoted exclusively to producing products for the Heinz picklers and canners, to be delivered in Heinz-owned freight and tank cars to his factories where they would be preserved in bottles manufactured by his own bottling plant.[18] Within a few years, his major competitors, Campbell's and Franco-American, were developing similar relationships with farmers and attempting to control all aspects of food production from seed hybridization to the price of the goods on grocery-store shelves.

Meanwhile, continued improvements in canning technology as well as the invention of various machines to speed the preparation of the foods for canning greatly increased the productivity of canners. By the turn of the century the rising output of cans whose tops were crimped, rather than soldered into place, signaled the end of the skilled can maker who, with the help of a "boy," could turn out 1500 cans a day. By 1910, a single machine could turn out 35,000 cans a day. When integrated into food processing lines using new machines to peel, shell, clean, slice, chop, and cook various foods this meant that companies with the requisite large investment could turn out canned food in an amount undreamed of a mere thirty years before. In 1910, ten years before the real heyday of American canning, processors employing more than 68,000 people turned out over 3 billion cans of food.[19]

By then, Heinz had been joined by some formidable competitors. When Van Camp's hit on the idea of adding pureed tomatoes to their canned salt pork and beans and promoting them as Van Camp's Pork and Beans in Tomato Sauce their product became a market leader. The Biardot family started the first commercial canned soup operation in New Jersey in 1887 and, trying to capitalize on the newly elevated status of French cooking, adopted the Franco-American label for their full line of canned soups (and, oddly enough, plum puddings as well), claiming that all of their recipes were those of French chefs. The giant of the industry, however, arose from the laboratory rather than the kitchen. In 1897, John T. Torrance, who had a Ph.D in chemistry, applied his scientific knowledge to the vexing problem of the bulkiness of the cans used by manufacturers of canned soups. When, in 1898, he came up with the solution—to condense the soup—he set up the Joseph P. Campbell Company of Camden, New Jersey, and ensured himself a hallowed spot in any future Food Processing Hall of Fame.[20]

By 1900, the American food processing industry became very big business indeed, accounting for 20 percent of the nation's manufacturing. Significantly, of the top four sectors of the industry—meat packing, flour milling, sugar refining, and baking—only fourth-ranked baking was not dominated by a few giant corporations, though its important cracker-baking sector already was.[21]

This growing domination of the American food processing industry by large corporations seems to have made quite an impression abroad, where electric Heinz pickle signs sprouted from London to Prague. News of the phenomenon even penetrated the court of Czar Nicholas II of Russia, likely through the derisive comments of Francophilic Russian aristocrats. The great Russian opera singer, Feodor Chaliapin, reported the following conversation with the Czar, after his return from a season with New York's Metropolitan Opera:

> CZAR: "I have heard the American kitchen is miserable. All the foods are prepared on a big scale and they have no individual taste or flavor. Is that true?
>
> CHALIAPIN: "Yes, Your Majesty, that is true. They have a flavor of American corporations and speculation." (I replied in an attempt at humor.)
>
> CZAR: "That I think is the drawback of the American conditions as far as I have heard. The trusts can manufacture iron and other industrial things on a big scale, but when it comes to the manufacture of food, there the commercial methods fail. As far as I have heard, they have commercialized literature and art, restaurants and homes. A man has to eat what the trust gives and has to be content with a home that another trust furnishes."[22]

Some of the smoke from the era's progressive crusade, with its attacks on the food and other trusts, had obviously wafted across to Russia. Yet if anything, this movement on behalf of the "little people" strengthened, rather than weakened, the large food processors. The very government regulations progressives hoped would remedy abuses in the food processing industry often paved the way for the elimination of smaller, more marginal producers and increased the concentration of economic power in a few hands.

This became evident early on, with the drive for federal meat inspection in the 1880s. Small eastern slaughterhouses and butchers found themselves unable to compete with the dressed beef being shipped in refrigerated cars by the large midwestern packers. Among other defensive measures, butchers' associations pressed state governments to require that dressed beef be inspected by state officials at least twenty-four hours before slaughter, something that would preclude the sale of beef slaughtered out of state. In response, the giant packers campaigned successfully for a federal meat inspection law, passed in 1891, which pre-empted these requirements and resulted in driving many local slaughterhouses out of business.[23] The large packers also hoped that the inspection law would head off restrictions on imports from America which competing European packers were demanding on the grounds that American meat was contaminated.[24]

The successful drive to reduce competition in the industry led Gustavus Swift to join with P. D. Armour and other large midwestern meat packers to absorb or drive out of business a host of other packers, and form what they called "the Big Five"—referred to by opponents as "the Beef Trust." This oligopoly divided the national market among themselves and managed with considerable success to control prices in that volatile industry, despite the fact that the capital outlay necessary for entry into the industry was relatively modest and competition kept surfacing on the local and regional levels.[25]

In 1906, it seemed that they had met a setback, however. Largely as a result of the uproar following the publication of Upton Sinclair's novel *The Jungle,* a striking exposé of working conditions in the Chicago slaughterhouses, a new, tougher, federal meat inspection law was enacted. Sinclair, a socialist, hoped to arouse public concern over the terrible conditions endured by workers in the plants. However, his descriptions of filth in the plants and stories of workers falling into vats and meat grinding machines and ending up in sausages that went to consumers' tables aroused the public, and the nefarious Beef Trust fell under a cloud of suspicion. (Sinclair is said to have commented ruefully: "I aimed at America's heart, but hit its stomach.")

Yet, while the new act meant stiffer inspection of the meat packing industry, the largest packers supported it. Not only would it provide better ammunition against European restrictions, it would also reassure the American public of the quality of their products. Their main concern was to have the government foot the bill for the elaborate system of inspection required by the law, something which they achieved. Although they were disappointed by the failure of the act to apply its regulations to meat that did not cross state lines, they ended up with something they could hardly find objectionable: a government-financed, government-run system to assure the public of the quality of their product.[26]

The Big Five were quick to use the new law for this purpose. "*The U.S. Inspection* stamp, on every pound and every package of Armour goods, guarantees purity, wholesomeness and honest labelling of *all Armour* food products," said one of that company's advertisements shortly after passage of the law. "To be *named* 'Extract of Beef,' it *must be* extract of *Beef*," it assured readers.[27]

Federal regulation also helped other food giants. In the early 1900s, "muckraking" journalists aroused public concern over dangerous food additives and food adulteration. As a result of a nationwide campaign in which many women's clubs supported the efforts of Dr. Harvey Wiley, Chief Chemist of the U.S. Department of Agriculture, to institute federal regulation of food additives and compulsory labeling of ingredients, the Pure Food and Drug Act was passed in 1906. Often regarded as a blow to the nefarious practices of big business, it too helped the giant food processors. Although initially dubious, they came to realize this in time to help push the legislation through Congress. Early in the campaign, H. J. Heinz saw that the unrestricted use of dangerous "canning powders" and other chemicals to preserve food was casting a cloud of suspicion over all canned and bottled products, including his own, which used only minimal amounts of chemical preservatives. He saw, correctly, that not only would the government stamp of approval assuage fears of processed foods, it would be particularly beneficial to large companies such as his which did not resort to the cost-cutting measures of the smaller, more marginal processors. These small-timers, unable to compete in advertising, sought a share of the market by lowering prices, and this often meant cutting costs in processing by using dangerous chemicals and inferior foods. By 1906, Heinz had converted the other large canners to the cause and the forerunner of the National Association of Canners came out in support of the pure food legislation.[28]

Years later, Wiley wrote that without Heinz's help he would have "lost the fight for pure food."[29] Crucial in persuading canners was a speech Wiley had made before their trade association in which he assured them that passage of the legislation would not only be of immense benefit to public health but also would increase their profits and protect them from competition.[30]

Yet within a few years even Wiley's generally benevolent attitude toward the large food processors had created too many enemies in high places and led to his being forced out of his job. One of his annoying *idées fixes*, which he was never able to prove, was that sodium benzoate, the preservative most commonly used by the respectable food processors, and practically the only one used by Heinz, was dangerous to human health. In 1913 his successor moved quickly to assuage fears that the Bureau of Chemistry was out to hinder the industry. Its job was not merely to punish food adulterers, he announced, but "to help honest manufacturers to discharge their duty to the community by supplying wholesome products. The Bureau of Chemistry belongs not only to the consumer but also to the manufacturer."[31]

Aside from deriving the same benefits from government approval of their products as the meat industry, the giants were able to use clever promotion and advertising to turn the pure-food scare to their advantage. Heinz's idea of allowing visitors to watch white-robed girls stuff pickle bottles swept the industry and suddenly, food processing plants across the nation were open to tourism. Kellogg's opened its Battle Creek plant to visitors in 1906 and kept it open until 1986, when it claimed the introduction of secret new processes forced its closure. In one 1906 issue of *Harper's Magazine,* Heinz reminded readers that its mincemeat was "the exemplification of purity" because it was prepared "by neat uniformed workers" in "model kitchens" which were always open to visitors. Franco-American Foods also declared its kitchens "always open to visitors," as did Blue Label Food Products, whose foods had "rich natural flavor" and were "prepared in clean kitchens under sanitary conditions." Perhaps the Armour packing company went further than it needed. Just months after two special federal commissioners, previously unfamiliar with the blood and gore of meat processing, had been appalled and physically sickened to discover that many of the conditions described in *The Jungle* did indeed exist, the company opened the doors of its slaughterhouses to the public.[32]

Others played variations on the cleanliness theme. Stacey's Forkdipt Chocolates were fork-dipped because "the fork is cleaner than the hand." Royal Baking Powder was "Absolutely Pure" and Bishop's California Preserves were "the only fruits in the world with a $1000 purity guarantee on every jar."[33] Even brewers felt compelled to reassure customers of their products' purity. Some months earlier, Schlitz had assured drinkers that it was "brewed in absolute cleanliness and cooled in filtered air." It was "sterilized after the bottle was sealed" and because of its purity "when your physician prescribes beer, it is always Schlitz beer."[34]

Concern over the purity of milk also led to the consolidation of the milk industry. When local and state governments passed laws ordaining that milk be pasteurized, thousands of small milk distributors, who had plied neighborhoods dipping milk out of cooled milk cans, were forced out of business. Only companies that could afford the considerable investment necessary to purchase pasteurizing equipment and a large inventory of bottles survived. In Detroit there were 158 milk dealers when the pasteurization law was passed in May, 1915. Within three months, the number declined to sixty-eight. Chicago's pasteurization regulations forced over 60 percent of its milk distributors out of business. In Boston, where settlement-house workers and the progressive Women's Municipal League led the fight for pure milk against the bitter opposition of the purveyors of milk, butter, and cheese, 1500 milk peddlers plied their trade in the 1880s. By 1914, the number declined to 200 and in 1923 it stood at 131. The number of distributors in Milwaukee decreased from 200 to 32 in the five years after a pasteurization ordinance was passed, setting the stage for the next phase of consolidation in the milk industry, when the city, like many others, would see 85 percent of its milk distribution network taken over by two giant national holding companies, Borden's and National Dairy Products (Sealtest).[35]

Between 1880 and World War I, the American food industry was radically transformed. Agriculture had always been the nation's biggest business, but now it was becoming big business in another sense, as new technology and the need for more capital investment were encouraging the creation of larger farms and the beginnings of more complex organizations to finance agricultural production. The effects of the revolution in technology and organization were even more striking after the food left the farm, for large new organizations now transported, processed, and marketed the farmer's products. Some sectors of the transformed food industry were dominated by giant new corporations: Swift, Armour, and Wilson in meat packing; Washburn-Crosby (Gold Medal Flour) and Pillsbury in flour milling; Heinz, Campbell's, and the California Fruit Grower's Exchange in canning. The tropical products boom brought whole countries into the American economic order, making the United and Standard Fruit Companies the arbiters of politics in much of Central America; American sugar producers the power-brokers in Cuba, the Dominican Republic, Puerto Rico, and Hawaii; and turning the ups and downs of American coffee consumption into the crucial events in the economies of countries such as Brazil, Colombia, and El Salvador.

On the other hand, the expansion of the food industry created new opportunities for thousands of smaller ventures. The grocery business, with a much greater variety of goods to sell and an urban community increasingly dependent on store-bought foods, was still a business for individuals and families. Even though the age of the chain store had begun, the chains, led by the Great Atlantic and Pacific Tea Stores company, were still networks of small stores, without self-service or meat counters. The meats shipped out by giant packers were still sold by family butchers, and the newly available fruits and vegetables were purchased by consumers from small stalls in urban markets, tiny neighborhood stores, or from itinerant peddlers who roamed residential neighborhoods with pushcarts.

Nevertheless, the rise of the giant processors marked the beginning of a momentous change in the history of food and diet, not just in America but in the world. Throughout human history food has been a primary item for exchange, barter, and sale, and people have amassed wealth by doing so. Wars have been fought and empires have risen and fallen in struggles for control of food supplies. But the fortunes and the struggles have arisen on the assumption that there was an existing market for the items involved, whether it was the spices of the Orient, the fisheries of the North Sea and North Atlantic, or the sugar of the West Indies. The Hanseatic League worked on the assumption that the market for salted herring was already there. Its aim was to gain control of supplying it, not to stimulate it. The Hanses never thought of subsidizing Christian missionaries in order to widen the market for fish created by meatless Fridays, Lent, and other days of fast.

Because of the rise of the giant food processing industries, by 1914 the United States was on the verge of becoming a country in which traditional rules no longer held. Pre-industrial food marketers dealt mainly in items the chief cost of which was transportation, followed by the cost of storage. Only in the case of a few luxury items, such as sugar, had the cost of processing played a major role. In the early 1870s, the food industry in America still centered on small, independent producers growing, raising, and processing their wares, sometimes marketing them themselves but more often selling them to local middlemen who sold them in bulk. By 1914, however, large corporations were playing a major role in almost all aspects of the system. Using new methods of capital formation to raise money for the technology of mass production, new organizational techniques to integrate their operations vertically, and new promotional methods as well as sheer size to market their products on a mass basis, these giants were now able to struggle against their greatest enemy, the forces of the uncontrolled marketplace. They now aspired not only to respond to consumer demands but to shape them.

Of course the attempt to control and stimulate demand for particular food products was by no means new in itself. In the past, when new products, such as coffee and tea, were introduced into foreign markets, individual importers would try to stimulate their use, often by claiming medicinal or aphrodisiacal properties. But the absence of mass communication restricted their efforts to what was, in effect, rumor-mongering among elites. Governments in search of revenue or power have tried to encourage or discourage the consumption of certain products, but this has usually been through coercive measures such as prohibitions, high taxes, and exorbitant duties. Only the emergence of large corporate entities profiting from mass markets for their mass produced foods allowed the mounting of large campaigns designed to change food habits through persuasion. The campaign of billboards and advertisements which flour millers began in 1915 encouraging Americans to "Eat More Wheat" would have been inconceivable a mere thirty years earlier, let alone three hundred years earlier. Monumental changes in agriculture and transportation effected fundamental changes in what Americans could produce. The great changes in business organization would play a major role in dictating what Americans would consume.

But the new food giants were not the only ones trying to persuade Americans to change their diets by substituting some foods for others. In the same decades of the later nineteenth century a new movement to reform the American diet which would ultimately claim its share of successes was also taking shape.

CHAPTER 4

The New England Kitchen and the Failure to Reform Working-Class Eating Habits

The 1870s were not good years for the American economy. The wartime and postwar boom had come to a spectacular end with the Panic of 1873, and the ensuing years were ones of nagging depression. Although the depression was mainly financial and agricultural in origin, it had grave effects on employment and wages among the new working class. In 1877, discontent over these and other issues erupted into violent strikes and riots in what was later dubbed the "Year of Violence." The Knights of Labor, the first working-class organization to achieve a mass following, rallied thousands of workers to its banners and began pressing for shorter hours and higher wages. By the early 1880s, many wealthier Americans were coming to realize that industrialization was creating immense social, economic, and political problems. As they looked at the swelling slums of the cities, at the festering factory towns, at armed conflicts between workers and the forces of capital, fears of social upheaval and an explosion from the lower classes became more than simply nightmares of the faint-hearted. Some sought protection in armed force, and armories were built in more developed areas of cities so that the propertied could assemble in their cavalry units to put down the next wave of riots. Others, perhaps more sophisticated, thought of putting out the fire at the source by improving the living conditions of the poor.

Of course, there were many ideas regarding how this could be done. Private philanthropy, public education, industrial training, arts and crafts, legislation to improve housing and sanitation, even trade unions—all had their advocates. However, most were undermined by the triumphant economic ideas of the day, those of the classical laissez-faire school which dictated that wages were set by natural forces that should not be interfered with. The normal wage for unskilled labor would inevitably settle at a level adequate to provide bare subsistence, but no more, said David Ricardo in his theory of the "Iron Law of Wages." It was wrongheaded to try to raise them above this, for higher wages would simply lead to higher birth rates among the workers and a surplus of labor which would soon drive wages down and pull living standards below the subsistence level until, after a period of real misery, they reached their natural level again. Any movement which tried to raise wages artificially, whether it be through government intervention or labor union activity, ran counter to these natural laws and contributed to the ultimate impoverishment of society as a whole.

Needless to say, this kind of thinking greatly restricted the scope of those who wanted to mitigate the condition of the poor. Even well-meaning philanthropists had to draw fine distinctions between the "deserving" and the "undeserving" poor, making it clear that only a minority could really be helped.

But "the poor will always be with us" was not a very satisfying slogan for those who continued to worry about their explosive potential. Many searched for other alternatives which, while not violating the laissez-faire canon, would still meliorate the living conditions of the poor. Among them were a remarkable trio, Edward Atkinson, Wilbur Atwater, and Ellen Richards, who fastened on to the workers' diets as the key to both the problem and its solution. In the experiment they undertook, and particularly in its ultimate failure, lie the origins of a major part of the movement which ultimately transformed the American diet.

Atkinson was a self-made Boston businessman who had achieved considerable success in the textile and fire insurance businesses. An active Democrat involved in the southern cotton trade, he was stoutly anti-tariff and laissez-faire to the bone. Like many of this ilk, he found himself caught between his belief that wages could not rise and his concern that the low living standards of the working class would lead to upheaval. A well-read man who thought seriously about economics, in 1886 and 1887 he came across two pieces of information which together seemed to him to mark a breakthrough from his conundrum: first, he read that new surveys of workers' living standards indicated that American and European workers' families spent between 40 and 50 percent of their budgets on food. Then he read a series of articles in *Century Magazine* by the chemist Wilbur O. Atwater arguing that Americans, especially the poor, spent much more on food than was necessary for proper nutrition. To Atkinson, the implications of these facts were clear and extraordinary: if workers could be shown how to spend less on food, a larger share of their wages could be devoted to better housing and clothes. In this way, the slums could be cleared, ragged children could be dressed, and workers could live a decent life without the need for raising wages.

The scientific underpinnings of Atwater's ideas came from Germany, where a new scientific approach to food had been pioneered earlier in the century. Until then, although various properties had always been attributed to specific foods, food itself had generally been regarded as an undifferentiated mass. Once food was ingested it was commonly thought the body did not differentiate between various substances. Thus, historically, there was never any concern about the poor living mainly on bread, "the staff of life." Problems arose only when they did not get enough of it, giving rise to the possibility of "bread riots." As for the rich, there were no compunctions against eating as much of any particular food as they liked and totally ignoring those which did not strike their fancy.

To mid-nineteenth-century man, much taken with the idea of the human body as an engine, food was seen mainly as fuel, and it mattered little whether it was composed of grains, meats, fruits, or vegetables. In summing up conventional medical wisdom on the topic in 1860 the *Ladies' Home Magazine* said simply that "the most useful articles of diet are the commonest," and concentrated on the total weight of food required by different people, ranging from 36 ounces per day for a prizefighter to 20 ounces for a woman.[1] Of course, people have always believed that eating certain foods brought specific health benefits or dangers (the *Ladies' Home Magazine* was a particular partisan of apples, for example),[2] but there was no proven scientific basis for these ideas and no overarching theory which broke the foods themselves down into a number of similar components.

Within a few years, however, thanks to the pioneering efforts of the great German scientist Justus von Liebig in the 1840s and 1850s, scientists were separating foods into protein, carbohydrates, fat, minerals, and water, and were concluding that each nutrient performed specific physiological functions. Carbohydrates and fats seemed to provide two different kinds of fuel while proteins repaired worn-out tissues. There was general puzzlement over the roles of minerals, but there was agreement that foods should contain those minerals which the body contained. These chemists, whose ideas formed the basis for what I will be calling the "New Nutrition," thus recommended that people select their foods on the basis of their chemical composition, rather than taste, appearance, or other considerations. In other words, they were telling people to eat "what was good for them" rather than "what they liked."

Until the late 1870s most American food research was devoted to analyzing animal rather than human food, but by the mid-1880s serious work on American food was well under way, especially at Wesleyan University in Connecticut. There Atwater, a dogged, humorless, and very ambitious researcher applying the German techniques to American food, became convinced that Americans had developed wasteful and unhealthy food habits, the result of abundance of the continent's food resources and their own "conceit" over economizing about food. Convinced that nutritionally inadequate diets produced moral as well as physical degradation, he warned that failure to mend America's "foodways" would bring the exhaustion of its resources and economic and moral decline.[3]

To Atwater, perhaps the most important ramification of the new science of food was that the distinction between cheap food and expensive food disintegrated under chemical analysis. Whatever food they came from, there was little perceptible difference in the way carbohydrates, fats, and most proteins were metabolized by the human body. The important thing was not, as most Americans thought, to ingest as large or small an amount of undifferentiated food as the body required, but to eat only as much of the necessary nutrients as were needed for these nutrients to perform their specific tasks.[4]

Most Americans ate more carbohydrates than they needed, especially in the form of sweets, said Atwater, and the poor ate too little protein. "People of small or moderate means" were the worst offenders when it came to waste. "Beset with false pride of show and the petty ambition to go ahead of their neighbors," they disdained economizing on food and purchased the finest flour and the best cuts of meat when cheaper grades of flour and meat, and alternative foods provided the same nutrients at less cost.[5] By spending their money more wisely, they could easily increase their intake of protein while decreasing their overall expenditure on food.

It is easy to see how Atwater's ideas excited Atkinson, for they were based on scientific evidence emanating from laboratory experiments, and were derived from the study of American foods and American conditions. Moreover, they contained specific recommendations for the kinds of lessons which those of modest means must be taught. Atkinson contacted Atwater and the chemist affirmed that they shared common ground. Not only was Atkinson correct in seeing the connection between adequate wages and an adequate food supply, he wrote, but wage rates were largely dependent on the "nutritive efficiency" of the food consumed. High protein and high energy (meaning high fat) diets meant that more work could be done and higher wages could be paid. It was the greater intake of protein and fat that made American workers more productive than their German counterparts, said Atwater.[6] This supported Atkinson's argument that even higher intakes of these nutrients, especially in cheaper forms, would improve labor productivity and allow higher standards of living.

To these reformers, the main obstacle to elevating the standard of living of American workers seemed to be the workers' own ignorance regarding food. Their blind prejudices were catered to by their equally ignorant wives who, taking pride in serving "only the best," wasted millions of dollars on expensive foods such as butter and beef tenderloin when other fats and cheaper cuts of meat could provide more food value at less cost. Disgusted by American workers' aversion to soups and stews, Atkinson lamented "they stigmatize simmered foods of the best kind under the name 'pig wash.'"[7]

This last prejudice struck a particularly sensitive chord with Atkinson, for his hope for reforming the eating habits of the poor rested on the Aladdin Oven, a slow-cooking oven he had invented in the late 1880s. Using a knowledge of heat resistant and conducting materials gained in his fire insurance business, he argued that the American way of cooking was all wrong. The standard kitchen ranges were made of iron and steel, materials which conducted rather than contained heat, so that the bulk of the energy burned in heating their ovens was wasted, dissipated through their shells. The Aladdin Oven, on the other hand, was a box made of wood or fiberboard lined with tin with a hole in the bottom into which was inserted the top of a kerosene lamp.[8] Although the savings in fuel were considerable, the Aladdin Oven took a long time to heat up (about 1½ hours to pass 200 degrees Fahrenheit) and never reached more than 350 degrees Fahrenheit when full; it often dropped below that for a considerable length of time after the door was opened. Atkinson's oven, therefore, took at least five hours to cook most meat dishes. Thus, the kinds of dishes for which it was most suitable were exactly the kinds of slow-cooked stews the American working man shunned. Although it attracted some interest from middle-class reformers and gadgeteers, Atkinson realized his oven would not penetrate the kitchens of the class he most wanted to change until they learned new habits of cooking and eating.

A chance to promote both slow cooking and cheap food among the working class came in 1889, when Atkinson joined with two scientists, Mary Hinman Abel and Ellen H. Richards, and linked the Aladdin Oven with something he and Atwater had not thought of: the public kitchen. Abel had been the winner of the American Public Health Association's Lomb Prize essay contest for 1888. Its donor, the Rochester lens manufacturer Henry Lomb, reflected the new interest in food reform by decreeing that the year's topic for the nationwide contest would be "Practical, Sanitary, and Economical Cooking Adapted to Persons of Moderate and Small Means." Abel was the wife of a professor of pharmacology who became familiar with German nutritional research while her husband studied in that country. Her essay, which the jury declared stood head and shoulders above all its competition, was a clear explication of the nature and functions of the components of food, interlarded with pleas that American housewives take more cues from their European counterparts by substituting cheese, beans, and cheaper cuts of meat for the all-pervasive beef tenderloin as sources of protein. It contained suggested weekly menus for families at three different levels of "moderate and small" means, including one for feeding a family of six for thirteen cents per person per day.[9]

One of the members of the Lomb Prize jury was the first female graduate of the Massachusetts Institute of Technology, Ellen H. Richards, a chemist who in 1884 became the first woman appointed to the university's faculty. Richards applied her skills in chemical analysis to a number of fields but was now involved in bringing the benefits of science and its methods to women and the home. She did research in the chemistry of cleaning and the adulteration of food, and was convinced that what was needed was scientific research aimed not simply at eliminating bad, adulterated food but at preparing good, nutritious food. She therefore suggested to Abel that they collaborate on research on changing the diets of Americans of limited means. When Abel accepted, Richards sought the aid of Atkinson, a member of the MIT Board of Trustees who was impressed with both women's work, in securing funding for the project. Atkinson tapped some business associates for several hundred dollars to underwrite research into the kind of slow cooking and bread baking which the Aladdin Oven was best suited for and to create recipes for cheap and nutritious homemade breads, stews, and soups.[10]

The promoters played adeptly on the belief, common among philanthropists and temperance advocates, that there was an intimate connection between poor food and working class intemperance: that workers drank alcohol as a substitute for good food.[11] Arguing, "Do not grumble about the saloon until you have put some soup in its place," they secured a contribution of several thousands of dollars from Pauline Agassiz Shaw, a Boston philanthropist, for the study of "the food and nutrition of the working men and its possible relation to the question of the use of intoxicating liquors."[12]

During a stint in Germany, Abel was much impressed by Berlin's *Volksküchen,* or "People's Kitchens," which served cheap, nourishing food to the city's working classes. Now the possibility of starting American counterparts seemed to be opening up. Richards, seizing upon the idea, persuaded Pauline Shaw that the connection between nourishing food and temperance could best be demonstrated by opening a public eating room, aimed mainly at men "as a rival to the saloon."[13]

The Rumford Food Laboratory went much further than the *Volksküchen* idea of soup kitchens for the poor. Count Rumford, the Massachusetts-born originator of the term "Science of Nutrition," had been an early nineteenth-century pioneer in applying science to the problem of cooking cheap, nourishing food for the poor, and the Rumford Food Laboratory was to be "an experiment station," resting "upon a scientific basis," using the latest scientific ideas and equipment to devise methods of cooking that would revolutionize the diets of the working class.[14] Unlike *Volksküchen,* its purpose was to be "education by every means," the best means being by example. Once accustomed to the food of the soon-renamed New England Kitchen (a grudging concession to the public's prejudice for homey rather than scientific names for eating places) the working classes would not only come to depend on its cheap food for much of their diet but would also want to learn how to cook that way for themselves.[15] Thus, although formal cooking lessons were not given, much of the Kitchen's cooking was done in full view of the patrons. This served Atkinson's purposes as well, and he donated five of his ovens to it. They were set up in prominent positions, and he was promised that they would be used as much as possible.[16] Abel, meanwhile, was persuaded to leave her husband at Johns Hopkins in Baltimore for six months while she went to Boston to supervise the exciting experiment "right among the poor sections."[17]

Abel and Richards thought that the *Volksküchen* idea had to be adapted to America in another way. The communitarian aspects of the cafés of Paris or the *Volksküchen* were not suited to "the free American," who liked to "be free in his selection of food," wrote Richards; "Home and family life are our strongholds," she said, and "the food must go to the families and not the people to the food."[18] The first New England Kitchen, therefore, was to be "take out."

The two women were cautious about opening the Kitchen's doors too soon—too cautious for Atkinson. He pressed them to open and fretted about their failure to develop the much-anticipated recipe for a three-cent loaf of bread baked in the Aladdin Oven.[19] But not until mid-1890, when they had developed, taste-tested, and chemically analyzed a number of basic dishes, including a slow-cooked beef broth made in the Aladdin Oven, did they begin public sale of their wares.

At first the Kitchen seemed successful. The Aladdin broth, which took twelve hours to reach the boiling point and exuded the flavor of raw meat, was a great favorite in sick rooms.[20] Within months, scores of doctors were recommending it to patients, and invalids were sending for it from near and far. Mary Abel returned to Baltimore after six months, but she left scientifically precise recipes for soups, stews, and chowders she and Richards developed. The kitchen workers were supervised by a former student of Richards's at MIT, a young Vassar graduate. For two hours each lunchtime the kitchen was abuzz with employees filling customers' pails and cans, many of which were sent off in muff boxes to teachers at local schools and employees in local businesses, at prices the founders thought equaled the cost of cooking the same foods at home. Although it was difficult to gauge its success in educating the poor in new ways, the reformers were gratified to note that after the first six months of operation there was a sharp rise in the standard of cleanliness of the dishes brought to be filled.[21]

In November 1891, with financial help arranged by Atkinson, an annex was opened across the street to bake and sell bread. Although it did not use the Aladdin Oven, it did make a point of using a recipe for "Health Bread" from Atkinson's treatise on nutrition.[22] The spring of 1892 brought what Abel and Richards thought of as "one of the crowning successes" of the Kitchen: with funds provided by another female philanthropist, they prepared and delivered hot school lunches which were varied, nutritive, and, they claimed, tasty, for fifteen cents each to a local high school with 300 students.[23] As a result of the success of its experiment, the New England Kitchen was rewarded with a contract to provide all nine Boston high schools with hot lunches beginning in 1894, the first such program in the country.[24]

Fortified by their apparent success, the founders looked to expansion. A branch was opened in the primarily black West End to serve food cooked on Pleasant Street. A separate Kitchen was opened in the ethnically variegated North End. Studies were made of the possibilities of opening in Olneyville, a manufacturing suburb of Providence, Rhode Island, to wean the largely Irish and French Canadian factory hands there (considered "the most incorrigible of all the communities") from their wayward food habits.[25]

Meanwhile, Atkinson was preaching the virtues of public kitchens and his oven in New York. In September 1890, his colleague in the Democratic reform movement, Abram Hewit, bought an Aladdin Oven and arranged for Atkinson to speak at the prestigious Cooper Union.[26] The speech and the demonstration so impressed Thomas Egleston, a Columbia University metallurgist involved in the settlement house movement, that he arranged for Atkinson to give a lecture in Columbia's largest lecture hall with the steel baron and philanthropist Andrew Carnegie in attendance.[27]

Egleston now threw himself into a frenzy of devotion to the new cause, securing a contribution of $5,000 from Thomas Havemeyer, a Wall Street financier, from the family which controlled the "Sugar Trust." The contribution enabled him to open a New York version of the New England Kitchen in December, 1891. Like Richards, Abel, and Atkinson, Egleston, Havemeyer, and Carnegie (who later contributed), all found it most attractive that the New England Kitchen was not a charitable soup kitchen but a scientific experiment station. Within two months of its opening, Egleston proclaimed the New York NEK a "great success."[28] Because it was not charity, and was ostensibly self-supporting, it soon became a standard stop on the tours of those investigating the achievements of the "New Philanthropy" in the United States.[29] Because it opened its doors to the poor where they lived, the NEK also aroused interest in the fledgling settlement house movement, whose social workers lived in residences among the poor, attempting to teach them proper living and work habits in their own environment. Fortified by another $5,000 contribution from Havemeyer, the New York Kitchen sailed into its second year with Egleston working to introduce its methods in the seven settlement house cooking schools upon whose boards he now served.[30]

The possibility of expansion to Chicago opened when Julia Lathrop, another student of Ellen Richards at MIT, accepted a post at Hull House, perhaps the most successful settlement house. Before Lathrop left for Chicago, Mary Abel trained her in the ways of the New England Kitchen, and at Hull House she opened a "people's kitchen" patterned on the New York and Boston ones.[31] The NEK message was brought to Philadelphia by two graduates of women's colleges who, after training at the Boston Kitchen, went to work in Philadelphia's College Settlement House, situated in a poor black and Jewish neighborhood.[32]

In 1893 the reformers set up a model workman's cottage in the Massachusetts pavilion at the Columbian Exposition. There they demonstrated how a worker could live and eat well on $500 a year. In their contiguous "Rumford Kitchen" they served thirty-cent meals cooked in an Aladdin-equipped kitchen to thousands of people from menus on which food values were noted.[33] Aladdins were distributed everywhere: to a Brooklyn Heights woman who Richards helped "personate" a workman's wife with four children living on $450 a year; and to the black educator Booker T. Washington, who wrote glowing testimonials to the Aladdins that Atkinson donated to Tuskegee College, the agricultural and industrial training school he headed in Alabama.[34]

But beneath the surface all was not well. Andrew Carnegie may have been impressed, but the new cooking and its message were failing to make a mark on those at whom they were mainly directed, the urban working classes. The NEK branch catering to Boston blacks never really got off the ground because of lack of support from that quarter. After two and one-half years of trying to attract the Italians, Jews, Slavs, and Portuguese of the North End, the kitchen there was abandoned as a failure.

The reformers began to realize that the prototypical "American worker" they had theorized about hardly existed, and that the food habits of the newer immigrants were resistant to "American" attempts to change them. By the time the New York NEK was ready to open, the Boston reformers were so discouraged by the response of most immigrants that they instructed that it be set up in a neighborhood of German and British immigrants. The mandate was difficult to follow, and the Hudson Street Kitchen was frustrated by the religious restrictions of Jews and the seemingly un-American demands of Italians. It never reached its promised goal of self-sufficiency and remained open mainly due to Havemeyer's contributions.

Similarly, the cooking school set up by the NEK graduates in the Philadelphia College Settlement House failed to attract enough students. Their public kitchen and coffee house failed to fulfill their promise of achieving financial independence and were set adrift by the hard-pressed settlement house in 1897 and allowed to expire quietly on their own.[35] The Hull House operation continued for thirty-two years, but the section which sold cooked foods at lunchtime to neighborhood factories was never popular. It was supported by the restaurant section which, converted to a coffee house, became a popular meeting place for local businessmen and schoolteachers.[36]

Even the flagship Boston restaurant could not break even on the working-class trade. Only the sales of broth to hospitals, school lunches to MIT, and, finally, the contract with the Boston School Committee kept it afloat. A small lunch room catering to neighborhood shop girls helped as well, but custom among the working class continued to disappoint. Part of the problem, the reformers thought, was technological, the result of Atkinson's failure to perfect a cheap system for delivering hot meals to homes and workplaces as well as a heatable worker's lunch pail. But it was also becoming apparent that the poor, of whatever ethnic origin, were simply not responding in sufficient numbers.

By 1894 Havemeyer was growing disillusioned, and Richards, Abel, and Atkinson began rethinking their attitudes toward reforming the food habits of the lower classes. Trying to convince the reluctant Havemeyer to continue supporting the project, Atkinson said that they now thought it "useless" to try to change the food habits of the "very poor" at the outset of reform. Their tastes were already too "depraved" and their prejudices in favor of high-priced flour and meat too fixed. However, wrote Atkinson, they have found a "field" in "a class considerably above the very poor . . . ," those living on small incomes who:

> *must* dress decently and cannot live in dirty or slummy quarters; shop girls, the lower grades of teachers, decorators, young men just starting life who possess intelligence but who earn very little money, &c, &c. This is the class that economises *unwisely,* often on food, in order to dress well, even without extravagance, and to occupy decent rooms.

The "jealous and suspicious working people in the lower grade" would be reached through the "sifting down of information" from these hard-working neighbors. Richards buttressed this, adding that for the "very poor" the problem of shelter overshadowed the food question. They "get enough to eat" and:

> have very decided preferences for the looks and flavor of food to which they have been accustomed. They will not try new things, and are exceedingly suspicious of any attempt to help them. But the great middle class of wage earners there are those whose ambition has been aroused, and who are ready to starve themselves for the sake of better clothes and better shelter. It is to this most worthy class that the Kitchen has been a great boon.[37]

Although Havemeyer agreed to continue subsidizing the New York Kitchen, fundamental problems remained. This class of upwardly mobile wage earners bought food in quantities too small to make cooking on the NEK scale economical unless it was served in large lunch rooms or taken to a network of smaller ones.[38]

By late 1894, Richards found additional reasons for abandoning the

direct assault on the poor. The poor comprised two classes, she wrote
Atkinson, "those who do not care for clean wholesome food" and "those
who know how to live cheaper than we can ever feed them." Their main
objective should still be to reach these "self-respecting wage-earners" and
their children, but it seemed clear that she regarded them as a distinct
minority.[39]

Meanwhile, the Aladdin Oven upon which Atkinson had pinned so
many hopes was not fulfilling its expectations. It was too expensive for the
working-class, required too much care and expertise to work, and continued to manifest various technical "bugs." A small one cost only $25 but
some kind of supplemental stove for heating water and frying was still
necessary. In addition the Aladdin Oven did not fulfill the most important
function of the stoves of the day: heating the kitchen in wintertime. It also
had to be "seasoned" for two weeks before it would function properly and
one had to use special recipes and techniques worked out by Atkinson and
the staff of the NEK. It could not be left unattended in the home for fear
that it might ignite and burn through the table it was set on, causing a
general conflagration.[40] In 1892, Egleston regretfully informed Atkinson
that all of the ovens sold as a result of Atkinson's lectures in New York
"failed entirely in use, although in the hands of exceptionally bright persons, because every one did something with it which made it impossible to
use."[41]

Despite experiments with glass ovens and asbestos lining, Atkinson was
never able to overcome the technological and intellectual barriers. If the
rich and well-educated could not master it, how much hope was there for
the poor? There was also growing despair over the ability of the poor to
master the rules of the New Nutrition. Some years later Richards quoted
the remark of a visitor to the Rumford Kitchen's $500-a-year workman's
cottage: "It will take a $5000 a year wife to do it."[42]

By late 1895, Havemeyer cut off his support and the New York Kitch-
en was on the verge of closing. Andrew Carnegie, who had already contributed $250 to the project, kept it going for another year, but seems to
have been more interested in it as a food laboratory than as a public
kitchen. By 1897 it too was closed.[43]

But the crusade to spread the message of the New Nutrition was by no
means over. Egleston and Carnegie had assumed that scientific research
for the project would remain in private hands, funded by philanthropists
such as Carnegie.[44] However, the active Democrat Atkinson seized upon
the opportunity presented by the election of fellow Democrat Grover
Cleveland to the presidency in 1892 and prevailed upon his "good friend"
Frederic Morton, the new Secretary of Agriculture, to set up laboratories
to study human food in the department's agricultural experiment stations.
In 1894, the first of these came into being, a laboratory at the experiment
station in Storrs, Connecticut, directed by Atkinson's associate Atwater.[45]

The federal government now seemed on its way to becoming the kind of center for food research and dissemination of nutritional information that the founders had hoped the New England Kitchen would become. Whatever the future benefits to the nation, the advantages to the reformer-scientists, at least in terms of scholarly respectability soon became manifest. Almost immediately, the Office of Experiment Stations began funding and publishing Abel's and Richards's studies.[46] Within a few years, Atwater, promoted to the newly created position of director of human nutrition studies of the Office of Experiment Stations, was able to employ a number of Richards's protégées whose research project results the Office subsequently published.

With the New England Kitchen displaced as a research center and its other goals seeming even more unattainable, the founders drifted away from active participation in its affairs and began re-evaluating their strategy.[47] The Boston NEK itself changed, de-emphasizing the hot food "take home" service and concentrating on the school lunch programs, as well as a new lunch room catering to secretaries, clerks, and other working girls. "It was quite a place for us college girls," a former patron recalled many years later,[48] but consequently not much of a place for working-class girls. In 1907, when it was taken over by the Women's Educational and Industrial Union, a middle-class philanthropic organization, its original role as the cutting edge of the New Nutrition among the working class had been all but forgotten.[49]

It is tempting to regard the founders of the Kitchen as they saw themselves: people of learning and vision frustrated by the ignorance and prejudices of the class they most wanted to help. After all, within decades, much of their message on nutrition had become part of the conventional wisdom. Yet to concentrate solely on the wisdom of their message would be to ignore their manifest failings. Like many reformers of the time, they went about their mission among the working class with the smug assurance that with "science" on their side, they were touting a way of life far superior to that worked out by millions of people in their daily struggle to survive. Once rejected, rather than re-examining their message and its audience, they dismissed the working-class as ignoramuses whose only hope lay in their propensity to imitate their betters. "I made one great mistake," wrote Atkinson in 1899, "I tried to work from below upward." Had he ignored the poor and demonstrated the Aladdin's superiority in cooking partridge, venison, and other game, he would have had more success, he explained, for "man is an imitative animal, especially woman."

Although they derided him as "Shinbone Atkinson" primarily out of ignorance, working-class hostility toward him was not without justification. Too often, Atkinson's pleas for cheaper eating were coupled with the argument that it would obviate wage raises.[50] His rabid antagonism toward trade unionism heightened suspicion of his message. Trade union leader and later Socialist presidential candidate Eugene V. Debs, who called him "probably more relentless in his hostility to trade unions than any other writer or speaker in the country," charged that his crusade was aimed at lowering, rather than raising, workers' standards of living. "He may teach men the science of the shinbone diet," wrote Debs, "and chuckle as he sees his degenerate disciples live on ten cents a day, and glory in his success in teaching Americans how to eat like Huns, but American workingmen are resolved not to be further degraded, scientifically or otherwise. . . ."[51]

The reference to Hun diets brings up another failing of the well-meaning reformers: their underestimation of the importance of the psychological role of food in American working-class families, native-born and immigrant. To most workers, eating better food, usually more meat and particularly more beefsteak, was one of the major rewards of hard work and a respectable job. To the reformers, this was simply a source of frustration, a product of the improvidence and ignorance of the working classes. Mary Abel, who often praised the "Hun cooking" Debs reviled, wrote with dismay of the American workers who "revel in unwonted luxury." Yet, as she and the others knew, Europeans ate less meat primarily because their incomes were lower. After all, the statistics they cited showed European workers spending about the same proportion of their incomes on food as Americans.[52] Abel herself underlined this point by quoting with disapproval an immigrant from Germany who rejoiced, "Where in the old country do you find a workman that can have meat on his table three times a day?" For this man, wrote Abel with ill-concealed disgust, "American freedom and prosperity had a very limited meaning."[53]

Reading Abel's homilies about the tyranny of "King Palate," whose reign brought an invasion of "impish creatures" named "Indigestion, Dyspepsia, Gout, Liver Disease, Delerium Tremens, and a hundred others, big and little,"[54] as well as the New England Kitchen founders' injunctions that it cook "cosmopolitan" food bland enough to offend no one, one suspects that they also suffered from the Achilles' heel of so many food reformers: bland palates and underdeveloped appreciations of the joy of eating. It was after tasting Kitchen food that the prototypical poor woman allegedly said: "I'd rather eat what I'd rather. I don't want to eat what's good for me."[55] Yet the reformers failed to devise recipes that were nutritious, cheap, and irresistible to King Palate. Despite their resolve to submit recipes to "community panels" for taste testing, their wares made no concession at all to the tastes and cooking methods of the large majority of immigrant customers. Along with beef broth, the core Kitchen menu was resolutely New England, featuring fish, clam, and corn chowders, "Pilgrim succotash," creamed codfish, pressed meat, corn mush, boiled hominy, oatmeal mush, cracked wheat, baked beans, and Indian pudding. It was hardly a bill of fare to attract Boston's Irish and French Canadians, not to mention Italians, Jews, and central and eastern Europeans.[56] At first, the founders would not even serve the mainstay working-class meat, pork. Only reluctantly, after they realized the clientele would not eat pea soup without pork and pepper were those ingredients added to it and the other dishes.[57] Moreover, as Abel herself recognized in her Lomb Prize essay, when it came to devising recipies for slow-cooked dishes that used meat economically and supplemented it with vegetable or other animal protein, the reformers had much to learn from the very immigrants they were trying to change. Yet they blamed their failure on the immigrants' conservatism with regard to food, rather than their own rigidity.

The great irony of this attempt to bring the benefits of science to the eating habits of the lower-class was that many of the things the reformers advocated were, by the light of today's nutritionists, both dangerous and unhealthy. As we have seen, one of the banes of the workingman's diet was the dearth of fresh vegetables and fruits. Yet, because they preached in the era before the discovery of vitamins, the New Nutritionists denigrated most fruits and vegetables, which emerged from the labs as mostly water and carbohydrates. Atwater urged Americans to eat more white flour and fewer potatoes because the former was a much cheaper source of carbohydrates. The bran of the wheat and the vitamin-packed skins of the potatoes were to be discarded as "refuse."[58] The tomato was dismissed as useful only in small quantities as a flavoring agent with no food value of its own. If one insisted on eating green vegetables, they were to be well boiled, to make them more digestible and lessen the waste of energy necessary to digest them. Only condensed milk, laced with sugar but deprived of Vitamins C and D, was used in the Kitchen. In short, if America turned *en masse* to follow their advice, rickets, beri-beri, scurvy, and other vitamin-deficiency diseases may have reached epidemic proportions.

Similarly, their calculations regarding protein and calorie requirements now seem quite incorrect. They urged the intake of over twice as much protein as is considered the maximum advisable burden on the kidneys.[59] The New Nutritionists' recommendations regarding quantities of food ingested were based not on laboratory experiments but on surveys of how much people actually ate. Thus, one of Atwater's contributions to the study of caloric intake was to revise upward the already high recommendations of the German scientist Voit. While Voit suggested 3,050 calories a day as the standard for a seventy-kilogram male engaged in moderate work, Atwater suggested 3,500 for Americans, citing the allegedly higher productivity of the American worker as the reason.[60] Atwater and his associates were also unaffected by our knowledge of the hazards of animal-derived fats, and recommended increased fat intakes to increase energy, telling housewives to buy the fattest cuts of meat and praising the virtues of lovely slices of fat from the tops or insides of various roasts.[61]

Thus, although acknowledging that modern scientific understanding of food and nutrition was still in its infancy, the reformers were nevertheless anxious to run off with incomplete knowledge and try to change one of the most important facets of human life. As Richard Cummings wrote over forty-five years ago, "The conclusions reached by the early American workers in the field of nutrition are excellent examples of the fact that 'a little knowledge may be a dangerous thing.'"[62]

But that was not the conclusion which the doughty reformers drew from the failure of the New England Kitchen experiment. After a few more years of desultory puttering with the Aladdin Oven, Atkinson drifted away from the food crusade, busying himself again with the tariff fight and joining the Anti-Imperialist League to head off the acquisition of colonies after the war with Spain. But Richards and Abel began to act on lessons drawn from the failed experiment. Atkinson himself had summed them up when he regretted not having promoted the Aladdin Oven for upper-class cooking, counting on the propensity of the lower class to emulate their betters. Richards and Abel came to similar conclusions. "It was unfortunate," wrote Richards to Atkinson in 1897, "that we began the food crusade from the point of view of cheap food. . . . I think if you had confined yourself to giving $2 or $5 dinners to your friends, of the very best materials, and instead of having a lunch room for your employees have had a very artistic room for your guests, that the thing might have gone much more rapidly than now."[63]

But whereas Atkinson blamed, among other things, the stubborness of cooks for the failure of new ideas to catch on, Richards saw hope in an alternative path. The real problem, she said, was that cooks were not "scientifically trained to take up new things and to conquer anything which has difficulties."[64] That this meant the abandonment of the lower classes as the object of conversion and the raising of the reformers' sights to those above them was made clear in a letter Richards wrote to a woman in 1899 in which she expressed a new eugenic concern for the future of the better-off. "I believe, with Professor S. H. Patten," she wrote, "that the well-to-do classes are being eliminated by their diet, to the detriment of social progress, and *they* and *not* the poor are most in need of missionary work." The solution to the problem lay in teaching a scientific approach to food and nutrition in the schools and colleges. "Education alone will bring the food question from the dark secluded corners of life to the sunlight of right thinking," she continued, "and therefore I am bending all my energies toward public school teaching of the right sort. Meanwhile I am waiting for the authorities of some college to show that they are up-to-date and are willing to put the food department on a level with the Greek or mathematics, by appointing a Professor of Hygiene and Sanitation."[65]

Richards was much closer to her goal than she could have dreamed at the time. Due to her efforts and those of Abel, people of similar convictions were already rallying to the newly upraised banner, not of Hygiene and Sanitation, but of Home Economics. She and Abel were instrumental in organizing a series of conferences at Lake Placid, New York, out of which grew the American Home Economics Association. With Richards as its first president and Abel as editor of its scholarly journal, the association had a definite scientific, scholarly thrust, seeking to attain status for the field by stimulating college training, research, publication, professional degrees, and teaching jobs for graduates in public schools or colleges. They were aided immensely by Atwater and his disciples, whose government agencies cooperated closely with the new professional home economists, providing them with outlets for publication and helping to cloak them in scientific respectability.

By 1900, then, a movement was growing which would direct much of its energies toward changing the diet of the middle class. Better-educated and more awed by modern scientific wisdom than the sullen workers who failed to respond to the New England Kitchen, middle-class Americans would be more easily impressed by the movement's aura of science and professionalism. More important, however, many of them had a very direct interest in the food question, as developments in their own homes made them very receptive to the New Nutritionists' message.

CHAPTER 5

The "Servant Problem" and Middle-Class Cookery

In the twenty-five years after 1880, the middle class had expanded tremendously in numbers and self-consciousness. Industrialization and urbanization created a host of new occupations, some of them managerial, others professional, and expanded the scope and profits of businesses which occupied the interstices between the giant new corporations and the traditional one- or two-man retail operations and artisanal workshops. As its self-confidence rose, so did its social aspirations. Soon this rising middle class, which in 1880 had tentatively begun to emulate the new styles in dining that had swept the upper class, became more serious about doing so.

But domestic service still posed the greatest barrier between upper-class habits and the life of the class below them, and, ultimately, middle-class hopes of imitating upper-class elegance in dining foundered on the rocks of this problem, which originated in the economics of dining and entertaining. Falling prices of previously exotic foods and continuing advances in the technology of food preservation, processing, and preparation expanded the culinary horizons of the middle class, allowing them to aspire to setting tables with a variety of foods which rivaled those of the upper class. Increasingly, then, in the 1880s and 1890s middle-class menus, particularly for entertaining, began to look like scaled-down versions of upper-class menus. They had fewer courses, less elaborate concoctions, and were less influenced by French cooking styles, but the order of dishes followed the same basic structure and diners were expected to eat about as much.

For middle-class "housekeepers," (the term used then to denote those who owned and managed households, rather than those who worked in them) the problem was to find servants capable of exploiting the new culinary opportunities. The housewife could, and often did, help with the preparation of food. But there was no way she could cook meals of the kind expected both by guests and family without the aid of at least one servant of considerable skill in the kitchen. A similar situation prevailed with regard to new methods of serving meals, making it necessary to have more servants, and more competent servants as well. While some etiquette books recommended *service à la Russe* to the middle classes of the 1880s and 1890s, this was impossible for most middle-class families. For it to be managed properly, according to etiquette writer Mary Sherwood, it was necessary to have at least one servant for every three guests, which generally meant hiring extra servants for dinner parties.[1] "Modified *service à la Russe*," the middle-class alternative, was never more than a partial solution to the problem, for while it removed carving—the most demanding skill—from the hands of the servants, it often placed it in the hands of hosts or hostesses, equally incompetent at carving. Moreover, "modified *service à la Russe*" did not mean dispensing with cooks and servants, it simply meant making do with less competent ones, leaving enormous scope for service *gaffes*. In her popular turn-of-the-century etiquette book Mary Sherwood extolled the "many simple little dinners given by young couples with small means which were far more enjoyable than the gold and silver 'diamond' dinners" given by the upper class. Yet her instructions for staging one still mandated "a good cook" (as opposed to "a French cook" for the dinners of the wealthier) and "a neat maid-servant in cap and apron" (as opposed to "several accomplished servants"). However, it is difficult to imagine a hostess of the period preparing and serving the kind of "simple dinner" recommended with only this level of help. It consisted of oysters, *Soupe à la Reine,* broiled fish, *Filet de Boeuf aux Champignons* or roast beef or mutton, roast partridges, tomato salad, cheese, ices, jellies, fruit, coffee, and liqueurs. The suggested wines were Chablis, hock (Rhinewine), Champagne, claret, Burgundy or Sherry, and liqueurs, although Sherwood admitted that lately it had been considered sufficient to serve champagne and claret through the whole dinner.[2]

To make matters worse, the middle-class housewife was expected to stage elaborate dinner parties with increasing frequency, for—as with the upper class—entertaining over food, and particularly at dinner parties, rapidly became one of the central features of middle-class social life. Luncheon and dinner clubs became popular. These met at members' homes and each member strove to surpass the others' presentations.[3] When guests were entertained, not only the food but the table, flower arrangements, silver, linens, china, and glass were expected to reflect the creativity and inventiveness of the hostess. Theme dinners, in which a single motif would dominate everything, were particular favorites. One very popular challenge in the early 1890s was to have "white dinners" or "green dinners" in which everything, including the food, would be in shades of the selected color.

Meanwhile, middle-class housekeepers were being swamped by other demands for food service. Breakfasts were expected to be large and include a number of cooked meats. Most husbands and schoolchildren still came home for lunch, and although the lunches were smaller, the nutritional ideas of the day dictated that they should be hot and substantial. Often, no sooner would the dishes from lunch have been cleared when preparations would have to be made for lady friends visiting for afternoon tea, the vogue for this modish repast having passed from the upper to the middle class in the 1880s and 1890s. Tea would be served at meetings of women's clubs, where middle-class ladies would meet in members' homes and sit in sharp-eyed judgement of the manner in which the dainty sandwiches, cakes, and beverages were prepared, displayed, and served. When, shortly after the meetings had dispersed, husband and children returned home, they again expected a hot meal, often consisting of four courses.

The cooking schools for middle-class women which proliferated in the 1880s and 1890s were ruled by "domestic scientists," who saw culinary salvation in the increased "refinement" of cooking and taught ridiculously complex methods of cookery and presentation which made cooking a more onerous, time-consuming process than ever.[4] Even for those who were not directly involved in much of the cooking, shopping was a formidable chore. The turn-of-the-century account books of Ella Lyman Cabot, a well-off Radcliffe graduate married to a doctor in Cambridge, show that she had to prepare detailed menus a week in advance, and deal directly with a number of merchants, including a butcher, fishmonger, egg man, milk man, a "provisioner" (for apples, butter, meats, and potatoes), and a grocer (S. S. Pierce, of course).[5]

In the face of these kinds of demands, it is easy to understand why by the 1890s middle-class women were becoming virtually obsessed by the "servant problem," for it seemed to be the main obstacle to fulfilling society's expectations of them. To these women, living primarily in the cities and large towns outside the South, the problem was twofold. On the one hand, it involved a servant shortage. It was difficult for service occupations to compete with the growing number of jobs available to females in other occupations in terms of working conditions, particularly in "free time." Native-born whites in particular were reluctant to take on full-time service positions, and immigrant girls drifted away from them as soon as job opportunities opened for them in factories or other occupations. On the other hand, the "problem" involved a competence crisis. This meant a dearth of servants able to cook and serve meals in the manner which employers demanded. Immigration had supplied the bulk of the servant population in the post-Civil War North, but in the 1880s and 1890s, as the nature of immigration into the country changed, so did the composition of the servant class. Northern European immigrants and farm girls, previously the backbone of the servant class outside the South (where black cooks and house servants continued to play their historic roles), were less interested in service. Speaking on the "Labor Problems in the Household" at a home economics conference in 1903, Mary Hinman Abel noted that:

> for fifty years the American-born white woman has hardly been considered as a source of supply for household service, and foreign emigration, formerly the reliance [*sic*], has entirely changed in character. In one case, out of 700 steerage passengers brought from South Germany by a North German Lloyd ship, 650 had their tickets already bought for them for the West, where they were to go into farming, and the remainder settled in the seaboard towns, going into shops or factories with former friends; and these figures can be duplicated at any immigration bureau. Very few are available for household service, as compared with the number such a shipload would have furnished 20 years ago.[6]

One of the conference participants, Mrs. Martha Van Renssalear, later a home economics professor at Cornell, told of how, desperate for domestic help, she drove to the country, thinking that farm girls would want a position. However, a man there "with considerable experience in that line" told her, "Never go to a country town to get a girl; they want to go to the city to work in a factory or to train themselves to be typewriters or schoolteachers."[7] Another woman complained that she had lost the services of a French-Canadian girl from Vermont who was a wonderful cook because she allowed her to become friendly with the neighborhood students who told her: "You're too good to do this work; you ought to learn to do typewriting and stenography."[8]

The Irish, German, and rural American servant girls had to be replaced by Eastern and Central Europeans, blacks from the South, and, in the West, Asians. This often meant that it was difficult for middle-class white Anglo-Saxon Protestants to find servants able to understand their orders, let alone understand their needs. Even in the days when English-speaking servants were the norm in kitchens, complaints about their incompetence were common. Now, grousing about them was the rule. The obvious solution was to pay higher wages, improve working conditions, and hire better-skilled and more highly motivated servants. It was apparent, after all, that the wealthy seemed hardly affected by the problem. Their households were run on the lines of the large English household, noted Mary Hinman Abel. Servants' hours and duties were "definite and seldom excessive" and they were accustomed to and enjoyed "the life among themselves." Most of them had been trained in Europe and "look forward to no change in their occupation. . . . The house service question is concerned with the small household only," she said.[9] But while some women did occasionally propose higher pay and better working conditions as a solution to the problem, the vast majority felt that they simply could not afford it, particularly for servants of the low level of competence they were forced to hire.

In the 1890s some middle-class women sought to break out of this conundrum by setting up programs for training servants, hoping that by turning cooking and serving for the middle classes into skilled occupations greater productivity could be matched by higher pay. When the National Household Economics Association was formed in 1893 two of its major goals were "to secure skilled labor in every major department in our homes" and to elevate domestic service to a more skilled level by organizing schools of household science and service and establishing employment bureaus for servants. Similar aims were proclaimed by the General Federation of Women's Clubs. Before the year was out women's clubs in Chicago, New York, and Philadelphia were organizing employment bureaus and planning training schools for domestics.[10] In Boston, the Women's Educational and Industrial Union set up a Domestic Reform League and mounted an ambitious program to train both master and servant in cooking and housekeeping.[11]

While the Boston school was hailed as "an effort to place the occupation of housekeeping on a strictly scientific and business basis,"[12] it was exactly the realities of housekeeping as a business that caused it and similar experiments in other cities to founder. Commenting on the failure of a similar cooking course for servants in Philadelphia, the famed cooking teacher Sarah Tyson Rorer put her finger on the economic realities which torpedoed all such ventures. They could never be self-supporting in societies with free markets in servants, she said, "as these poor souls have not the wherewithal to pay." Yet "housewives can rarely pay for them, as they frequently leave as soon as they are trained."[13] "All are agreed that it is vain to talk of training schools or model employment bureaus while there is practically nothing to train or distribute," said Mary Hinman Abel in 1903.[14]

Another proposed solution was bringing service into the world of modern capitalism by putting it on a contract basis, specifying hours of work, tasks to be fulfilled, and so on. Mary Hinman Abel and other home economists were attracted to this because it smacked of division of labor and specialization, which they regarded as the keys to America's industrial progress. They experimented with setting up a bureau which would send out specialists in cooking, laundry, and other household chores on an hourly or daily basis.[15] But this approach was suited for day work, not for live-in help.[16] While it might have sufficed for employers looking for charwomen and laundresses, it could not supply girls who would be up at the crack of dawn to light the stoves and begin breakfast and then stay late into the night to cook, clear, and clean the dinner dishes.

The failure of these experiments lent credence to another kind of solution: cooperative kitchens. Perhaps their best-known advocate was Edward Bellamy, whose utopian novel *Looking Backward* had evoked immense public interest. In 1889, the editors of *Good Housekeeping* magazine sensed correctly that, while the bulk of their middle-class readership would hardly sympathize with his socialism, they would find his ideas on solving the "servant problem" of great interest. They therefore commissioned an article in which he elaborated on the system of cooperative housekeeping described in his novel. Perhaps in deference to the editors' political predilections, Bellamy eliminated the potentially statist aspects, which had housekeeping done by female members of the "Industrial Army," and emphasized instead the idea of cooperative housekeeping as a solution to the servant problem.

"What can be done with the Servant girl?" Bellamy asked. "Nothing," he replied. "What can be done without her? Everything." There was no future for domestic service in America, he argued. It ran counter to "the democratic spirit of the Age" and "but for foreign importations . . . would have become extinct in America" long before. Even the immigrants could not remain immune from the democratic spirit for long, for "the rich gloss of inherited servility which had taken a dozen centuries to grow, wore threadbare, as a rule, at the end of six months on this side of the water." What was needed, said Bellamy, was to follow the direction which the evolution of the household had been taking for many years: to have an increasing number of its functions contracted to outside agencies. Large cooperative laundries and non-profit employment agencies could do housecleaning. Cooperative kitchens, working on fixed contracts to provide a certain minimum number of meals and service, could take over cooking and scullion work. One of the benefits of cooperative cooking would be the elevation of American cooking from the abysmal level to which it had fallen in the past twenty-five years, since mother making her pie and Aunt Jane dressing her turkey had been replaced in the kitchens of well-to-do families by a "succession of casual employees, of whom it might be said in defense that their cooking is quite as good as people deserve who tolerate a system which produces such cooking."[17]

Bellamy's article spurred middle-class interest in cooperative kitchens. "Bellamy Clubs" such as that in Kansas City, Missouri, tried them, and women in a number of cities and towns in the Northeast and Midwest joined together to share food preparation and dining facilities in a number of different ways.[18] Some months after Bellamy's article appeared, *Good Housekeeping* ran a glowing article on cooperation which cited an unnamed cooperative eating arrangement in which some families "of comfortable incomes" had rented a house, hired servants to staff it, and ate their family meals there. "One cook, of better quality than usual, had done for 50 people what ten incompetent cooks had formerly tried to do for ten separate families."[19]

The major theme in this and other reports on cooperative eating arrangements was that they enabled middle-class people to escape what Catherine Selden, writing in the prestigious *North American Review,* called "The Tyranny of the Kitchen." By this she meant, not the person chained to her pots, pans, and stove but the housewife at the mercy of the incompetents she was forced to hire to use those utensils. While sharing "certain defects of character which belong to the human race in general," those who entered domestic service also suffered from "deficiencies peculiar to the class itself." Servant girls would not train themselves. "The housekeeper must continue to teach her ignorant employee, and at the same time pay her the price which is due skilled labor." Servants' wages would continue to rise and their hours of work diminish. Thus, "the advantages lie almost exclusively with the class which we are in the habit of regarding as one of the least intelligent in the community: a class, however, which has shown itself capable of being both aggressive and tyrannical." The only solution, she concluded, lay in cooperative housekeeping arrangements, particularly with regard to food.[20]

Employers were not the only ones who saw cooperative kitchens as a direct attack on the power of servants. So did servants. When forty upper-middle-class families in Evanston, Illinois, formed a cooperative kitchen and laundering arrangement and fired their cooks and laundresses, the maids, who they retained to do the remaining housekeeping, struck, both in support of the fired servants and in protest against the extra burdens being placed on them. A servants' league even drew up a blacklist of employers.[21]

Selden recommended that the growing network of women's clubs put the organization of cooperative kitchens on their agenda, and many of them did. The idea became a popular topic for discussion and the fledgling home economics movement made it a standard part of its curricula for schools and colleges. But few of the experiments lasted very long. Selden warned that the organization of the cooperatives should be left in the hands of men, who were accustomed to organizing large enterprises and would lend them "the prestige which comes from past success."[22] But others saw the problem with cooperatives as having nothing to do with the feminine role in directing them. Instead, they regarded them as basically incompatible with the American ideal of family life. Indeed, this had been the gist of much of the criticism aimed at Bellamy's proposals. His scheme would "destroy the homelikeness of the home," wrote one *Good Housekeeping* reader. "The home is the unit whose integrity it behooves us to protect against every danger," especially against "the socialist doctrine of collectivism and cooperation." The editors of *Good Housekeeping* were themselves cautious about the collectivist implications of cooperative housekeeping. Cooperation had worked in some spheres, they noted, but it should not go too far. "Too much cooperative housekeeping would stand in danger of making households like so many peas in a pod—all alike—and crush out those specialities that all good housekeepers have in the way of cooking," they warned.[23] Ellen Richards would not allow the New England Kitchen to be a cooperative, or even to have a dining room, arguing that "home and family life are our strongholds. The food must go to the families and not the people to the food."[24]

There were also concerns that, by eliminating their supervisory role in the kitchen, cooperative dining might, in *Good Housekeeping*'s words, "make the lives of housewives too full of idleness and deprive them of healthful care."[25] A Congregationalist church magazine, while welcoming anything which might "lessen existing evils in this domestic problem," warned that in the same way as God had ordained that men develop character through struggle and responsibility so did women "attain their moral breadth and balance in the exercise of those functions necessary to the administration of a true home."[26]

Advocates of cooperative cooking and dining tried to assuage fears that they represented some kind of recrudescence of antebellum experiments in communal living. "The conspicuous cooperating ventures of history have frequently been those whose members gave themselves up to voluntary poverty, with community of goods and daily employment," said one advocate disapprovingly. "The *successful* ones of the future will be those organized for mutual thrift, on a self-supporting basis, but leaving intact the individual home in its most important features."[27] The secretary of one cooperative wrote that rather than undermining the individual middle-class home they were attempting to preserve its high standards in the face of the servant shortage and rising costs.[28]

Ultimately, the promise of higher-quality food for less money was not enough to sustain most of the cooperatives over the next thirty years. Some were destroyed by the failure of women to agree on how the cooperatives were to be run. Cooperative kitchens were doomed to failure because middle-class Americans were too individualistic, said Melusina Fay Peirce, a Cambridge, Massachusetts, woman who campaigned for cooperative housekeeping without much success. There was nothing in the lives of middle-class housewives to prepare them for the experience of cooperation.[29] The president of the Wisconsin federation of women's clubs reported in 1908 that a promising cooperative in her home town of Green Bay, set up by a "woman of ability" in a rented house "in a cookless neighborhood" had been very successful for a time until "each woman thought she had something better to suggest, each wanting to have her own finger in the pie and the thing soon went to pieces."[30]

Many cooperators thought that their main weakness was their inability to provide the privacy and the "individuality" of the middle-class home, and some went to considerable lengths to overcome this. The cooperative in Carthage, Missouri, which managed to keep going for four years, from 1907 to 1911, tried to ensure a "home-like atmosphere" by having members sit at tables set with their own china and condiments, situated far enough apart to ensure privacy of conversation.[31] In others members provided their own linens as well, and one experimenter even specified separate dining rooms as essential for success.[32] None, however, had an acceptable solution to the problem of how to fulfill the current expectations for entertaining dinner guests.

But there seemed to be a more obvious solution to the problem of privacy, and that was to have families take home or have delivered to them food that had been prepared by skilled cooks at a central source. Ellen Richards saw this as the best hope for the working classes, helping to develop in them the reverence for family life upon which American civilization rested. In 1893, Catherine Selden had suggested having community kitchens cook for private homes "to combine the conveniences and organization of commercial life with the privacy of home and the independence of the individual."[33] This idea inspired the feminist Charlotte Perkins Gilman as well. Five years later, in her book *Women and Economics,* she proposed the construction of large blocks of kitchenless apartments, to be served by central kitchens run by professionals. She rejected cooperation on the grounds that it meant "the union of families for the better performance of their supposed functions. The process fails because . . . cooking and cleaning are not family functions. We do not have a family mouth, a family stomach. . . . Eating is an individual function. Cooking is a social function. Neither is in the faintest degree a family function. . . ." Convinced that cooking and eating had to be made "scientific" and "efficient," Gilman saw no hope in training either housewives or ordinary domestic servants. "It is permanently impossible that half the world, acting as amateur cooks for the other half, can attain any high degree of scientific accuracy or technical skill," she wrote. "The development of any human labor requires specialization, and specialization is forbidden by our cook-by-nature-system. . . . Science has shown us what we need, and how and when we need it, but the affectionate labor of wife and mother is little touched by these advances." Domestic servants were part of the problem, not the solution, for they brought to cooking "an even lower degree of training and a narrower experience."[34]

Although few previous proposals for apartment blocks with common kitchens and laundries came anywhere near fruition, Gilman proposed that the kitchens be located within the complex because the "take-home" solution faced two formidable technological obstacles: slow transportation, which meant that communal kitchens had to be very close to dining facilities in order for the food to arrive hot, and the absence of convenient containers in which food could be shipped and still arrive hot at the home.[35] Reheating previously cooked food on a home stove was not a particularly viable solution, for starting the wood, coal, or oil stoves of the day was a long, tedious, and filthy process, normally reserved for the very servants who communal kitchens were to replace.

Gilman's reverence for specialization and efficiency, along with her despair over the possibility of untrained housewives and servant girls mastering culinary science, reflected much of the thinking of the new generation of professional home economists emerging from the colleges and universities of the country. So did her rejection of cooperative kitchens. Her friend, Helen Campbell, head of the school of Home Economics at the University of Wisconsin, saw no hope for cooperative kitchens. "Evolution" was already pointing the way out of the kitchen in the form of restaurants, bakeries, pickle factories, and "the long list of industries contributing to the household life of man. It is not cooperation that has brought them to their present stage of development, but business pure and simple." The very forces of capitalism which had transformed so much of American life would now certainly "take the simple, profitable step that is to follow" and, along with the home economics movement, modernize American eating and housekeeping.[36]

Some older home economists were not ready to abandon the cooperative dream for business principles with such alacrity. Caroline Hunt remarked that "most business enterprises lead to dissension, warfare, and selfishness, while the home leads in the opposite direction. Institutions which are the exponents of self-sacrifice and love cultivate self-sacrifice and love. . . . We should find some way of cooperation which will bring out the best which is in us. Business enterprises furnish us with much that is harmful, such as adulterated food and cloth."[37] Nevertheless, by the early 1900s, hope in cooperatives was fading, shunted aside by possible solutions to the domestic crisis which seemed more in tune with the new forces of competitive capitalism. To many of those intrigued by specialization, efficiency, and the application of scientific principles and technology to social and economic problems "take-home" foods now seemed to present themselves as the modern solution to the problem.

In 1901, the Boston's Women's Education and Industrial Union and the Association of Collegiate Alumnae published the results of a two-year experiment with take-home foods for the middle class. The study concluded that although a service which prepared food to be taken or delivered to homes could not sell the food for less than the cost of producing it, "prepared meals" still represented a preferable alternative to home-cooked meals. Not only was the quality of the food high (presumably better than that produced by incompetent servants), but when the savings in labor of housewife and servant were taken into account, the added expense was not significant. Moreover, they reported, home delivery of food was in keeping with the long-run evolution of the home: "In so far as it is in line with the general impulse by which industrial and social forces are shaping the world, it is inevitable. Failure to recognize the tendency can only prolong present friction and discomfort; attempts to thwart it can only result in defeat."[38] Thus, confident that evolution was on its side, the WEIU set up a system for delivering hot dinners from its working girls' lunch room (formerly the New England Kitchen) to patrons in their homes. While everybody complained about the shortage of competent servants and the high wages demanded by them, the WEIU boldly announced, it was finally doing something about it.[39]

The WEIU experiment lasted about three years before fading quietly from the scene. What caused its demise is not known, but the fact that the lunch room to which it was attached continued to function for many years would indicate that the problem lay not so much with the food as with the way it arrived at homes. Within a few years, however, soaring production of automobiles seemed to have provided the breakthrough. By 1910, a cooperative in Evanston, Illinois, began to give its members the option of eating their meals in the communal dining room or having them delivered to their homes by automobile.[40] Charlotte Perkins Gilman was among the first to recognize the new possibilities for home delivery of hot food created by cheaper automobiles. In her 1912 novel, *What Diantha Did,* first published serially in 1910, her heroine's company of skilled domestic workers used a small van to deliver hot meals to the homes of the well-to-do and tourists. Her solution to the heat-retention problem was to have the food delivered in asbestos-lined boxes with compartments for hot and cold foods and (aluminum) service for five. "Mrs. Rae enjoyed every mouthful of her meal," says the narrator. "The soup was hot. The salad was crisp and the ice cream hard. . . . The coffee was perfect and almost burned her tongue." Significantly, at one stage she even exclaims "Why—why—it's like Paris."[41]

Alas, food-delivery services set up in the following years were by no means "like Paris." One of the most successful of the communal dining experiments, in Montclair, New Jersey, added home delivery of its food (by liveried black waiters) to its services, and the Evanston co-op members seemed to respond favorably, but these experiments, which lasted only a few years, and others which were even more ephemeral, were based on a valid but premature idea. The fact that, like Diantha's service, they served mainly an upper-middle-class clientele is a clue to their great weakness: they were simply too expensive to operate. In large part this was due to the nature of the meals they delivered: standard three-course meals consisting of a variety of foodstuffs from a menu that changed every day. Ultimately home delivery of food would become economical when based on the delivery of one major item, most often pizza. This, with a beverage, would be regarded as a complete meal by later generations of Americans.

[margin handwritten note: take-out cuisine]

But prewar middle-class concepts of what constituted a proper meal could never accommodate such eating habits. Only when these ideas changed would the possibility of liberation from the "servant problem" arise.

Bellamy suggested, tongue-in-cheek, that the servant problem remained insoluble because "a large proportion of American women derive their pin-money from articles furnished to magazines and Sunday papers on the servant question, and thus have a pecuniary interest in keeping it an open one."[42] In fact, though, the crux of the problem was as much social and intellectual as it was pecuniary. Simply put, the prewar middle class was unable to solve the "servant problem" while retaining its conception of what constituted proper eating. Sooner or later, something had to give. As repeated experiments to replace the servant girl failed and alternative job opportunities for her multiplied, it slowly became apparent that it was middle-class expectations of the kitchen, rather than its performance, that needed to change.

CHAPTER 6

The New Nutritionists Assault the Middle Classes

In the aftermath of the failure of the New England Kitchen experiment most New Nutritionists had turned their backs on direct intervention into the lives of the poor. "The attempts to furnish restaurants for wage earners . . . with food of a strictly wholesome and nutritious character" had failed, Ellen Richards wrote in 1899, and "reluctantly the plans have one after another been given up." But this did not mean abandoning the crusade. Rather, it meant a shift in focus. The campaign for "the education of public sentiment," would continue, but now its main objective would be the middle and upper-middle classes.[1]

Richards's major work, *The Cost of Living,* published the following year, reflected this new orientation. A summary of the economic wisdom of the New Nutritionists and home economists, it was intended "for the educated young people of the land," especially for those about to begin life on an annual income of $1500 to $3000.[2] Most other leading home economists joined her in adopting a "trickle down" attitude toward changing the working-class diet. The poor would change only after their betters set the example. In the words of one leading home economist, the struggle to improve the home "is undertaken by the interested few, its results if successful to be superimposed on the inert and as yet indifferent many."[3] The "interested few" were led by the new breed of "scientific" home economists. Desperate to gain acceptance of their field as a respected scholarly discipline, they received valuable support from the chemist

72

Wilbur Atwater, who had been determinedly constructing a nutritional research empire for himself.

In 1887, when Congress appropriated funds to set up experiment stations in each state to help advance useful agricultural knowledge, the only kind of nutrition research envisaged was that dealing with better animal fodder. But under Atwater, its first director, and his successor, Alfred C. True, his former research assistant at Wesleyan, the federal Office of Experiment Stations also funded research on human nutrition. Not surprisingly, the office was particularly enthusiastic about Atwater's work, and he assumed the directorship of the Connecticut state experiment station in nearby Storrs when he returned to his academic post in Middletown.[4] In 1893, Atwater's endeavors received a boost when Edward Atkinson persuaded J. Sterling Morton, the new Secretary of Agriculture, to support a special appropriation of $15,000 for human nutrition research in the state experiment stations.

There was one minor problem: the federal government did not normally fund "pure" theoretical research. Atkinson's proposal had been received favorably by the President and cabinet mainly because it combined research with instruction in new principles of nutrition. The assumption was that the money would further research of the kind being undertaken by the New England Kitchen (itself praised as an "experiment station"), and that replicas of the Kitchen would be set up in state experiment stations across the country to develop recipes for and to instruct the poor.[5] However, by the time Congress approved the appropriation, the NEK was failing, and the money was easily redirected toward "pure" research, into a project designed to thrust Atwater, and the OES, into the vanguard of human nutrition research: the construction of America's first respiration calorimeter.

Until the early 1890s, the only way to estimate basic nutritional requirements was to record the foods consumed by people engaged in various activities and then calculate the number of calories and amounts of the various food elements these foods had contained. The respiration calorimeter, an elaborate air-tight chamber in which men or animals could live for days with their intake and output of food and heat measured, enabled scientists to calculate the exact number of calories actually burned under various circumstances, and to measure more accurately the consumption of other nutrients. Although the agriculture department's human nutrition appropriation for 1894 was cut to $10,000 by a somewhat skeptical Congress, Atwater succeeded in constructing one of these expensive contraptions in his laboratory at Wesleyan.[6]

Government funding put a high premium on Atwater's now well-honed political skills; he needed an effective lobby to support this expensive new venture. Unforeseen technical bugs delayed construction of the calorimeter and raised the expected costs of running it to about $10,000 a year.[7] It seemed that continued government support would be forthcoming only if Atwater could link what was plainly a venture into "pure" research with the NEK ideal of educating the masses in the ideas of the New Nutrition. In 1895, an adept lobbying campaign emphasizing the educational aspect of the project to key members of the congressional agricultural committees paid off and the $15,000 budget was restored. The same argument also persuaded the governor and assembly of Connecticut to contribute funds for the calorimeter. "Any information that enables the laborer to select his food according to its nutritive value, and to prepare it in the most advantageous manner, must result in much saving of his hard-earned money," said the governor in true NEK style.[8]

In 1896, however, when the calorimeter was finally put to work and the possibility of dazzling scientific discoveries loomed on the horizon, Atwater began to distance himself from direct intervention. As word of experiments being carried out behind closed doors in Middletown leaked out, newspapers and magazines ran excited stories of the glory which was to accrue to American science while politicians worried over whether adequate due was being given for their support.[9]

Atwater now "came out of the closet," as it were, to assume his role as one of America's foremost "pure" scientists. In October 1896 he rejected the proposal of Carroll D. Wright, the U.S. Commissioner of Labor, that they cooperate in a program to survey and change the diets of urban slum-dwellers. As Commissioner of Labor in Massachusetts in the mid-1880s Wright, a friend of Atkinson, had supported Atwater when he had conducted the country's first systematic dietary surveys and continued his support from Washington. He also supported the New England Kitchen and its exhibit at the Chicago exposition. Now, Atwater told him, they had "come to a parting of the ways." There were now "two definite and measurably distinct lines of inquiry; one, which is more especially statistical and sociological, is peculiarly appropriate to the Department of Labor. The other, which is more chemical and sociological but of course has economic purpose, comes equally well within the province of the Department of Agriculture." Atwater's meaning seems quite clear: he would leave the studies and surveys which underlay direct intervention to improve the lot of the working class to the likes of Wright and his fellow reformers. But this did not mean leaving to them all "sociological" inquiry and consideration of "economic purpose," for it was exactly this kind of concern that brought support from government.[10]

The focus of the dietary surveys Atwater continued to supervise for the OES now began to shift from the lower to the middle and upper-middle classes. By 1901 he had developed a macro-research project, a "comparative nutrition of mankind," which left the old concern for the American working class submerged in a sea of data from the respiration calorimeter and dietary surveys of Eskimos, Filipinos, Chinese, and any other national group whose diets could be quantified.[11] When applying for funding for his research he would trot out its original selling point, the improvement of labor productivity,[12] but few of the Americans studied used physical productive power. In 1907, when the results of the 320 dietary surveys done in America under Atwater's supervision were summarized by his assistant, Charles Langworthy, only fifteen dealt with "very poor working people."[13]

Atwater's turn away from the working class for research purposes complemented the shift of Richards and the home economists toward the middle and upper class as the primary object for conversion, helping to strengthen the bonds first forged in the New England Kitchen experiment. Richards had come to terms with the fact that she was, in the words of an admiring biographer, "tempermentally unsuited for the routine details of pure science,"[14] but she and Abel realized that cooperation with Atwater and his circle would lend an invaluable aura of science to their struggling young field.

Academic respectability was particularly important to home economists because theirs was one of the few fields open to women who wanted careers in science. While a significant number of women had begun attending college in the 1870s, and science was often a part of the undergraduate curriculum, they were discouraged from aspiring to scientific careers. When she graduated from Vassar in the mid-1870s wishing to pursue a career in chemistry, Richards found that the only aspects of science which seemed open to women were those directly related to what was regarded as women's proper sphere, the home and family. Only by studying the purity of water for the home, domestic sanitation, and the chemistry of food could she go on to postgraduate study. Helen Campbell, later head of home economics at the University of Wisconsin, was allowed to study medicine, but mainly because she studied it as related to food.[15] In 1889, when Isabel Bevier graduated from Case Western Reserve in chemistry and wanted to go on for graduate work her professor sent her to work under Atwater, telling her, she recalled, "that the place for women in chemistry was in work in foods, and that the big universities in the Middle West, like Michigan, Wisconsin and Illinois, would one day have some kind of department for foods work with women in it, and I should get ready."[16] The scientific study of home economics thus held out hope for the creation of a kind of separate but equal sphere for women in a male-dominated academic world. As one of its advocates wrote in 1896, "No one can deny that in this way lies a legitimate field in which women may earn a living. Complaint of unfair competition here cannot be raised; the home and what pertains to it constitute women's true sphere of activity. . . . Higher education and special training will win for women the right to places of equal rank with men."[17]

Aware that the home economists could be an effective lobby for

expanding the powers and budget of the OES, Atwater, True, and Langworthy were more than happy to help them in their struggle to achieve
academic legitimacy. Atwater and Langworthy appeared at home economists' meetings, delivering scholarly summaries of the latest scientific
research in human nutrition. Langworthy was made vice president of the
new American Home Economics Association and Alfred C. True a member of its council. True and Atwater assigned young college graduates
seeking careers in home economics to OES-funded research projects. One
of Atwater's research assistants, Isabel Bevier, became the head of home
economics at the University of Illinois.[18] Caroline Hunt, her counterpart
at the University of Wisconsin, was also a former Atwater assistant and
later moved to Washington as Langworthy's assistant.[19] Another Atwater
research assistant, Martha Van Renssalear, went on to become the head of
home economics at Cornell and shared the vice presidency of the AHEA
with Langworthy.[20] Mary Hinman Abel, the editor of its journal, was also,
of course, an Atwater disciple.

The OES also provided an outlet for the *sine qua non* of academic
respectability, scholarly publication. One of the aims of the first Lake
Placid Conference on Home Economics, held in 1898, out of which the
American Home Economics Association eventually emerged, was "the
preparation of a series of papers or brochures on domestic science, which
the government may publish as it now does bulletins on food and nutrition
through the department of agriculture."[21] Works such as Richards's studies of the costs of various foods and Abel's *Sugar as Food* were published as
Bulletins of the OES. The OES's publication of the results of the dietary
surveys she did for Atwater in Pittsburgh in 1894–96 helped pave the way
for Isabel Bevier's rise to the deanship of the University of Illinois's new
school of home economics.[22]

Atwater, meanwhile, pointed out to the home economists that increased
budget appropriations for the OES would allow the publication of even
more of their work, and encouraged them to lobby Congress for increased
funding for human nutrition studies. The home economists responded
enthusiastically, writing members of Congress and encouraging university
administrators to point out the importance of nutrition research to their
representatives.[23]

The nutritional scientists also helped scientific home economists to
compete with the older conception of home economics which constituted
the most serious obstacle to professionalizing the field. Many of those who
taught "domestic science" and cooking in the schools were concerned only
with teaching the practical aspects of housekeeping. Indeed, the first
women's colleges to venture into the field, Vassar, Mount Holyoke, and
Wellesley, had experimented with various forms of work-sharing and
practical training in the 1870s and 1880s. In the Midwest and West, the
domestic science courses of the land grant colleges and universities were

expected to teach future farmers' wives cooking and housekeeping. And there were hundreds of teachers of "domestic science" and "domestic economy" working for normal and high schools, state agricultural extension bureaus, farm bureaus and farmers' institutes who were more concerned with teaching better methods of home canning than the latest theories about the metabolism of protein. Typically, while Richards, Abel, Bevier, and Campbell were most proud of their connections with science, Emma Ewing, one of the great pioneers of domestic science, who set up the domestic economy programs in a host of midwestern colleges and institutions, built her reputation on a new method for baking bread.[24]

The scientific home economists thus saw themselves as part of "an age-old conflict between cooking and sewing school adherents and those who believed in the scientific approach to the teaching of household science."[25] The former's unscientific cooking lessons were dismissed as "empirical," the result of trial and error techniques. In contrast, the scientific home economists advocated the "inductive method in cookery," which emphasized the chemistry of cooking and nutrition, the economics of the household, and the history of the home and family. Only this theoretical grounding, they argued, would allow students to deal with the myriad of situations which arise in the household daily, giving them the flexibility to go beyond a few memorized recipes.[26]

Thanks to their friends in the OES, the scientific home economists received strong backing from the U.S. Department of Agriculture. In his annual report for 1897 the Secretary of Agriculture noted that while "cooking and sewing are now commonly taught in the public schools. . . . this teaching needs a scientific basis if it is to be thoroughly useful." Medicine and engineering had recently passed beyond training which was "largely empirical" to teaching the underlying scientific theories, and it was necessary for domestic science to do the same.[27] As administrator of funds destined for the land grant colleges and provider of much of the funding for the agricultural extension services, both of which employed large numbers of cooking teachers, the department's view on this issue was not easily ignored.

In 1896, home economists were pleased to note that what Ellen Richards called the "trade school" conceptions of their field seemed to have foundered in the elite colleges ("by divine appointment," according to Helen Campbell).[28] Most important, the cooking school teachers were now being shunted aside by apostles of the new scientific approach in the land grant institutions. By 1896, the Iowa Agricultural College course set up by Ewing the bread baker had been declared a failure, as had a similar one at the University of Illinois. The year before, the scientific approach was introduced at the University of Wisconsin in an environment far removed from the oven: in the lecture hall of Richard T. Ely, the well-known Progressive economist, who devoted twelve lectures to the subject

in one of his courses. Illinois soon began constructing a new home economics program around that approach, using eight of Ely's lectures.[29]

The wide ranging lectures may have been fascinating,[30] but the scientific approach left home economists open to the charge that they were not
teaching girls anything of practical value. Land grant colleges and universities were particularly vulnerable, as they were usually connected to colleges of agriculture and their extension services which were expected to
provide practical advice to the states' farmers. Bevier, for example, came
under intense attack from Illinois's farmers' institutes for being "too the-
oretically inclined." It was Bevier's luck that, upon hiring her the university president said he was concerned mainly with "results from the labs
and classrooms which would bring prestige to the university," and an
endorsement of her scientific prowess from True helped her weather the
storm.[31] True, as head of a branch of the Department of Agriculture,
could also help scientific home economists at land grant institutions by
publishing their research. In turn, when justifying the OES program of
research and publication on human nutrition to Congress, True could
connect it to agriculture by citing the needs of the home economists in the
land grant colleges.[32] Congress supported True, appropriating substantial
sums to the OES and widening its powers. In 1906, the Adams Act
mandated the Department of Agriculture to carry out original scientific
research. Drafted by True, it put the OES in charge of directing this work,
and a large portion of the funding went to work on human nutrition.[33]

Still, the nagging problem remained: the OES Bulletins, standard fare
for undergraduate teaching and widely circulated to women's clubs by the
home economists, were of little use in cooking. Dietary surveys and scientific treatises on the digestibility of various foods may have looked all right
on scholarly *curricula vitae,* but their relevance to the kitchen seemed
tenuous indeed. "Not one of these bulletins tells you how to get a meal of
victuals," a disgruntled woman told Isabel Bevier, who conceded that "at
first glance the connection between the bulletins and the work of the
teacher of cookery is not apparent." Yet, Bevier assured readers of the
American Kitchen Magazine, "while the ordinary housewife is apt to be
confused by the terms 'nutrients,' 'protein,' 'calories,' and to find the
arithmetic of the dietary quite unintelligible," Director True was confident that general principles of human nutrition were emerging from these
theoretical studies. These were counterparts to the principles used to feed
livestock: guides which could be adapted to individual circumstances and
different environments, rather than fixed recipes for feeding all.[34] But
these guidelines still told cooks little about how to cook. Indeed, despite
her understanding of human nutrition, like many of her colleagues, Isabel
Bevier remained a notoriously poor cook. "Fine cooking was not in my
repertoire," she recalled toward the end of her life.[35]

But fine cooking was not what scientific home economists intended to propogate; rather, they set out to preach the gospel of the New Nutrition. Among their first successes were the cooking courses in urban schools. Cookery instruction in the schools had originated as a female counterpart to manual training for boys in industrial schools. Both were expected to improve students' job prospects upon graduation at age twelve, to prepare them to set up their own households, and to instill respect for the dignity of manual labor. In the mid-1880s, however, grammar schools, whose students spanned a wider class spectrum, began to teach the subject as well.[36] But a strange thing happened to the cookery courses when they moved to the grammar schools: they became more scientific and less practical. It seemed with the acceptance of courses being taught in an academic setting, school boards demanded professional credentials that could be provided only by those committed to the scientific approach to the kitchen.[37] Home economists were brought in to supervise and provide an aura of academic respectability.[38]

So, in the 1890s, what had originated as courses to teach working-class children how to cook were transformed into courses on the chemistry of food and its composition, even in the earliest grades. In 1898, Atwater wrote True that fortunately the man in charge of implementing the new home economics program in New York City in 1897–98 thought it "essential . . . that the instruction be made less empirical. It does not suffice to teach girls the art of cooking. What is wanted is the fundamentals of the science of nutrition." The OES bulletins would be particularly useful to him, Atwater thought, because he wished to "utilize the best data and highest authority."[39] A subsequent OES report on home economics in the city's grammar schools noted with satisfaction that "the real object of the study has been kept carefully in view, and the understanding of food values, chemical changes, hygenic influences, and the physiological truths has not been sacrificed for the simple ability to make palatable dishes."[40]

By 1900, however, public high school systems were expanding rapidly, and much of the cookery training, including instruction in the New Nutrition, became concentrated there. Since a majority of working-class and immigrant school girls tended to drop out at about age fourteen, for the most part the message reached native-born middle-class children.

A perusal of the stupifying high school domestic science textbooks of the time might fuel skepticism regarding how much of the New Nutrition these students could really retain. However, it can be assumed that many imbibed at least the basic stance toward food: that one was supposed to "eat to live rather than live to eat"; that food was composed of various "nutrients," including proteins, carbohydrates, and fats; and that foods contained varying amounts of calories, which had something to do with energy. Superficial as this knowledge might have been, home economists in the schools played an important part in making these terms part of the middle-class lexicon. By the time of World War I, thousands of mainly middle-class female graduates of the nation's public school system had some knowledge of the basics of the New Nutrition. When stimulated by advertising and other forces, the attitudes embodied in this knowledge could form the basis for changing eating habits.

One of the reasons for the rise of home economics in the high schools and colleges was that it seemed to represent a solution to the crisis of the middle-class kitchen and dining room. As the experiments with communal kitchens faltered and the schools for servants closed, home economics, with its attempt to apply Science to the household, seemed to hold out hope for salvation from the "tyranny of the kitchen."

It was largely for this reason that the scientific home economists garnered impressive support from the women's clubs of America. The membership of these middle and upper-middle-class clubs had mushroomed in the 1890s and early 1900s, as homemakers found an interesting, socially-acceptable focus for activities outside the home. They involved themselves in temperance activities, supported pure food legislation, debated suffrage, but also, it seems, devoted much of their time to wrestling with the problem of maintaining the expected standards of the middle-class home. This made them particularly receptive to the scientific home economists and to the new attitudes towards food.

Ellen Richards had been advocating scientific cooking as a solution to the "servant crisis" as early as 1886.[41] At the Women's Congress, which met at Chicago's Columbian Exposition in 1893, representatives of a number of women's clubs agreed that the solution to the problems of the middle-class household lay in putting it on a scientific basis. They subsequently formed the National Household Economics Association, whose organizing manifesto expressed two main objectives, both of which tackled the "servant crisis." The first was to organize "schools of household science and service" and establish employment bureaus for servants. The second was "to promote among members of the association a more scientific knowledge of the economic value of various foods and fuels" as well as "the importance of proper sanitation and plumbing in the home."[42]

The General Federation of Women's Clubs was excited about the NHEA's program and urged every women's club to establish a household economics section to study and carry out this program.[43] The club women responded enthusiastically, assigning the writings of Atwater, Richards, Abel, and others in the OES stable for discussion and underwriting experiments in simplified cooking and feeding. In New Jersey, club women searching for solutions to the "servant problem" successfully pushed Rutgers into teaching home economics.[44]

The new emphasis on science in the kitchen represented a distinct turn away from the Victorian ideal of domesticity which saw the home, presided over by a moral and loving woman, as a haven from the jungle of the outside world. Increasingly, home economists talked of bringing the home into step with the modern industrial world. Swimming with, rather than against, the tide of industrial change seemed to lead in a number of promising directions, in particular, transferring production from the home to outside the home. In the 1880s and early 1890s this had aroused ambivalent feelings among home economists who sanctified the home, apotheosizing housewives who could bake perfect loaves of bread and condemning the poor for buying it at the baker. However, after the turn of the century they began to regard the products of the canner, the bottler, and eventually, even the baker, with increasing favor, seeing in them partial solutions, at least, to the nagging labor problem.[45]

Frederick W. Taylor, the *guru* of the "Scientific Management" movement, was one of the middle-class culture heros of the day, and his use of time-and-motion studies to break complex tasks down into simple ones seemed to have an obvious bearing on the kitchen: many home economists thought that the root of the servant problem lay in inefficient organization of kitchen labor. Taylor himself was excited by the prospect that his ideas might revolutionize home life. When a suburban New Jersey club woman wrote the first book to apply his ideas to the home, he wrote in its introduction that "in a smaller way perhaps she is doing a pioneer work similar to that of Leonardo da Vinci in his 'Il Codice Atlantico,' Newton in his 'Principia,' and Darwin in his 'Origin of Species.'. . . I am not sure that this new branch of engineering is not destined to do almost as much for mankind as the work of either of [*sic*] these great men mentioned."[46]

Of course, there were "experts" who advocated taking the new approach to absurd lengths, and time-and-motion studies proved irresistible to many would-be reformers in the kitchen. Throughout the country thousands of middle-class women, encouraged by the home economics committees of their women's clubs, followed their servants carrying stop watches and clipboards, breaking down the simplest domestic functions into even simpler components in search of elusive labor-saving methods in the kitchen. Among the more zealous were the Brueres, a Connecticut professor and his wife, who wrote a popular column on home efficiency for *Collier's* magazine. "The middle class servant is obsolescent," they said, "being in the reprehensible act of vanishing into her own home, on the one hand, and into the factory, on the other." They therefore turned their home in Darien into a "Housekeeping Experiment Station" (another favorite device) to devise ways of escaping dependence on servants.[47] The following account of one of their experiments—typical of much that appeared in household economics texts of the time—compared the time and motion consumed when a servant cooked three eggs on a stove to that expended when an insulated fireless cooker—in this case a fireless egg coddler—was used.

1. Place the three eggs in boiling water.	1. With right hand lift the cover from the coddler.
2. Watch the clock. After three minutes,	2. Omit.
	3. Place cover on table.
3. Take serving dish in left,	4. With left hand lift kettle of hot water at same time.
3(a) spoon in right hand.	
4. Lift one egg out of water.	5. Lift egg rack from coddler with right hand.
5. Place in serving dish.	
6. Place spoon on top of stove.	6. Pour a little hot water into the coddler.
7. Carry service dish to breakfast room.	
	7. Omit.
8. Place egg in cup before right person.	8. Omit.
	9. Omit.
9. Return to stove.	10. Omit.
10. Place serving dish on stove.	11. Omit.
11. Look at clock. After one minute,	12. Rinse out coddler. Pour water in sink.
12. Lift second egg from water with spoon with same movement as 3, 4, 5, and 6.	
	13. Return coddler to table.
13. Repeat No. 7.	14. With right hand place eggs in rack.
14. Repeat No. 8.	15. Place rack in coddler.
15. Repeat No. 9.	16. With left hand lift kettle. Fill coddler to three-egg mark.
16. Repeat No. 10.	
17. Look at clock. After one minute,	17. Omit.
18. Repeat 3, 4, 5, 6, 7.	18. Place kettle on stove.
19. Repeat No. 8.	19. With right hand put cover on coddler.
20. Return to kitchen.	
21.	20. Carry coddler to breakfast table.
22.	21. Place before mistress.
	22. Return to kitchen.

Total motions, 37.

Trips to breakfast room, 3

Time, six minutes.

Total motions, 15.

Trips to breakfast room, 1.

Time, 50 seconds[48]

This chart seems to indicate that most of the time was saved by cooking three eggs in the egg coddler at the same time, while, for some unexplained reason, the cook only served one at a time from the stove. It also shows that Taylorism did not necessarily save enough time and labor to dispense altogether with that bane of the middle class, the servant girl herself. Yet, by 1912, when this book was published, the realization of the awful truth of what Edward Bellamy had said over forty years before—that the middle-class housewife would never be free until she freed herself from dependence on cooks and servants—was taking hold on the middle-class.

Freedom from the cares of the home *was* what middle-class women wanted. In their women's clubs, at their teas, they continued to conspire and experiment with ways to free themselves from the terrible burdens of the home while at the same time continuing to fulfill society's expectations of them. Finally, when neither social experimentation nor Taylorism provided the solution, they helped change society's expectations of them and their kitchens. By adopting the new concepts of nutrition they managed to downgrade both the quantity and quality of what was expected from their kitchens. It was in this realm, rather than in the fantasies of Taylorism, that the home economists had their greatest effect on middle-class foodways.

The home economists had always condemned overeating. Too much fuel clogged the human machine, said the pioneers. It overtaxed the digestive system, said the more sophisticated. Ellen Richards even warned that overfeeding imperiled the survival of the white race: "In all the discussion of the infertility of the higher branches of the human race," she wrote, "how little attention is paid to the weakening effect of the pampered appetite."[49] The difficulty, of course, was in defining what constituted an excessive intake of food. As long as they stuck by Atwater's inflated standards, they did not have much leeway in reducing the quantity of food ingested. They could disapprove of excesses induced by serving too many courses, and this they did, but until 1905 they adhered to Atwater's recommendations.

However, they could do something about the nature of food in the "pampered diet." The fact was that food prepared by following basic scientific principles was invariably simple. Elaborate methods of food preparation and dazzling combinations of ingredients were anathema to those who wanted to develop easy recipes whose nutritional content could be calculated. Since even the most imaginative cook would have trouble inventing more than a few truly unique dishes, let alone a whole new cuisine, the home economists naturally fell back on what they knew: a variant of the British cuisine dominant in New England before the upper class began experimenting with French cuisine. For this reason they thought the name "New England Kitchen" was an attractive one, and they were right. Cookbook authors sensed this too, and schemed to include "Boston" and "New England" in their titles. Here was a simple, straightforward cuisine, revolving around boiled, broiled, and roasted meats and potatoes, which native-born Americans were accustomed to and liked. All that need be done was make it even simpler.

Maria Parloa, the first principal of the Boston Cooking School and author of the first cookbook to promote this connection, was a close associate of Richards and Abel and an enthusiastic supporter of the New England Kitchen. Her more famous successor, Fanny Merritt Farmer, prefaced her 1896 *Boston Cooking School Cook Book,* whose various editions would become one of the most popular cookbooks in American history, with an implied admonition against those miscreants who lived to eat. Thanks to the scientific advances of the last decade, she wrote, "the time is not far distant when knowledge of the principles of diet will be an essential part of one's education. Then mankind will eat to live, will be able to do better mental and physical work, and disease will be less frequent." She hoped that "through its condensed scientific knowledge," her cookbook would lead to "deeper thought and broader study of what to eat."[50]

Although she was inclined toward interesting and rather elaborate concoctions and included instructions for a twelve-course dinner, most of Farmer's recommended menus for family dinners and luncheons were quite simple: soup, meat or fish, potatoes (sixteen of the eighteen dinner menus included potatoes and the remaining two suggested sweet potatoes), two vegetables, dessert, cheese, and coffee. The menus in the home economists' favorite food magazine of the later 1890s, the *American Kitchen Magazine* (successor to the *New England Kitchen Magazine*), were often even simpler. The two main meals of the day were usually two-course affairs: meat or fish plus potatoes or rice, a vegetable, and dessert. The dishes themselves were also simple: stews, or those New England standbys, "scalloped" fish, oysters, chicken, and so on, accompanied by boiled, mashed, or baked potatoes, rolls, and boiled vegetables. Even Sunday dinners offered little to challenge a cook: typically mutton stew, boiled potatoes, and turnips followed by jelly, wafers, and cheese.[51] Neither the *Boston Cooking School Cook Book* nor the *American Kitchen Magazine* cut down appreciably on breakfast recommendations. These continued to feature meats—such as steak and pork chops—carbohydrates, and fats in multitudinous forms. A typical suggestion in Farmer's book called for oranges, wheat germ with sugar and cream, "warmed over lamb," French fried potatoes, raised biscuits, buckwheat cakes with maple syrup, and coffee.[52]

Sara Tyson Rorer, the flamboyant and imperious Philadelphia cooking school director who became food editor of the *Ladies Home Journal* in 1897, devoted increasing attention to the servantless home. She traveled the country demonstrating tableside cookery, done with her own jewel-encrusted chafing dish, for those poor unfortunates who did not have a maid. She soon began recommending simpler meals for everyone, and

Mrs. Rorer's Menu Book, published in 1905, recommended meals that were significantly lighter than those she had suggested in the 1890s.[53]

Thus, by 1905, the groundwork was being laid for a shift by middle-class America toward smaller and less elaborate meals. Together, scientists in the forefront of the study of human nutrition and those responsible for the development of the pseudo-science of home economics were playing important roles in reshaping middle-class attitudes toward food. Their ideas were being propagated among the middle classes in schools, colleges, and universities, by women's clubs, women's magazines, and cookbooks. Additional support was now about to come from an unlikely alliance of a new generation of nutritional scientists and banner-bearers of the grand old American tradition of food faddism.

CHAPTER 7

Scientists, Pseudoscientists, and Faddists

On both sides of the Atlantic, the decades that straddled the turn of the century constituted a veritable Golden Age of food faddism. An unusually large array of vegetarians (who subdivided themselves like amoebae into fruitarians, nutarians, lacto-ovarians, and argued among themselves about whether fish was as harmful as meat) faced spirited challenges from aggressive meat-eaters who swore by regimens such as the Salisbury all-beef diet. ("Whatever merits vegetarians may claim for their diet, they cannot produce a single talented or handsome vegetarian, born of vegetarian parents in England, America, or Germany," wrote a typical meat advocate.)[1] "Raw foodists" refused to eat anything that had been heated, while others abjured fermented foods. A "no breakfast fad" flew in the face of the traditional belief in the importance of that meal, while a multitude of methods were proposed for dealing with the "poisonous" bacteria science had recently discovered congregating in the nation's colons.

Whatever the fad, advocates of drastic dietary change usually shared a common characteristic: they bore personal witness to its efficacy. Almost invariably, proponents would tell of their own devastating health problems, miraculously cured by the proposed diet—mysterious or common physical or psychological ailments that had defied the greatest of modern medical minds had disappeared once certain foods were added or deleted from the diet. Of course, this had always been so, but it had been up to individuals to judge for themselves. However, now that scientists were

86

perfecting ways of studying the chemistry of foods and human beings in laboratories, it was possible to subject them to impersonal scientific testing. These tests, it was thought, represented a higher form of verification, for they would remove the subjective factor and either "prove" or "disprove" the various claims.

His ability to ingratiate himself into the realm of "pure" laboratory science differentiated the turn-of-the-century American faddist Horace Fletcher from most of his competitors. Although he had no scientific training, the links he forged with some of the world's most respected scientists enabled this wealthy retired businessman, who lived in a magnificent thirteenth-century *palazzo* on Venice's Grand Canal, to play a major role in converting America, and indeed the Western world, to lower-protein diets. This would help push the middle class seeking freedom from the "tyranny of the kitchen," towards eating less food and simplifying their meals.

Although right thinking may have played a role in Fletcher's success, it was clearly not an important factor, for his main interest, "thorough mastication," was both ridiculous and tedious. Fletcher thought that there was a mechanism in the back of the mouth whose "filter function" performed much of the digestive process. He therefore recommended chewing each mouthful of food until it had absolutely no taste and was involuntarily swallowed, which normally meant chewing at least one hundred times.[2] (There was no need to specify an exact number of chews, he said, for once the technique was mastered, food not thoroughly masticated would be automatically regurgitated.) Liquids were to be swished about the mouth for at least thirty seconds before allowed to pass down the gullet, and overall food intake would be reduced by eating only when hungry.[3]

Although Fletcher carried it to lengths previously undreamed of, the idea of prolonged chewing was by no means new; nor was there any novelty in Fletcher's claim that reducing his food intake had cured him of a severe case of dyspepsia and other internal disorders. The (literally) bloated well-to-do of the Western world were well accustomed to tales of how illnesses had been cured by restricting diets. Nor was his wealth a particularly distinguishing factor. Indeed, John D. Rockefeller had recently claimed to have conquered a serious illness by reducing his food consumption and in 1904 he announced to a less-than-stunned world that cheese was a healthful food.[4]

Two things about Fletcher's claims made him stand out from the rest. Although his explanation of why and how was rather cockeyed, when combined with his dietary regimen,[5] the end result of "thorough mastication" was often a drastically reduced intake of protein, which coincided with what some prominent "pure" scientists were beginning to suspect would lead to better health. Second (and most important in a field where the cost of equipment such as respiration calorimeters was upping the research ante), Fletcher seemed willing to devote a substantial portion of his wealth to subsidizing scientists who wished to test his theories.

Fletcher first came to international scientific attention in 1901, when his personal physician, Ernest Van Someren, read a paper to the British Medical Association claiming that by thoroughly masticating his food, Fletcher had drastically reduced his intake of protein and yet significantly increased his "subjective and objective well-being."[6] The thirty-year-old doctor also testified that, thanks to thorough mastication, he himself had been cured of "gout, incapacitating headaches, frequent colds, boils on the neck and face, chronic eczema of the toes, . . . frequent acid dyspepsia" and, "worse still," loss of interest "in life and in my work."[7] When Britain's leading physiologist, Sir Michael Foster of Cambridge University, learned that Fletcher was interested in setting up a Nutrition Institute for research into food and physiology, he quickly invited Fletcher to Cambridge, where a few volunteers practiced chewing in the Fletcher fashion. Foster claimed to be duly impressed. "More than one person [here] has joined the chewing set," he wrote Henry P. Bowditch, the prominent professor of physiology at Harvard.[8] But Foster was most enthusiastic about Fletcher's plans for the nutrition institute, which would put at his disposal costly apparati such as the respiration calorimeter. He wrote a very favorable report on the experiment, but concluded that although it was clear that further study was "urgently called for . . . the Cambridge laboratories do not possess at present either the necessary equipment or the funds to provide it." Elaborate and expensive equipment would be required, he noted, and it was clear where he thought the funds for it would come from.[9]

Delays in setting up the institute and suspicion of Fletcher among the trustees of the new Carnegie Institution, which was about to dole out undreamed of sums for scientific research, soon cooled British ardor for Fletcher.[10] But by then Fletcher had little need of Foster or a nutrition institute of his own, for he was now attracting considerable attention in the United States. In part this came from performing physical feats unusual for a man of his fifty years. In December 1902, for example, the five-foot-six Fletcher climbed the 854 steps of the Washington Monument and then bounded down them without resting. The next winter, not having skated for thirty-five years, he went for three hours straight and claimed to feel no soreness.[11]

More important, though, Fletcher was now working with prominent American scientists and funding their experiments to test his own ideas. The most distinguished, the physiologist Russell H. Chittenden, who was the first director of Yale University's prestigious Sheffield School of Science, had recently undergone a personal conversion to the cause. Until recently, Chittenden had been in the forefront of the anti-vegetarian campaign. Meats, he had written, had "certain stimulating properties which distinguish them from the grosser vegetable foods." Along with tea and coffee, they stimulated the brain and nerves. For this reason, he said, Sir William Roberts was correct when he noted that in the struggle for existence, which is "almost exclusively a brain struggle," it is the meat eaters who prevail.[12]

However, Chittenden was plagued by some nagging ailments, and, apparently at Bowditch's suggestion, he invited Fletcher to his lab. There, he carefully monitored Fletcher's ingestions and excretions (noting with regard to the latter, as all observers did, the remarkable absence of odor) and concluded that Fletcher was able to survive on far less food intake than Voit or Atwater recommended and still maintain his weight at 165 pounds. Most significant, where Voit had dictated that a man of Fletcher's size needed 118 grams of protein a day and Atwater had suggested 125 grams for good health, Chittenden calculated that Fletcher consumed less than 45 grams of protein a day with no signs of ill-health. In fact, the director of the Yale gymnasium was amazed at the ease with which Fletcher, who claimed to indulge in no regimen of exercises, was able to perform exercises normally given only to the varsity crew. When Chittenden cut down his own protein intake to Fletcher's levels he found that the rheumatic pain his his knee virtually disappeared, his headaches went away, and although he lost fourteen pounds, he felt stronger than ever.[13]

With Fletcher's financial support, Chittenden embarked on more extensive testing. Three groups of men were subjected to the Fletcher regimen and thorough mastication. Chittenden, his associate, Lafayette Mendel (later in the forefront of vitamin research), and three graduate research assistants served as representative "brain workers" in sedentary occupations. Members of the varsity crew were recruited as hard workers. For the group in the middle, men with a moderate daily expenditure of energy, Fletcher managed to secure the services of a platoon of the U.S. Army.

The army's interest in food and nutrition had been jogged by the "embalmed beef" scandal of the Spanish-American War, in which it was charged that thousands of cans of rotten beef were served to the troops in Cuba. In response to the subsequent uproar and investigations, the army brought in the New Nutritionists. In 1902, it announced that a new emergency ration for men in the field had been developed which had been "figured out by physiological mathematicians to a nicety which reduces to grams and calories the protein, the fats, the carbohydrates, and fuel value of the ration."[14] Fletcher's ideas piqued the interest of the Army chief of staff, General Leonard Wood, likely because a reduction in the standard ration would bring enormous benefits. "Your claims are all right, and as soon as your plans for practical application are organized *everybody must help*," he told Fletcher.[15] The commandant of the military academy at West Point became a convert to thorough mastication, urging it on his cadets,[16] and in 1904 a twenty-man unit was sent to Yale in an attempt to prove that they could subsist on one-third the normal military ration with no impairment of physical capability. Although three of the disgruntled squad soon deserted and four more were discharged after being caught devouring the free lunch at a nearby saloon, the remaining thirteen, supervised by Yale's physical education instructors, were pronounced in excellent physical shape, as were the other participants in the experiment.[17]

Chittenden was diplomatic about "Fletcherizing," as "thorough mastication" was coming to be called. While declaring that Fletcher's odorless stools (which Fletcher would send to him and others through the mails) did indeed indicate that prolonged chewing aided the complete digestion of food, he avoided Fletcher's physiological hokum about digestion in the rear of the mouth. Yet he played along with Fletcher, lamenting that the place where the "filter function" took place was too "opaque" to appear on x-rays, and that it was a dangerous locale to have x-rayed. He also praised Fletcherizing as a method for reducing food intake.[18] But he recognized from the start that the real breakthrough was the new protein requirement.

Chittenden regarded the new evidence in much the same light as Atwater: from the standpoint of physiological economy and health. But where Atwater had originally stressed the economic benefits of dietary reform, Chittenden emphasized good health over economy. "The taking of an excess of food," he wrote, "is just as harmful as insufficient nourishment, involving as it does not only wasteful expenditure, but what is of even greater moment, an expenditure of energy in the part of the body which may in the long run prove disastrous. . . . If our standards are now unnecessarily high, then surely we are not only practicing an uneconomical method of sustaining life, but we are subjecting ourselves to conditions the reverse of physiological, and which must of necessity be inimical to our well being."[19] This kind of message would have much more impact on a middle- and upper-class audience than would appeals to economies in the kitchen.

Understandably, Chittenden's standards faced considerable opposition. The suggestion of reducing protein intake by almost two-thirds was not easily heeded. After all, the father of modern nutritional science von Liebig himself had labeled protein the muscle-building substance and declared it absolutely necessary for human strength. Not only had Atwater and the New Nutritionists equated protein with strength and productivity, so too had the thousands of people involved in sports. Participants and spectators alike knew that atheletes performed best having eaten meat three times a day. Their "training tables" included at least two kinds of meat, and huge slabs of beef were the *sine qua non* of peak physical performance. "White bread, red meat, and blue blood make the tricolor flag of conquest," wrote a New York City doctor, denouncing advocates of a low-protein diet in *Cosmopolitan* magazine.[20]

Much of the scientific opposition sprang from Atwater's disciples. The OES, now headed by Langworthy and supervised by True, continued to adhere to Atwater standards. Atwater's successor as Director of the Nutrition Laboratory of the Carnegie Institution in Boston, his ex-student Francis Benedict, argued that much of Chittenden's evidence was not convincing because it consisted merely of the testimony of subjects who said they felt better.[21]

But Benedict could not counter Chittenden's greatest selling point, Fletcher's undoubted physical achievements. His ability to lift a 300-pound weight 350 times in rapid succession using his calf muscles alone—double the record of any Yale athlete—was verified by third parties, including the Yale director of physical education.[22] Fletcher enthralled the annual convention of home economists with a letter recounting how, thanks to his regime, he had braved eighteen months in the Orient, where there was "an ever-changing food supply ranging from the riz-tave of Dutch Java to the curries of British India, from the fruits and vegetables of the Philippines to those of Upper Burmah and the Vale of Kashmir." Among those who could attest to Fletcher's physical endurance was none other than General Wood, for the two had spent nine hours "breaking our way through the tropical jungle of a volcanic island in the Philippines." Luckily for Wood, he was not present when Fletcher was "caught in a blizzard at 8500 feet elevation in the Himalayas . . . and was compelled to wade in deep snow for some 11 miles for nearly as many hours." In Fletcher's eyes, though, perhaps his diet's greatest achievement was to cure him of painful writer's cramp, and he ended his letter with a touching reference to this remarkable feat:

> Through my own search for and discovery of the natural protection which the mouth affords, I have brought the human wreck Fletcher of New Orleans out of the depths of his infirmities, off the scrap heap of modern club and social life, and have secured his recuperation as shown in the endurance tests just now completed and by this letter which he is writing by hand at the dictation of a new Fletcher.[23]

Fletcher's flair for self-promotion and his physical prowess, buttressed by a monumental ego, made him one of the two best known food faddists of the day. Many well-known personalities, including socialist author Upton Sinclair and anti-socialist Yale professor of economics Irving Fisher—who brought Fletcher's ideas into the eugenics movement—became ardent "chewers."[24] Henry James became a thoroughgoing disciple of Fletcher, whom he addressed as "my dear friend and benefactor." Fletcherizing had caused his *malaise* to disappear, he wrote Fletcher in September 1905, and "all my serenity and improvement return."[25] His faith in Fletcher was reinforced three years later when Fletcher pinpointed the cause of "all that sinister heartburn, . . . or ravage of the 'alimentary canal'": "the abuse of too drastic mouthwashes . . . Listerine in parti-cular."[26]

Henry's brother, the brilliant Harvard philosopher William James, was valued even more highly as a convert, for he seemed to have accommo-dated moral philosophy to modern experimental science, and Fletcher was well aware of the benefits of support from a man so esteemed by the scientific community. In November 1905, James wrote to the Harvard *Crimson* urging the Harvard community to attend a lecture by Fletcher, whose "teaching and example have been of such vital benefit to certain persons whom I know." James declared that "if his observations on diet, confirmed already on a limited scale, should prove true on a universal scale, it is impossible to overestimate their revolutionary import." Fletcher's joy knew no bounds. "It gives me tons of courage, acres of strength and, as a respected authority, it clears the track for my campaign," he wrote James. "Fletcherism" was "advancing the same cause as Prag-matism," he later assured the philosopher.[27] Because of the seriousness with which he was taken by men like William and Henry James, Fletcher was able to bridge the gap between such scientists as Chittenden and Mendel and that famous heir of the great nineteenth-century religious health-food tradition, Dr. John Harvey Kellogg, probably the only food faddist of the Progressive era to outshine Fletcher.[28]

Kellogg's Battle Creek "Sanitorium" began as a small Seventh-Day Adventist affair, serving vegetarian food mandated to that sect by its founder Ellen White. Although White received her orders through per-sonal encounters with God, her views on diet bore a striking resemblance to those circulating in the 1830s, particularly those of William Sylvester Graham, the teetotaling vegetarian who reviled meat and spicy foods for their supposed aphrodisiacal qualities, and a lesser known philosopher of health, Larken Coles.[29] The sanitorium had been foundering when Kel-logg took it over in 1876, but the dynamism of the robust, fast-talking crusader (who, in his later years, with his white hair, white goatee, and white suits, came to bear a rather striking resemblance to another dynamo of the food business, Colonel Sanders) soon brought the institute to life, expanding its clientele far beyond the followers of White. Patients were put on individualized diets designed to cure their particular problems. The underweight were subjected to twenty-six feedings a day and forced to lie motionless in bed with sandbags on their bellies to aid the absorption of nutrients. They were forbidden physical activity of any kind, even brush-ing their teeth, for this would burn up valuable calories. Patients with high blood pressure were put on a diet of grapes, and nothing but grapes: from ten to fourteen pounds of them a day.[30]

By the early twentieth century, although his scientific credentials were non-existent and his medical ones hardly impressive, Kellogg was widely accepted as one of the leaders of American science and medicine. He conferred with Pavlov in his Russian laboratory, discussed the contribution of protein to the proliferation of bacteria in the colon with experts at France's Pasteur Institute, corresponded with scientists throughout the world, and published his pseudo-scientific condemnations of meat and masturbation (consumption of the former encouraged the latter) in his own medical journals.[31] By then, not only was the "San" attracting thousands of middle- and upper-middle-class Americans to its "cures," it also counted many members of the elite among its patrons, including John D. Rockefeller and Theodore Roosevelt.[32] Indeed, in 1906, when Henry Bowditch, who was a physician as well as the Professor of Physiology at Harvard, was struck by illness he too sought out Kellogg and his "San,"[33] though he acknowledged that Kellogg was "looked at askance by many in the regular profession."[34]

Kellogg was greatly impressed by Fletcher when the Great Masticator visited the San in 1902. Although he had always advocated chewing food well, Kellogg never thought of taking it to Fletcher's lengths. "You are the founder of a new and wonderful movement," he told Fletcher.[35] He coined the term "Fletcherize" and hung a huge banner in the San's Grand Dining Room admonishing patients to do so. He even wrote an entertaining "Chewing Song" to be sung at meals to encourage Fletcherizing. Although Fletcher did not adopt Kellogg's vegetarianism, he often manifested great disdain for meat and supported Kellogg's attacks on protein, as well as his assertions that "the decline of a nation commences when gourmandizing begins."[36]

Like Fletcher, Kellogg developed close contacts with the scientific home economists and lent some glitter to their rather dull annual conferences by giving or sending papers on the latest in nutrition research. In 1907, he announced new discoveries by the scientist Metchnikoff, whom he had just visited at the Pasteur Institute in Paris, which seemed to confirm that aging and degenerative disease were caused by "poisons produced by parasitic bacteria living in the intestine, particularly in the colon." These bacteria, 300 to 400 million of which were present in a gram of meat, could be starved out by greatly reducing consumption of the protein they fed on. Furthermore, it seemed, "the work of extermination" could be "greatly accelerated" by eating "a Bulgarian milk preparation, known as yogurt."[37] At their 1908 conference in the great revivalist complex at Chautauqua, New York, a veritable capital of temperance, gastronomic restraint, and moral uplift, both Kellogg and Fletcher were featured speakers, and both presented evidence to support the growing belief among home economists that Americans should reduce their food consumption.[38] At last a scientific basis for smaller meals was emerging.

The new scientific ideas were soon reflected in home economics courses and textbooks, as well as cookbooks and cookery columns. Sara Tyson Rorer, a Kellogg admirer who regularly propounded the ideas of the New

Nutritionists in her *Ladies Home Journal* column, had recently been warning that eating foods that took a lot of energy to digest produced "nervous
prostration" and headaches.[39] Now, with protein identified as the most
indigestible element, she joined in the anti-protein crusade. Americans ate
too much meat, she proclaimed in 1909 and henceforth her menus would
no longer include meat three times a day.[40] Prestigious upper-middle-
class journals such as the *Scientific American* joined in as well, popularizing
and seeming to endorse the calls of Fletcher and Chittenden for Americans to eat less.[41]

Chittenden published his most influential book on the subject, *The
Nutrition of Man,* in 1907, but the controversy over protein requirements
raged for many years and indeed still continues. For home economists,
though, the major blow for lower protein requirements was struck by one
of their own, Professor Henry C. Sherman, a Columbia University chemist who held a joint appointment at Teachers College, by then an imperial
center of home economics just entering its most expansive phase. His
1911 book, *The Chemistry of Food and Nutrition,* showed protein requirements between that of Chittenden, who had settled on 60 grams as his
requirement, and Atwater's 125-gram requirement, recommending 75
grams per day as safe for those wishing to undertake a low-protein diet and
100 grams for an average diet (whatever that was). The upshot was a
considerable erosion of the Atwater standard and support for less food
consumption.[42] Sherman's book rapidly became the new Bible of home
economics and dietetics courses. Three years later, in his textbook analyzing various foods, he recommended that Americans halve their present
consumption of meat.[43] That same year, Fletcher wrote to Irving Fisher
that Atwater had become a "discredited authority" who had "fallen from
his very high protein perch."[44]

For some years, Langworthy and other Atwater students continued to
hew to the higher standards, although in 1911 Langworthy did grudgingly
concede that under certain circumstances 100 grams per day of protein
might be an adequate minimum.[45] In 1918, however, after subjecting
some subjects to low-protein diets with no apparent ill-effects, Benedict
deserted the high-protein cause.[46] But by that time nutritional science was
already taking a sharp turn: in other laboratories chemists were experimenting, not with humans in gymnasia or calorimeters but with mice in
cages, and the discovery of vitamins would again revolutionize concepts of
the nature of food.[47]

By then the first generation of New Nutritionists had passed from the
scene. Atkinson was felled by a heart attack in 1905, while walking to his
Boston office. Atwater succumbed to cancer in 1907, just as his new
Carnegie-financed laboratory in Boston was finally getting under way.
Ellen Richards, who had abandoned her laboratory in favor of propagation
of the faith, spent her declining years teaching at MIT, traveling with her

mining engineer husband, and entertaining her students and other home economists with grace and dignity in her home in Brookline until her death at age sixty-eight in 1911.[48] The paeans which followed each of their deaths naturally emphasized their contributions to certain fields: Atkinson's to fire insurance and economics, Atwater's to chemistry, and Richards as the founder of the home economics profession. The obituary writers of the day could not, of course, see that together they had also played a major role in creating the basis for changing American eating habits.

As for the next half-generation, both Kellogg and Chittenden continued to function as living testimony to their own dietary recommendations. Kellogg lived an active, exercise-filled life until 1943, when he died at age ninety-one, and Chittenden outlived most of his high-protein critics, dying in the same year at age eighty-seven. Fletcher was not so fortunate. By 1919, when he succumbed to a heart attack at age sixty-eight, interest in Fletcherizing was dwindling. William James, who, in Henry's words, had always Fletcherized "less devoutedly—not to say fanatically," than Henry, drifted away from it in 1908.[49] Henry abandoned it in 1909, apparently because surviving on so little food made him miserable.[50] Although Kellogg kept preaching it into the early 1920s, and Irving Fisher managed to interest some eugenists in his ideas, it soon slipped into the interstices of the faddist world. Middle-class mothers continued to urge their children, as they always had, to chew their food well, but with no thought for the filter function in the back of the mouth and no warnings that failure to do so would bring regurgitation.

The demise of Fletcherizing was an event of some significance, for among other things it symbolized that at that stage, at least, middle-class America was unwilling to de-socialize the act of eating by subordinating taste and social interaction to concerns over health. And anti-social it was. The vegetarian superstar Bernarr McFadden, another apostle of thorough mastication, specifically forbade conversation at mealtime because this "diversion" interfered with proper chewing.[51] According to Francis W. Crowinshield, the last of the "great arbiters" of New York society, Fletcherizing "added a new horror to dining out," because "these strange creatures seldom repay attention. The best that can be expected from them is the tense and awful silence that always accompanies their excruciating tortures of mastication."[52] Perhaps only in a country such as America, with its earlier tradition of silent, grim determination at the dinner table, could Fletcherizing have gained even a toehold.

The extent to which Fletcher, Kellogg, Chittenden and the rest were victorious against the dreaded "Gluttony" and "gourmandizing" can be overstated, for most prewar middle-class people remained robust eaters. Studies of the amounts of food consumed in college dormitories, boarding houses, and fraternity houses showed them continuing to tuck back impressive amounts of food. Students in a boarding house at the University of Minnesota in 1910 were typical: they consumed an average of 3,715 calories and 105 grams of protein per person per day, and this does not include food and beverages consumed outside the boarding house.[53]

Moreover, conspicuous consumption, particularly of French food, seemed as popular as ever in the trend-setting upper circles. While the middle classes were beginning to re-examine their kitchens and tables, their social superiors continued on their expansive way, undaunted by Chittenden, home economists, and warnings against protein. The dining room of the Waldorf Hotel in New York ascended to the pinnacle of that city's *beau monde* thanks to the snobbery of Oscar Tschirky, its francophilic *maître d' hôtel,* who assured the elite that everything there was as fine as in Paris. In 1911, when the owner of the Forum Hotel in Oakland made a successful bid to establish his dining room as a mecca for the Bay Area elite he did so by bringing in a French chef who had worked with Escoffier.[54] In April 1913, when Frank W. Woolworth hosted a dinner in the newly opened Woolworth Building in New York City to honor Cass Gilbert, the architect, even Mrs. Astor would have found the menu more than adequate. More to the point, she would have found it little changed from similar situations in the 1880s. Caviar, oysters, turtle soup, Turban of Pompano with Austrian potatoes, breast of guinea hen with Nesselrode sauce, Terrapin Baltimore style, Royal Punch, Roast squab, walnut and grapefruit salad, frozen *bombe,* fancy cakes, coffee, and a splendid array of wines graced the table. Perhaps only a diminution in the number of French dishes and terms on the menu distinguished it from those which had been the norm for well over thirty years. This by no means implied waning status for French food. Even the dinner staged by the city's Mexican community that year at the Hotel Astor to celebrate the centennial of Mexican independence was French, as was the annual dinner of a prosaic New York City Forester's Lodge at a more declassé hotel.[55]

But diligent home economists were assiduously working to undermine this way of dining. The scientific home economists in Washington reaped a reward for their adept lobbying in 1914, when the Smith-Lever Act effectively transferred responsibility for home economics extension work from the farmers' bureaus and state extension offices to the home economists of the land grant colleges and universities. The next year, the Office of Experiment Stations was renamed the States Relations Office and a special Bureau of Home Economics was created within it to conduct and disseminate the results of home economics research. In 1917, the Smith-Hughes Act gave the *coup de grace* to the old "cooking and sewing school" adherents by providing land grant colleges with funds for training teachers of home economics, giving the scientific home economists who ran their departments effective control over the teaching of home economics in the public schools of most states. The scientific home economists were now able to spread the message of the New Nutrition virtually unimpeded by miscreants concerned about the taste, rather than the economy and health, of food.

By then as well, the New Nutritionist network had become a wide one indeed. Agencies of state and local governments across the nation reproduced USDA pamphlets on nutrition by the thousands, distributing them to farmers, housewives, and schoolchildren. Private interest groups pitched in too. In 1916 alone, the Metropolitan Life Insurance Company distributed 300,000 copies of "Food Facts," a pamphlet outlining the principles of the New Nutrition.[56] By then, the message of the home economists and New Nutritionists had also become a standard feature of middle-class cookbooks. Atwater's charts on the protein, carbohydrate, fat, and calorie content of foods were well-nigh ubiquitous, as were admonitions to cook simply.

Still, most foods were to be prepared and served separately, and this required a lot of time for preparation, as well as pots, pans, and serving dishes to clean. Although there was much talk of "labor-saving" utensils developed for the kitchen in the past twenty years, wrote Maria Parloa in 1908, they had in fact done little to reduce the labor needed in the kitchen.[57] Furthermore, availability of kitchen help was shrinking. In the North in particular, the number of live-in servants declined sharply after 1900, as the supply of immigrant girls was not enough to replenish the numbers of women who left service for marriage and factory jobs.[58] Savings in labor thus had to come from reducing the number of ingredients in dishes, the steps in their preparation, and the number of courses. The result was aptly summed up in the stern admonition of one of the more popular cookbooks of the day: "Avoid fancy cooking."[59]

CHAPTER 8

New Reformers and
New Immigrants

Those reformers who had redirected their efforts from the working-class toward the middle-class diet chose wisely, for, as we have seen, the middle class offered a peculiarly fertile field for their message. Still, particularly as the rise of a progressive impulse after the turn of the century jogged both conscience and self-interest to make the middle classes more aware of the plight of the poor, others were prepared to step into their shoes. The newly trained home economists who found inspiration in the New England Kitchen experiment and hoped that new techniques might bring about the revolution in working-class eating habits that eluded the pioneers were joined by a new breed of professionals: full-time social workers employed by private or government agencies. These experts in dealing with the poor shunted aside volunteers who tried to uplift the poor through instructive visits to their households. Their agencies replaced capricious philanthropists who doled out charity to those individuals they discerned to be the "deserving poor."

Like the New England Kitchen generation, the new professionals thought indoctrination in the New Nutrition would cure workers of their uneconomical food habits. In 1913, when experts from the New York School Lunch Committee investigated the homes of the "malnourished" they declared "it was found to be more ignorance than poverty that was the cause of this condition."[1] The director of the nation's largest private relief agency, the New York Association for Improving the Condition of the Poor, agreed, declaring in 1917 that ignorance, not poverty, was the cause of malnutrition.[2] NYAICP pamphlets told slum-dwellers that many did not get enough to eat simply because they did not spend their food dollars wisely. "Buy the right things with the money you spend," was their message.[3] By the 1910s relief agencies distributing food to the poor commonly dispensed the lessons of the New Nutritionists along with it. In 1916 a New York City nutrition worker estimated that in that city alone there were hundreds of organizations trying to combat malnutrition among the poor "by what may be called nutritional guidance."[4]

Some professionals followed the debates in nutritional science closely and tried to adjust their message accordingly, particularly with the emergence of new low-protein theories.[5] As a result, in addition to criticizing workers for purchasing expensive cuts of meat when cheaper ones would do, some health reformers now accused workingmen of eating too much meat of any kind. A common theme was that pride and the desire to emulate their betters—not bodily requirements—was what led workers to eat more meat than needed.[6] "Overeating is as Harmful as Undereating" was the theme of one NYAICP campaign in the slums.[7] However, perhaps because of a professional predisposition toward painting a grim picture of the life of those they wished to help, most social workers and health reformers were slow to adopt the new lower standards and emphasized that the poor were undernourished, not overfed.

Food reform for the working classes drew support from prohibitionists and temperance advocates who agreed with Sara Tyson Rorer that "the hankering of the ill-fed stomach drives men to drink."[8] The idea received impressive backing in 1896 when a committee of the American Public Health Association blamed drunkenness on "bad cooking, unpalatable meals, and the extravagant use of ice" and called for the establishment of people's kitchens of the New England Kitchen mold to teach economical cooking in the slums.[9] A few years earlier, Jacob Riis, the journalist whose photographs and articles helped arouse middle-class concern over living conditions in New York City's slums, wrote that "half the drunkenness that makes so many homes miserable is at least encouraged, if not directly caused, by mismanagement and bad cooking at home."[10] Riis thought home economics courses for tenement girls and their families could cure the problem and home economists were not averse to encouraging this idea. They cited saloon keepers (always anonymous) who swore that nothing had hurt their business so much as the teaching of home economics in the public schools.[11]

Some encouraged the consumption of coffee as an antidote to alcohol. The American Public Health Association supported this, claiming there was "a physiological antagonism between coffee and alcohol, as well as between coffee and opium" and called coffee a healthy "stimulative" ("much favored by brain workers") as well as an anti-malarial agent.[12]

Chittenden, Fletcher, and other experts on nutrition agreed that coffee was indeed brain food. This benign view of coffee prompted reformers to suggest founding coffee houses in the slums to displace saloons. The popularity of coffee houses among Jews and Italians, two groups of note-worthy sobriety when compared to most other immigrant groups, lent weight to this idea. Jane Addams extolled their cafés as the "Salons of the Ghetto. . . . performing a function somewhat between the eighteenth cen-tury coffee house and the Parisian cafe."[13] The NYAICP actually opened a coffee house in an ex-saloon on New York's tough West Side, hoping in vain, as it turned out, that retaining the bar and many of the saloon's furnishings would help lure hard-drinking Irish longshoremen away from the real saloons.[14]

However, faith in coffee as a form of Antabuse was by no means univer-sal. The Committee of Fifty medical and scientific experts assembled to investigate and combat the alcohol problem declared that "fried foods and strong coffee form the bulk of the American workingman's diet. This causes indigestion and of itself fosters a thirst for stimulants which the saloon readily supplies."[15] Other experts thought that, like alcohol, the stimulative properties of coffee and tea encouraged crime. One of the era's most prominent experts on juvenile delinquency wrote "the unset-tling of the nervous system which occurs in young people by the excessive use of these stimulants is a direct factor making for delinquency in many environments."[16]

Unlike their Kitchen predecessors, the new generation of scientific housekeepers were trained to meet the problem of immigrant cooking and eating habits head on. The wave of "New Immigrants" that began in the 1880s and 1890s became a flood after the turn of the century.[17] Most of these people were drawn not to America's farms but to its cities and industrial towns.

This vast movement reinforced a social pattern which was already dis-cernible in the 1880s: a bifurcated working class. Now, the division between the relatively well-off skilled and semi-skilled and the struggling unskilled was reinforced by ethnic differences, for most "New Immi-grants" were in the latter category. Peter Shergold's study of the standard of living of the working class in Pittsburgh in this period depicts a striking contrast between the living conditions of the upper sector, mainly white native-born Americans or immigrants of Anglo-Saxon, Celtic, and north-ern European ancestry, and the central, eastern, and southern Europeans who comprised the bulk of the unskilled:

> At the top of the wage pyramid were those high-skilled, high-income workers able to purchase their own homes, to wash in indoor bathrooms, buy hand-rolled stogies or the *National Labor Tribune,* or, occasionally, watch the Pirates at Forbes Field or arrange an excursion to Kennywood Park. . . . At the broad base of the pyramid was the city's large laboring population,

crowded into hastily converted tenements and rapidly deteriorating wooden constructs, sharing outside toilet facilities and a communal faucet, living next to the noise, glare, and stench of the mills and furnaces. Here were children fighting imaginary battles along the unpaved streets and open sewers and workers to whom leisure was sleep, to whom recreation was a half hour at the nickelodeon, or a drink in the saloon after work, to whom contentment was a full pipe of tobacco, or a Sunday afternoon gambling at cards.[18]

Since most of the unskilled were "New Immigrants" of diverse origins, generalizations about what these workers ate are fraught with danger. However, it is clear that, as in the 1880s, there were substantial differences between the two worlds. The upper strata fully reflected the remarkable new opportunities for variety in diet created by the transportation and preservation revolutions. Ample supplies of beefsteak, fruits, and vegetables graced their tables, constituting the "reefs of roast beef and apple pie" upon which the German sociologist Werner Sombart saw the dreams of American socialists dashed.[19] This class of skilled or semi-skilled workers, mainly of British origin, ate much better than their relatives across the ocean. A British Board of Trade comparison with their counterparts in the United Kingdom concluded that on virtually every score the native-born, British-born, Canadian-born, and northern European-born (mainly German) Americans ate much better. The Americans ate more meat of all kinds, more eggs, more potatoes, and much more fruit and vegetables, particularly of the canned variety. There was relative equality in amounts of sugar and fresh milk, and the British surpassed the Americans only in consumption of cheese and bread.[20] The conclusion was inescapable: the diet of the "American-British-Northern European Group" of American families was "more varied and more liberal than that of families that as nearly correspond to them in the United Kingdom."[21]

We have a description of what seems to be a relatively typical bill of fare of the families of semi-skilled English-speaking steel workers from a 1910 study of workers' lives in the steel-making town of Homestead, near Pittsburgh, Pennsylvania. The lunches were relatively light because the man did not come home for lunch that week, but the investigator noted elsewhere that women normally prided themselves in the varied and elaborate lunches they prepared for their men:

MONDAY

Breakfast: Oatmeal and milk, eggs and bacon, bread, butter, jelly and coffee.
Dinner: Soup, bread, fruit.
Supper: Meat, beans, potatoes, fruit, red beets, pickles.

TUESDAY

Breakfast: Chocolate, eggs, bread, butter, jelly.
Dinner: Spinach, potatoes, pickles, warmed over meat, fruits, bread, butter.
Supper: Meat, sweet potatoes, carrots, beans, tomatoes, tea, bread, butter, and fruit.

WEDNESDAY

Breakfast: Eggs, corncakes, potatoes, coffee, rhubarb, bread, butter.
Dinner: Soup, bread, butter.
Supper: Lamb stew with dumplings, cucumber, eggplant, beans, corn, coffee,
   bread and butter, fruit.[22]

These were bills of fare of an amplitude and variety that most of their British counterparts could not afford. They also compare favorably with what was typical for semi-skilled steelworkers of thirty years before, particularly in the greater consumption of fruits and vegetables.

Foods consumed in the other working-class world also reflected new opportunities, but not to quite the same extent. Generally, less money to spend on food meant less variety on the dinner table and a greater dependence on the seasonality of foods. Except during the summer months, when fruit and vegetables were relatively cheap, it was normally a world of large loaves of crusty bread, stewed meats, potatoes, onions, and cabbage, accompanied by large quantities of pickles and other stimulating condiments. A study of anthracite coal mining communities showed Slavic families spending only an average of $2.68 per capita per month on groceries while the average English-speaking family, with a much higher income, spent over twice as much, allowing them to achieve greater variety in their diets. The Slavs purchased flour, barley, salt pork, potatoes, cabbages, barrel pickles, garlic, coffee, sardines, eggs, and some butter and sugar. The English-speakers purchased these items plus ham, onions, bottled pickles, tea, lard, dried beef, spices, cakes or crackers, mackerel, canned tomatoes, peaches, apricots, cherries, lemons, cheese, and salmon.[23]

Markedly lower expenditures on food among the immigrants by no means reflected a lower regard for its importance than among the native and British-born. Indeed, quite the opposite was true, for native and British-born families tended to spend a considerably smaller proportion of their income on food (and more on rent) than most other ethnic groups on the same economic level.[24] Moreover, immigrant women often took great pride, not just in their cooking skills, but in their ability to cook economically. These skills were an important part of the armory that defended the central role of Italian and Jewish mothers in their families. A native-born investigator in Homestead, with its many Slavs, reported that "many women show a genuine pride in their skill at buying and in utilizing different cuts of meat. . . . I shall not soon forget the enthusiasm with which one young wife described a special potato meat pie, her husband's favorite dish, which she made from the ends of steak too tough to use in any other way. These women are anxious not only to practice economies, but to conceal them by good choosing and skillful cooking."[25]

If there were real dietary problems, they arose not so much from ignorance of the New Nutrition as from the ups-and-downs of working class lives in a boom-and-bust economy with little in the way of an economic "safety net." Frequent bouts of unemployment, or the serious injury, illness, or death of the major breadwinner would wreak havoc on family budgets, and the amount devoted to food was usually slashed. This usually meant sharply reduced expenditures for what we now think are some of the most important foods: milk, fruit, and vegetables.

Despite evidence that the real problem was not so much cooking methods as economic insecurity, the new generation of social workers, public health workers, and dietary reformers continued the assault on the supposedly inferior manner in which food, particularly that of the immigrants, was chosen, prepared and served. Some felt that the American-born worker's diet was fine, and the problem was simply to help the foreign-born adopt this diet. One settlement house worker's study of wage earners' budgets concluded that they "illustrate what English and foreign economic writers have recognized, i.e., that the ordinary diet of the American workingman's family, compared with that of other countries, is abundant and varied. While foreigners bring their 'macaroni,' 'bologna,' or 'potato and tea' standards to this country, the different conditions of labor and climate soon modify and enlarge this diet." What was needed, she concluded, was to teach the immigrants how to Americanize their diets in an economical fashion.[26] By 1910, just a few years after this was written, how to do this was being taught in a number of colleges and universities.[27]

The new professionals studied assiduously the food habits of the immigrants they confronted. But they sought not to learn from them but to learn how to change them. When, after years of research, Winifred Gibbs, Columbia Teachers College's expert in changing immigrant diets, published a book of recipes for "economical cooking," it contained *none* of the many economical and nourishing European dishes whose savory smells wafted through neighborhoods not far from her Morningside Heights demonstration kitchen.[28]

This kind of attitude was all the more remarkable because home economists were not smug and self-satisfied about their own culture's food. Indeed, they spent much of their time denouncing their countrymen's eating habits. Their narrowness stemmed from their determination to learn only from science and not from the accumulated experience of millions of Europeans forced to economize on food. Nutritional science told them that the essence of European economical cooking: the *minestras* and *pasta-fagioles* of Italy, the *borschts*, *gulyashen*, and *cholents* of Eastern Europe were uneconomical because they were mixtures of foods and therefore required uneconomical expenditures of energy to digest. Strong seasonings that made bland but cheap foods tasty were denounced for overworking the digestive process and stimulating cravings for alcohol. Nutritional science reinforced what their palates and stomachs already told them: that any cuisine as coarse, overspiced, "garlicky," and indelicate-looking as the food of central, eastern, and southern Europe must be unhealthy as well. To most of these native-born daughters of the middle and upper class, who preferred their own food awash in a sea of bland white sauce and for whom "dainty" was the greatest compliment one could bestow on food, one whiff of the pungent air in the tenements or a glance into the stew pots was enough to confirm that the contents must wreak havoc on the human digestive system.

Home economists, social workers, and visiting nurses tried valiantly to discourage immigrants from eating spicy, mixed foods. In 1904, Robert Woods, head of one of Boston's most important settlement houses, blamed an apparent increase in death rates from first to second generation Italians who settled in New England in part on their "overstimulating and innutritious diet" and wrote that changing their diets was "the chief step in bringing about the adaption of the Italian type of life to America."[29] An NYAICP exhibit designed to demonstrate deficiencies of their food habits to Italian immigrants in lower Manhattan condemned the "complexity of combinations" in the most common Italian dishes as "a real tax on digestion." Although the American foods the exhibit proposed were only of equal food value yet cost five cents a meal more, they were proclaimed to be superior because the food value of the Italian menu "was theoretical only, with too little attention paid to strict assimilation." (This reflected the belief that when foods were mixed together in one dish a higher proportion of the nutrients were excreted as waste.) Among the lessons to be learned were "separation of one elaborate dish into three simple ones."[30] Immigrants from rural Poland faced similar criticisms. Not only did they eat the same dish for one meal, they also ate it from the same bowl. They therefore had to be taught to serve food on separate plates, as well as to separate the ingredients.[31]

Support came from those who sought to "Americanize" the new immigrants for social and political reasons. Many of these "Americanizers" were convinced that the immigrants could never be weaned from their old-country attitudes toward work, society, and politics until they abandoned their old-country ways of living and eating. The acrid smells of garlic and onions wafting through the immigrant quarters seemed to provide unpleasant evidence that their inhabitants found American ways unappealing; that they continued to find foreign (and dangerous) ideas as palatable as their foreign food. Thus, when the International Harvester farm equipment company set up its pioneer "Americanization" program in its midwestern plants, an important feature was a "model workingman's home" in which immigrant workers' wives were taught American methods of cooking.[32] The National Civic Federation, which united business leaders and anti-socialist trade unionists in an effort to head off social upheaval, sponsored homemaking courses for immigrant girls in Boston settlement houses and fitted out a complete apartment in which immigrant girls were taught cooking, cleaning, child care, and "business ethics."[33] Jane Addams was enthusiastic about public school cooking lessons because they would help immigrant girls "connect the entire family with American food and household habits."[34] For these assimilationists, food preferences often became the touchstone of Americanization. "Still eating spaghetti, not yet assimilated," noted a social worker after visiting an Italian household.[35]

The immigrants' apparent indifference to the presumed importance of the large American breakfast aroused great concern. The habit of breakfasting only on coffee and breads and giving children the same drew particular fire. An NYAICP nutritionist proudly told of the medical inspector and nurse in an immigrant school who asked the children what they had for breakfast. "From a large number came the reply 'Coffee and bread,' 'Coffee and bread' with an occasional 'Bread and tea' until the monotony was relieved by 'cocoa and cereal.' The two inquirers looked at each other in surprise, then the nurse asked the child's name and commented, 'Oh that's one of the A.I.C.P. families! I wish those above the relief line could have the same instruction.'"[36] Even freshness in the morning's bread and rolls met disapproval. Mabel Hyde Kittredge, who set up a series of "housekeeping centers" in tenement houses for New York City settlement houses, bemoaned the tenement dwellers' European habit of sending the children out each morning to purchase fresh bread and rolls for breakfast. "Poor little tenement girl," she wrote, "she does not know that in the well-managed home breakfast is bought the day before."[37]

Americanizing table manners was regarded as almost as important as Americanizing cooking. When genteel Boston ladies formed a Louisa May Alcott Club for little immigrant girls and furnished a demonstration apartment to teach them the American way of housekeeping, one of the first things they did was to give the seven-year-olds lessons in proper table manners. "Neither time nor thought has been given to the proper use of knife and fork," one of its organiziers lamented, "and in most of the homes a napkin is an unheard of quantity."[38] Eva White, a Brahmin who headed Boston's Peabody House settlement, taught "dining room etiquette" in special classes for immigrant girls.[39] Those fortunate enough to go on to high school would then read in their home economics text that dainty afternoon teas were now a popular way to entertain friends who drop in for an "afternoon call."[40]

Immigrant food shopping came under fire as well. Reformers fretted over the many small food stores in immigrant neighborhoods whose prices were higher than those "downtown." That these stores allowed payment be deferred to pay day or until periods of joblessness were over, carried foreign foods unavailable downtown, enabled women to deal in their native language, and functioned as neighborhood social centers counted little to them. They also ignored the fact that the savings to be garnered from shopping at large stores were significant only to those who could buy in bulk, and few immigrants had enough storage space to do so.[41] Yet Eva White lamented that it was difficult to teach them to cook economically because "no matter what inducements the larger stores of the city offer, they will trade with none but their own people."[42] Others warned against patronizing small merchants for health reasons. The Boston Women's Municipal League circulated flyers warning immigrants against buying food from street markets or from small stores which lacked proper sanitation and allowed in dogs and cats.[43] The NYAICP circulated similar leaflets in Italian, warning that food purchased from ambulatory vendors and open-air stalls was invariably germ-laden. The pamphlets also advised against shopping in delicatessens because their salami, sausages, pickles, and potato salads damaged the stomach without providing any sustenance.[44] The taste for imported Italian ingredients came under particular fire. Teachers College investigators, oblivious to the economical ways in which Italian immigrants used these crucial ingredients, lamented finding poor Italian immigrant families "suffering from cold and lack of food, buying one or two ounces of Roman cheese and small quantitites of olive oil . . . The investigators found many homes in which housewifes bought no milk at all because they thought it too expensive and at the same time were buying a small piece of cheese at $1.25 a pound."[45]

Immigrants' resistance to formal and informal pressures to Americanize their food habits varied. Only the most frugal could resist taking advantage of the greater availability of high-status foods which had rarely graced their tables in Europe. They commonly ate more meat in America, particularly beef but also poultry, lamb, and pork. They also indulged more in sweets, particularly sweet cakes and rolls, something many regarded as a peculiarly American habit.[46] Coffee drinking, which perplexed reformers, was in most cases an American-acquired habit. In much of central, eastern, and southern Europe coffee was a high status drink which the poor, especially the peasants, could hardly afford. Slavic immigrants seem to have manifested a particular weakness for coffee. In their homes it was customary to have a pot of coffee on the stove all day long, with members of the family helping themselves at will. Asked if she had changed her diet upon coming to America, a Polish woman replied, "Naturally, at home everyone had soup for breakfast, and here everyone has coffee and bread."[47] A Czech immigrant who arrived in 1914 perhaps exemplified the most common attitude toward the presence of all of these old-country luxuries on the table when he recalled that his family thought that in America "we ate like kings compared to what we had over there. Oh, it was really heaven."[48]

Many immigrant women took advantage of the increased availability of fruits and vegetables in summer and fall and preserved them for consumption in the off-seasons. Meanwhile, lower prices for canned goods, still expensive, high-status items in the 1880s and 1890s, made them afford-able to native-born women, and they became a symbol of Americaniza-tion. A Croatian immigrant to an industrial town in Iowa recalled that in 1914, "foreign-born people used to make disparaging remarks about the native American women sitting in the shade in the summer heat fanning themselves while the foreign-born women sweated in their kitchens put-ting up hundreds of jars of beans, tomatoes, preserves, jellies, pickles, beets, fruits of all kinds. Instead of putting up vegetables, meat, etc., for the winter native Americans bought canned goods from the store. None of the foreign-born women would be caught dead with store bread on the table."[49]

The foreign-born tended to take in boarders, which naturally affected the way they ate. Often they squeezed an enormous number of people from their home districts, mainly single men, into overcrowded apart-ments and workingmen's cottages across the nation. A 1914 survey of Polish and Lithuanian families in Chicago's stockyard district, many of whom lived in rented flats of four rooms or less, turned up an average of 4.12 lodgers per family.[50] This arrangement encouraged methods of cook-ing brought over from the old country: stewing multi-food dishes, served with large loaves of crusty bread.

Various groups responded to other aspects of the new culinary environ-ment in distinctive fashions. Most were from cultures where bread had deep-rooted symbolic importance, and they would patronize only bakeries run by their countrymen. Italians, complaining that the quality, variety, and availability of fresh fruits and vegetables did not match that of their *paesi,* constructed vast networks linking truck farms around the major cities, large fruit and vegetable operations in California, and the wholesale and retail markets of the major cities. Lithuanians, on the other hand, seem to have ignored fresh produce in favor of canned.[51] Italians also demonstrated a remarkable ability to grow their own fruits and vegetables in almost any available plot of land or window box, while Jews, who contented themselves with buying produce from street peddlers, were not averse to having live poultry share their living quarters. (It was not unheard-of for other immigrants to keep an occasional goat in their inner-city tenements.) Jews and Italians increased their consumption of veal, while Jews indulged more in beef: boiled, stewed, corned, or smoked and highly spiced in the fashion introduced by Rumanian Jews, as pastrami. Italians sent fishing boats into the waters off both coasts in search of shellfish, squid, and the other salt-water denizens they valued, while Jews and other central and eastern Europeans created a large new market for the smoked and fresh fish of the upper Great Lakes.

Immigrants differed in the importance they attached to food and the amount of income and time they were willing to devote to it. For Italians, particularly those from the South, preparing and sharing food was the central ritual of a closely knit family. Despite their legendary frugality, Italian immigrants imported vast amounts of pasta, olive oil, and cheese from Italy, fearing that to use inferior American substitutes would be regarded as a sign of not caring for the family. For Jews, food also had important family functions and was often used to strengthen the bond between mother and son. Hungarians, Bohemians, and Croatians placed great store on the mother's skill in food preparation and women prided themselves in the many hours they devoted to preparing their specialities. On the other hand, Poles, Lithuanians, Russians, and Ukrainians were less attached to old-country culinary ways and more amenable to Americanizing influences, perhaps because cooking was less important to the mother's role in the family or because they had somewhat less sophisticated heritages of old-country cooking to preserve.[52] Yet, even among these groups, old-country food tastes persisted. Consulted about settlement house cooking demonstrations for Polish women, a Polish woman advised that the secret of success was: "Whatever you do, make it taste Polish. Put cabbage in."[53]

Despite occasional successes, most efforts of the early-twentieth-century food reformers to change working-class food habits, particularly those of immigrants, had little more impact than those of Richards and the New England Kitchen pioneers. This is not to say that working-class food habits had not changed in the years between 1880 and the outbreak of World War I. Indeed, they had changed markedly, but mainly as the result of revolutions in transportation and distribution. Fresh meats replaced salted meats, and milk, fresh fruits, and vegetables came to play much more important roles in workers' diets. "There can be little doubt," said an article in the *American Journal of Public Health* regarding the prewar changes, "that the introduction of Southern fresh vegetables and fruits during the long winter of the North has proved beneficial to that large class of workers to whom variety in their food has always proved difficult owing to expense."[54] However, these were not changes the reformers were interested in promoting. While they were beginning to admit that variety in diet seemed to be a healthful thing, they remained fixated on the economics of working-class food habits, particularly those of immigrants. In the long run, the Americanizers would win out, for the passing of the first generation of immigrants and the growing impact of a changing middle-class culture would inevitably accomplish much of what the prewar reformers failed to do. But not before other assaults were resisted.

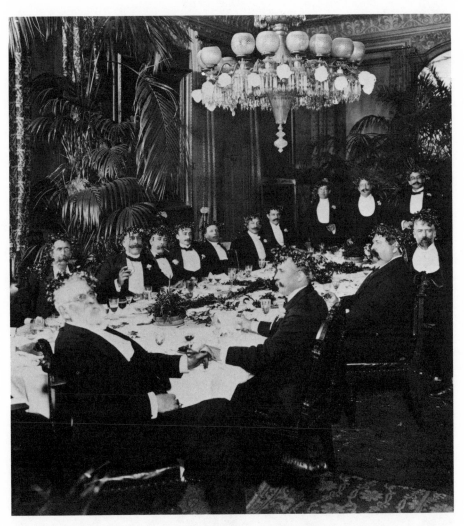

Laurel-leaf-bedecked men enjoying after-dinner port and cigars, perhaps after a "theme" dinner, in New York City, 1901. *(Museum of the City of New York)*

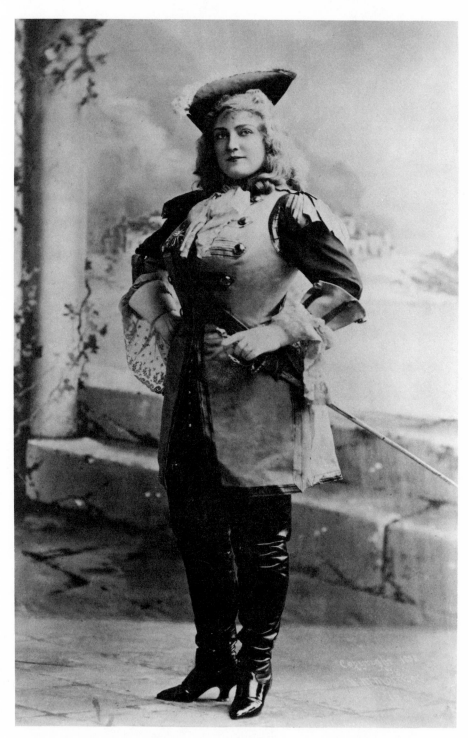

Actress Lillian Russell, the "American Beauty" whose "airy, fairy" looks slew many a late-nineteenth-century man, in the early 1890s, *before* she put on weight. *(Photographic Division, Library of Congress)*

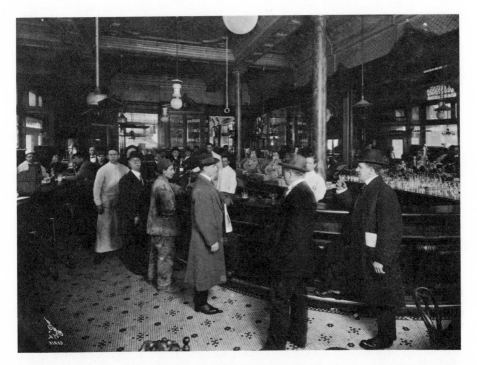

A prewar bar (Fitzgerald's, in New York City) with the "free" lunch counter on the left. The cash register would indicate that, like most "free lunches," there was a nominal fee, ostensibly to deter the totally indigent. *(Museum of the City of New York)*

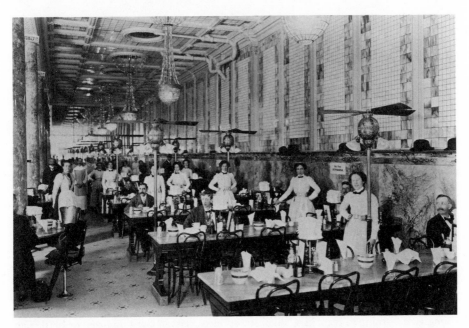

A New York City outlet of Child's restaurants, one of the new chains that arose at the turn of the century to serve quick meals in hygienic-looking surroundings to the growing number of white-collar workers. *(Museum of the City of New York)*

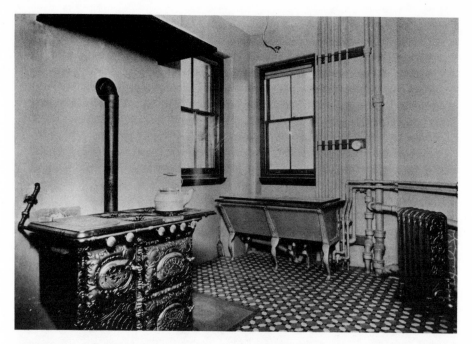

The kitchen of a well-off middle-class family in New York's Upper West Side in the 1890s. The monster stove, attached to a hot water heater, burned coal or wood, and the messy job of lighting, stoking, refueling, and cleaning it was almost certainly the task of an immigrant servant girl. *(Museum of the City of New York)*

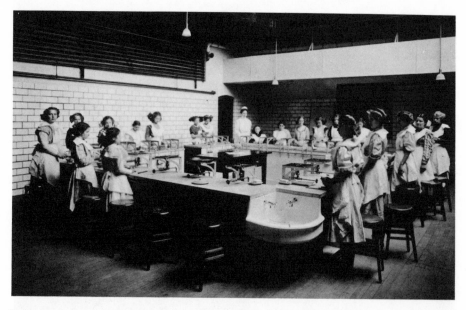

Young girls learning to cook in a "domestic science" class in Gary, Indiana, in 1910. The absence of charts giving the chemical composition of foods would indicate that the instructor was of the old "cooking and sewing school" kind, much maligned by the newer "scientific" home economists. *(Photographic Division, Library of Congress)*

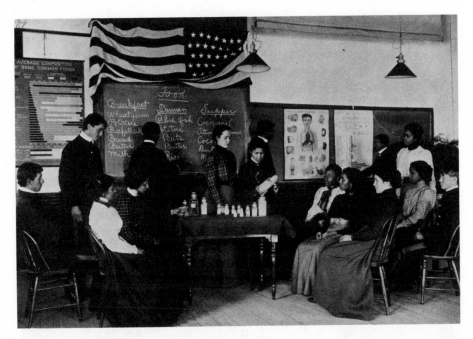

Students in Tuskegee Institute, the Alabama Negro college headed by Booker T. Washington, which cooperated closely with the "New Nutritionists," studying the chemist Wilbur Atwater's food principles in "Hygiene" class. *(Photographic Division, Library of Congress)*

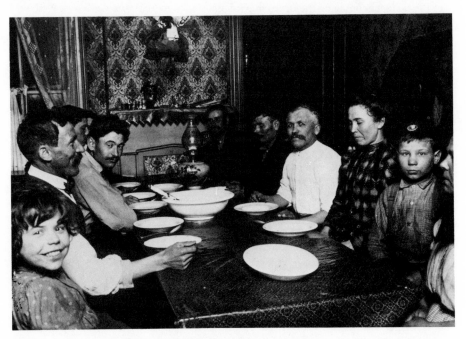

Slavic immigrants in a New York City boarding house awaiting the kind of stewed one-dish dinner which reformers regarded as unhealthy. *(Lewis Hine Collection, New York City Public Library)*

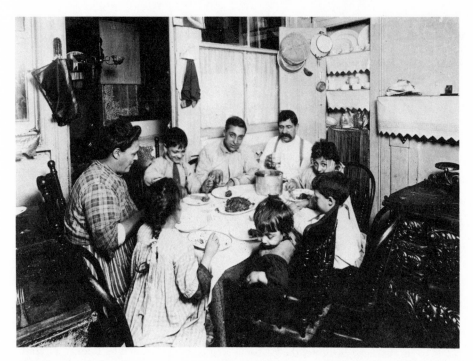

An Italian immigrant family. The mother, whose role in preparing and serving food was of paramount importance in maintaining strong family ties, probably sat down at this, the initial stage of the meal, only for the benefit of the camera. Normally she would hover over the table, encouraging the males in particular to eat more. *(Hine Collection, New York City Public Library)*

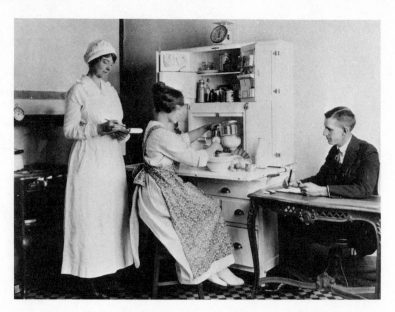

Researchers pushing out the frontiers of "Scientific Housekeeping" by conducting a time-and-motion study of a woman using an egg-beater at the "Appleton Experiment Station," Connecticut, 1912. *(Schlesinger Library, Radcliffe College)*

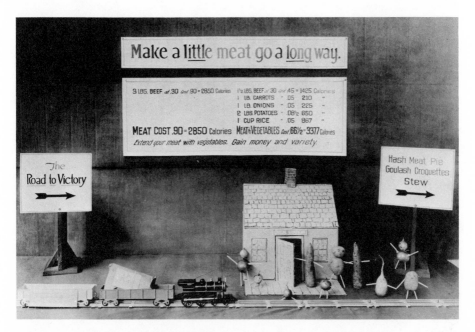

A traveling exhibit of the U.S. Food Administration discouraging consumption of meat by teaching the principles of the New Nutrition. *(Library of Congress)*

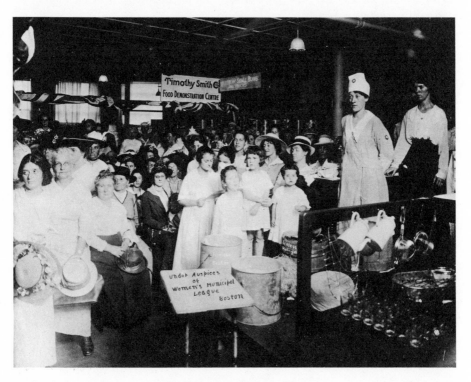

Food Administration conservation lessons in a Boston department store, given by the kind of native-born middle- and upper-middle-class women who responded most enthusiastically to the conservation message. *(Library of Congress)*

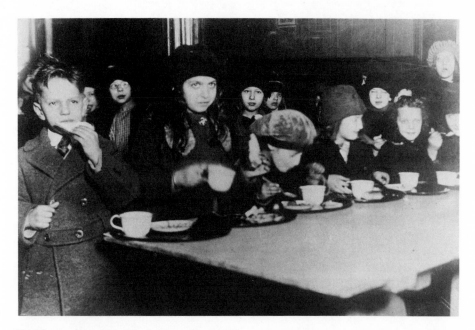

Healthy-looking New York City schoolchildren who, largely due to experts' misinformation, were adjudged malnourished, eating one of the three-cent hot lunches in a Manhattan school, provided by the New York Association for Improving the Condition of the Poor, 1918. *(Library of Congress)*

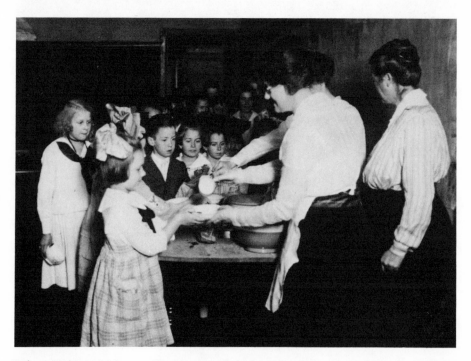

Robust-looking children in Washington, D.C., being served a hot "penny lunch" by the Red Cross after an investigation revealed "many cases" of malnutrition. *(Library of Congress)*

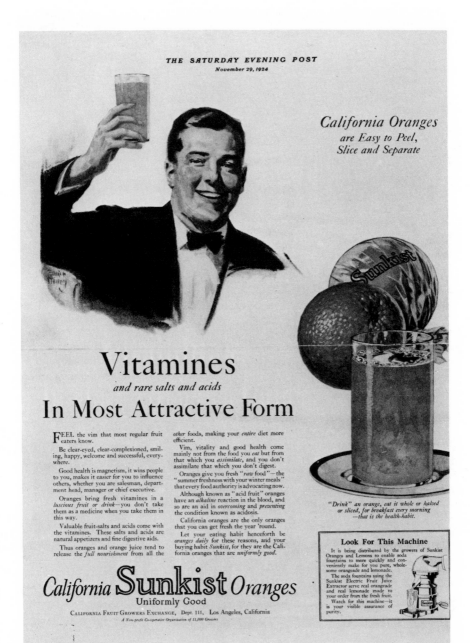

The California Fruit Growers Association stimulating vitamin-consciousness in 1924. Note the vagueness regarding exactly what vitamins did, how much of them was required, and the reference to the dreaded affliction "acidosis," a non-existent ailment "discovered" by Elmer McCollum, the great American pioneer in vitamin research. (*Library of Congress*)

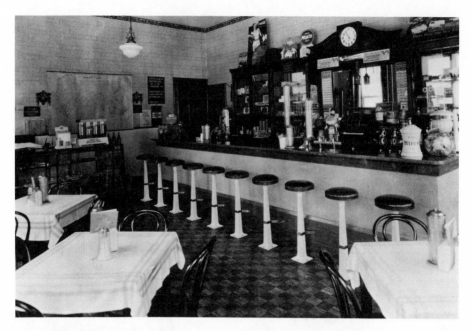

Lunch room and soda fountain at the Hotel Frantz, Myerston, Pa., 1925. Prohibition practically killed the hotel dining room trade, forcing many such hotels to convert their bars into soda fountains and to open restaurants serving light fare to compete with the coffee shops, cafeterias, and drug store lunch counters which were proliferating around them. *(Library of Congress)*

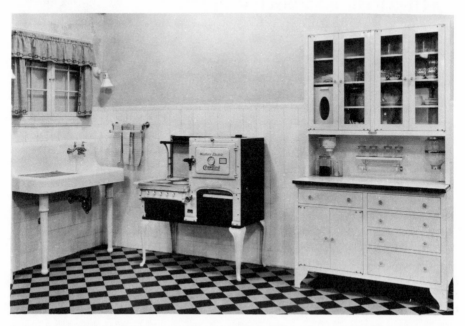

A "model kitchen," 1924. Its clean lines, uncluttered by prewar contraptions, and electric stove reflect the new expectation that the housewife would spend as little time as possible in the (now servantless) kitchen. *(Library of Congress)*

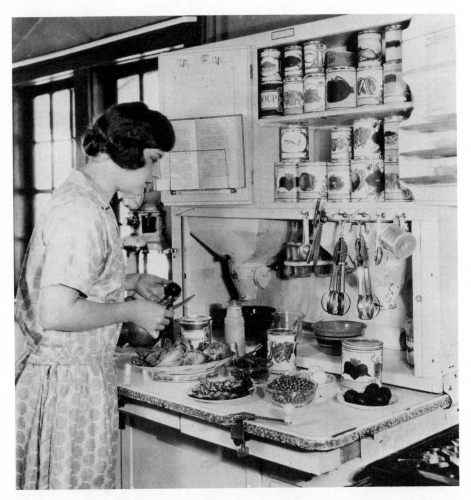

Home economist Christine Frederick preparing a salad at her Appleton Experiment Station in 1925. Note that, with the exception of the lettuce, all the ingredients are canned. *(Schlesinger Library, Radcliffe College)*

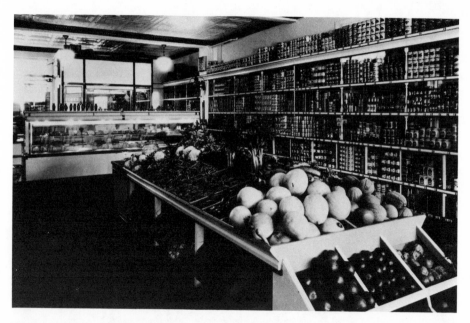

The interior of a chain grocery store in Washington, D.C., in 1920. Although the canning industry was on the threshold of another great wave of expansion, note the large proportion of space already devoted to canned and bottled goods. *(Library of Congress)*

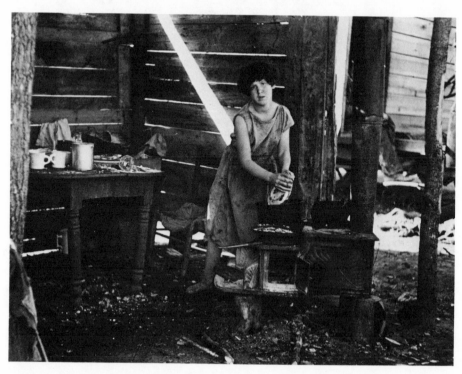

A twelve-year-old girl cooking a meal for a family of nine in a hut on U.S. 70 in Tennessee, March 1936. *(Farm Security Administration Collection, Library of Congress)*

CHAPTER 9

The Great Malnutrition Scare, 1907–1921

The industrial depressions of 1907 and 1914–15 were relatively short, but they were severe, and led to concern over the effects of wage cuts and layoffs on workers' standards of living. Rising food prices after 1910 added to the concern, for the nation had been lulled by decades of stable or falling food prices, and much of the attention focused on the effects of economic instability on workers' diets. A spate of books and articles painted alarming pictures of workers' families desperately trying to keep their heads above water in an economy with no mechanism for keeping wages abreast of rising living costs.[1] Yet food prices continued to climb. After rising sharply in 1912 and 1913 and at a slower pace in the next two years, in 1916 they jumped 19 percent as crop shortfalls, shortages of railway cars, and increased demand from the warring Allies put particular pressure on the price of many of the foods essential to the working-class diet: bread, potatoes, onions, and cabbage. One alarmed social worker called it "the worst food convulsion ever experienced."[2]

Within three months, however, the situation was much worse, as prices of these and other popular items nearly doubled. In February 1917, food riots broke out in New York City, Boston, and Philadelphia. The New York rioters attacked food shops and burned pedlars' pushcarts in the lower East Side and in the Brownsville and Williamsburg sections of Brooklyn. Demonstrators marched on the Waldorf Hotel in an attempt to confront the governor. A delegation of protesters accosted the mayor in his office demanding the seizure of all stored foods and the establishment of municipal food shops and markets. Retailers disclaimed responsibility and blamed wholesalers. Six thousand kosher poultry shops and 130 kosher poultry slaughterhouses closed down just before the Passover holiday season in protest against the wholesalers, whom they charged with cornering the market in Kosher poultry.[3]

Meanwhile, in Boston, three hundred men and women crying "We must have food" and "We want potatoes" stormed J. Lipsky's grocery store in the West End, and guards had to be placed around a potato-laden schooner recently in from Nova Scotia. A meeting of West End mothers voted to bar social workers from their homes and demanded that the money used to support settlement houses be turned over for a breakfast fund for school children.[4] In Philadelphia, food riots erupted in the aftermath of a demonstration by wives of striking sugar refinery employees in which one man was killed and several injured.[5] In Congress, noting that "in the same paper that tells of starvation in New York there is a whole page devoted to a sumptuous entertainment at the Riding and Hunt Club . . . and long accounts of stately repasts by men in public life," Senator George Norris said he would like to "throttle" those who conspired to hold back food from the people. Others proposed that the federal government appropriate $50 million "to feed the poor threatened with starvation."[6]

Earlier rises in food prices prompted a variety of responses. In 1912 and 1913 committees of the U.S. Senate, state legislatures, and private charitable agencies launched investigations seeking to discover who was to blame. In urban areas, where much of the suspicion focused on wholesalers and retailers, prominent reformers attempted to organize consumer cooperatives to deal directly with growers and processors.[7] During the 1916–17 crisis George W. Perkins, a Progressive Wall Street lawyer who headed New York City's emergency food committee, suggested cooperative distribution of foods as a solution, as did reformers in Philadelphia and other cities.[8] But the seeds of consumer cooperatives fell on barren ground in urban America and, with no cooperatives to deal with, Perkins's committee had to sell its carloads of beans and fish to retailers who merely promised to sell them to the poor at cost.[9] The professional social workers at the NYAICP were dubious about cooperatives; the NYAICP ran nonprofit "people's stores" selling food inexpensively by eliminating the retailer's profit. But the stores could not provide the credit and other services of the small immigrant grocery store. Nor could they compete with the prices of the proliferating "chain stores." They closed in 1918.[10]

Naturally, there were some who thought the New Nutrition would help solve the problem. Municipal authorities and private agencies in a number of cities distributed copies of Atwater's tables of food values in the slums and recommended milk as a substitute for eggs and meat.[11] Chicago's municipal institutions managed to replace the potatoes on their menus with rice, but the new York City Health Department's campaign to persuade workers to substitute rice for potatoes brought denunciations of the "rice diet" from women in Brownsville and protests that they were trying to foist "food for Chinamen" on the American workingman.[12] The crises also prompted a revival of the idea of public kitchens for the poor. During the depression of 1914–15 a number of wealthy New York City women, led by Mrs. James Burden and Mrs. William K. Vanderbilt, offered to help the NYAICP set up public kitchens. Burden and Vanderbilt were particularly enthusiastic about the project because the customer was "not the recipient of charity." The kitchen's aim was to "enhance the value of the workingman's dollar" by providing him with wholesome food at minimum cost.[13] Bailey Burritt, the NYAICP director (impressed that Burden and Vanderbilt seemed "to be in touch with an enthusiastic and loose pursed group") encouraged them to set one up on the city's Lower West Side, where unemployment among sailors and longshoremen was particularly high.[14]

Although it originated as a relief measure, the project soon took on many of the trappings of the NEK. The kitchen disseminated knowledge "regarding sanitary, dietary, economic, and culinary food values." Professor Henry C. Sherman and Dr. Graham Lusk, a prominent nutrition researcher, were brought in to help with "the development of the kitchen as an educational factor as well as a food distribution center."[15] The menus were emblazoned with the slogan "A penny saved is a penny earned," and the walls were plastered with placards listing calorific values and other themes of the New Nutrition. Winifred Gibbs herself was lured down from Teachers College to give lessons on how people of "moderate means" could cook "model meals."[16]

The founders avoided some of the ethnic problems faced by the NEK by selecting a neighborhood of Irish and northern Europeans who would feel quite at home with the kitchen's menu of mutton broth, roast lamb, corned beef and cabbage, pork and beans, hash and beans, and the like. However, after a spectacularly successful opening day in February 1915, business trailed off.[17] The first three years' losses were made up by Mrs. Burden and her committee, who raised money with the rather unwieldy but all-inclusive slogan "A Business Enterprise with a Social Purpose, to Sell at Cost Good Hot Food for Consumption in Homes Where It Is Impracticable to Prepare Meals and to Inculcate Wholesome Food Habits."[18]

As the slogan indicated, the kitchen, like the NEK, was mainly intended to serve food to be taken home. Indeed, like Ellen Richards, the ladies were sensitive to the threat eating out seemed to pose to the family. Criticisms from the head of the New York State Federation of Labor who warned that "instituting a movement of this kind would have quite a tendency towards effecting neglect in many of the households" did nothing to alleviate this concern.[19] However, it was the kitchen's sit-down restaurant which garnered the most patronage, and the take-home service had to be discontinued.

Although it broke even in 1918, the kitchen failed to spawn, as its founders had hoped, a network of similar establishments. Nor was it effective in changing the eating habits of neighborhood residents. Instead, except perhaps for the strange slogans on the wall and more care for cleanliness, there was little to distinguish it from other working-class eateries. In 1919 and 1920 its financial footing was weakened by the opening of a money-losing coffee shop in an ex-saloon, and in 1921 it quietly folded.[20]

Clearly, most deliberate attempts to change working-class eating habits failed miserably. Cooperatives, peoples' stores, exhortations to eat rice, and public kitchens had no real impact. Indeed, of all the measures which emerged from the food crises of 1907–17 only one was at all successful: school lunch programs. Their development was intimately linked with one of the more fascinating phenomena of the period, what might be called the Great Malnutrition Scare of 1907–21.

The first phase of the scare was anchored in the cost of living studies precipitated by the food crises. Because they used Atwater's over-estimates of nutritional requirements, they almost invariably produced alarming statistics on malnutrition. Previously, the inflated protein and calorie requirements had tended to generate pessimistic conclusions regarding the diets of the poor, but any generalizations were limited by the small number of case studies undertaken. The exact amounts of each nutrient individuals or families ingested had to be calculated, which meant keeping detailed records of all food purchased, eaten, and discarded. Few of the families most in need could master this kind of nutritional bookkeeping.

Then, in 1907, a different approach emerged. Robert Chapin, a New York City reformer writing an exposé of the poor living conditions of the city's workers, asked Frank Underhill, a chemist, to estimate how much money a hypothetical workingman's family of five would have to spend to provide themselves with a nutritionally adequate diet. Although he was an assistant professor in Chittenden's laboratory, Underhill used not Chittenden's emerging standards but a composite of the older and higher standards of Atwater and others.[21] He then calculated that a minimum nutritionally adequate diet would require the expenditure of at least twenty-two cents per adult male per day.[22]

Underhill's estimate provided useful ammunition for those who argued that the standard of living of American workers was terribly low. Chapin labeled an alarming proportion of the New York City families he studied "under-fed," including 22 percent of those whose family incomes were the equivalent of $800 to $900 for a family of five, a sum heretofore considered more than adequate by most experts.[23] In 1911, Frank Streightoff used Underhill's calculations to conclude that "at least one-third of all industrial families in the United States are underfed."[24] The author of the 1911 study of steelworkers in Homestead used Underhill's standard and concluded that even the best-off English-speaking workers were only slightly above the underfed level; most of the rest were below it. Although clearly puzzled by their healthy appearance and the apparent adequacy of the food on most tables, she did not question the standard.[25]

Although no one seemed to quarrel with its reliance on Atwater's standards,[26] there were other shortcomings to the Underhill approach. The fact that people spent more than a certain amount on food did not mean that they spent it properly. Nor did it mean that the nourishing food was shared equally within the family. While global estimates were useful to those such as Chapin who argued for higher wages, they were of little use to those who wished to identify and cure the individual cases of malnutrition.[27] Thus, by 1912, other methods for determining who was "under-fed" were coming into fashion. First, the word "under-fed" began to give way to the terms "under-nourished" and "malnourished," which reflected the New Nutritionist belief that it was the quality of food, rather than the quantity, that counted. Also, in line with growing concern over the welfare of children and the future of the race, the search for malnutrition came to focus very much on the young.

Then, the great anthropometric craze of the time held out tantalizing possibilities for new methods for diagnosing malnutrition. Physicians, psychologists, anthropologists, and criminologists seemed to be making remarkable advances by avidly measuring all parts of the human body, finding in the cephalic indices of the shape of the cranium the key to the superiority of the Nordic race, discovering in characteristics of the brow ridge and the distance between eyes tell-tale signs of criminality, and so on. It seemed inevitable that some would search for signs of malnutrition in the measurements of the body. Thousands of children were now measured and weighed, averages calculated, and charts compiled listing what was thought to be the normal height and weight of well-nourished children at each age. But the charts were based almost entirely on native-born children, with a disproportionate number from upper-middle-class private schools, and there was no way to distinguish between the roles of nutrition and heredity in determining stature.[28] This was of particular importance for immigrants' children, for many were from parts of Europe where a combination of the two had historically produced people of short stature.[29] Not surprisingly, in the mid-1910s experts applying height/weight/age ratios to New York City's one million schoolchildren, a high proportion of whom were immigrants, estimated that 225,000 were undernourished.[30] (One can imagine the dismay with which thousands of doting Jewish and Italian mothers who hovered over their children at dinnertime refilling their plates received the news that school authorities had declared their little boys malnourished.[31])

Some social workers and public health officials were troubled by the high proportion of Italians and Jews labeled malnourished and wrestled in vain with the statistics, trying to figure out how much could be ascribed to heredity.[32] Some experts pointed out that children matured at different paces, and eliminated age from the calculation, using only the ratio of height to weight in determining who was malnourished. While this did tend to produce lower estimates than those that included age,[33] it also had a tendency to produce results that seemed to run counter to common sense, including an alarming tendency to show tall, thin, middle-class native-born children as the most malnourished group.[34] A survey of students at two private prep schools indicated that 10 to 20 percent were underweight for their height, twice the proportion found in a school in New York City's impoverished Lower East Side![35]

The problem was that height/weight ratios are of use only in determining severe cases of malnutrition. They are used today by public health relief agencies, but mainly in parts of the world suffering from severe famines. Stature is a good indicator of nutritional status, but only when used to measure changes over time among large numbers of people. It is useless as the only tool for diagnosing individual cases of malnutrition. An alternative was to regard certain physical defects and ailments as signs of malnutrition. By 1910, the most commonly cited tell-tale signs were poor teeth, swollen adenoids, and hypertrophied tonsils.[36] Rickets was also widely regarded as connected with low standards of living, but there was considerable disagreement over whether and how it was related to poor nutrition. The same was true for poor eyesight.

The confusion that reigned over the diagnosis of malnutrition might not have been of great consequence had it not been a time in which systems of medical inspection of students were being inaugurated and expanded in the public school systems of the nation. One of the major roles of the medical inspectors was to identify cases of malnutrition so that they could be dealt with by the expanding network of social agencies concerned with nutrition. With no universally accepted standards and hundreds of children to examine each day, the doctors and nurses naturally tended to use subjective assessments based primarily on physical appearance to identify the malnourished. This made them susceptible to pressure to find the many cases of malnutrition described by such experts as Chapin and Streightoff.

New York City furnished a good example of what could happen under these circumstances. There, the zealous new head of the city's department of health, Dr. Josephine Baker, was convinced, perhaps by studies such as

Chapin's, that malnutrition was "the most serious and widespread physical defect found among school children." Several times in 1912, she accused her department's school medical inspectors of overlooking many cases of malnutrition. While the occasional case of malnutrition stood out clearly in the better-off schools, she argued, "in sections where children come from crowded tenement homes we sometimes find that nearly all of the children are below par physically, and after we have worked with them for some time it seems as though they are a common type rather than a physical disability." Heeding this advice, they dutifully discovered more malnutrition cases that year than ever before.[37] The number of cases diagnosed increased again in each of the next two years but still remained far below experts' estimates of how many there should be. Calculations using Chapin's figures led to estimates that about 25 percent of the city's students were malnourished, while those employing Streightoff's figures concluded that this category should comprise about half the student population.[38] Despite Baker's urging, in the 1914–15 school year her department's inspectors managed to diagnose only 4 percent of the city's school children as "undernourished," a figure which crept up to 5 percent the next year.[39]

In 1915, however, a new method of diagnosing malnutrition emerged, elevating the number of malnutrition cases diagnosed to alarming proportions. Developed by an expert at the Carnegie Institution in Dumferline, Scotland (Andrew Carnegie's birthplace), it used height, weight, eyesight, breathing, muscularity, mental alertness, and rosiness of complexion as the key indicators of nutritional status. Taking all of these into account, examiners would classify children's nutrition in four categories: 1) excellent, 2) adequate, 3) needs attention and supervision, and 4) requires immediate hospitalization. While all of this may have looked good on paper, and may have made sense to the rosy-cheeked British, the problems in applying these criteria to immigrant children in America should have been apparent from the outset. Not only were they subjective or irrelevant, they were also ethnocentrically biased. Again, Italian, Jewish, and other Mediterranean children emerged as undernourished because they tended to be shorter and less rosy in complexion.[40] Jews also had a greater than average propensity to be near-sighted,[41] and those forced to attend Hebrew school at the end of each school day did not have the same opportunities to develop muscularity as children who played on the streets after school.[42]

The greatest problem with the Dumferline Scale, however, was that the lines between the four categories were extremely vague. Since the first category was labeled "excellent," it could be implied that there was something inadequate about the nutrition of those in the second category, even though it was labeled "nutritionally adequate." Moreover, because there was no clear distinction between the second category and the third one, "needs attention," there was a natural tendency to play it safe and slot children into the third category. They could then be merged with the small number in the fourth category ("requires immediate hospitalization") as the "undernourished" or "malnourished" to produce alarming statistics.

Despite its manifest inadequacies, the Dumferline Scale was adopted by New York City's Health Department in December 1915, and a number of other major cities followed suit. The results were predictable: a growing number of reports from public health authorities that malnutrition was rife and rising. In the first year after the adoption of the scale in New York City, the number of "undernourished" (now those in the two lowest Dumferline categories) more than doubled from the previous year, to 110,000, or over 10 percent of the public school population.[43] As a result, nutrition clinics were set up by public and private agencies in New York City, Boston, and Philadelphia. Public schools offered "nutrition classes," where the undernourished were segregated and encouraged to compete with each other in weight gain, using a method pioneered by Dr. William Emerson, a Boston physician. But nutrition clinics handling patients on a one-to-one basis were expensive to operate, and while Emerson claimed to have met with great success in Boston, the nutrition class method failed rather miserably in its first year in New York City.[44] Many of those concerned about child welfare now came to regard school lunch programs as their best hope for combating this growing scourge.

The first major program had started in some Boston high schools in 1894, in large part due to Ellen Richards and Edward Atkinson. The New England Kitchen ran the program as a "private enterpise" that paid for itself many times over.[45] Although the lunches never became the effective instruments for teaching the New Nutrition the founders had envisaged, by the early twentieth century they were praised for providing nutritionally sound meals at low prices to children who would not normally have them, and this became the main justification for similar lunch programs in other cities.[46] By 1912, over forty cities had lunch programs in their elementary schools.[47]

The growing concern over malnutrition among children spurred on these endeavors. In early 1913 Elizabeth Milbank Anderson, the Progressive daughter of a wealthy corporation lawyer, became so alarmed about malnutrition among schoolchildren that she endowed the NYAICP with a large trust fund, a large part of which was to be used to expand the city's school lunch program. Fourteen schools were to be chosen "from those most sorely in need of proper nourishment," and the NYAICP was to serve 600,000 meals a year for only one penny a meal.[48]

But private agencies could not afford to subsidize the programs on the scale thought necessary, particularly in the face of rising food prices. Even the well-endowed NYAICP program had to charge a penny a portion rather than a penny a meal.[49] Various reformers took up the call for municipal support for school lunch programs. In April 1913, after watching school lunches being served to students in a Manhattan elementary school, ex-President Theodore Roosevelt gave the idea his benediction.[50] Social service agencies in a number of cities also began pressing for municipal subsidies for lunch programs.[51] Home economists rallied to the cause, a course of action they had long favored. In a 1913 article in the *Journal of Home Ecomomics,* C. F. Langworthy wrote that school lunch programs provided excellent laboratories for teaching the ideas of the New Nutrition, particularly to boys who were untouched by home economics classes.[52]

In New York City, the board of education would finance only some of the necessary equipment for the program, which after two years served but 35 of the city's 500 schools.[53] That is, until Josephine Baker weighed into the battle with new and ever-more-shocking statistics. In December 1917, calling for the expansion of the lunch program to include all city schools, she warned that "the buying power of the dollar has not kept pace with the cost of food and for the last eighteen months the children of the city have been underfed. . . . Are we going to wait until we see the tuberculosis statistics going up before before we do anything?"[54] Despite her alarmist warnings, the tuberculosis statistics did not rise. But using the Dumferline Scale, Baker's estimates for malnutrition certainly did. At hearings on the bill to have the city take over financing of school lunches, she deftly merged those children in Dumferline categories three and four into cases of "severe malnutrition" and declared that there were 225,000 schoolchildren in this category. She also labelled the 611,000 children in category two as "below normal standard."[55]

While social workers in the NYAICP, which ran much of the school lunch program, were encouraged by Baker's support, they became concerned that her escalating estimates of the extent of the problem would undermine their credibility.[56] Bailey Burritt, the director, wrote Baker questioning her assertion that over 600,000 children were "below normal standard" when it seemed clear that those in category two (adequate nutrition) were considered "above the normal line." "I am a bit afraid that the case of defective nutrition which we are all so vitally interested in is a bit in danger of suffering from overstatement," he wrote. "If, for example, we point out that only 17 percent of New York City children are normal then we give a new meaning to the word normal."[57]

Opponents of school lunches on the board of education did not find Baker's statistics particularly compelling. Pointing out that a large majority of principals and district superintendents saw little if any need for school lunch programs and that five had already been closed for lack of patronage, a board subcommittee reported that "inspired sensational reports of great need for a luncheon service are not substantiated by facts submitted to the district superintendents. Almost the sole urging for the establishment of such a system comes from outside the schools, largely from people interested in having the City relieve private agencies from doing the work they have been doing for some years."[58] But Baker was not to be deterred. Late in 1919 she announced that preliminary figures indicated that there were 300,000 undernourished children in the city. Burritt remarked wryly to a colleague that "obviously we are not dealing with stable standards." The inspections, he said, in which one inspector would examine 500 children in a morning, were so cursory as to encourage doubt about any conclusions drawn from them. He attributed the rising number to "increased community thinking about nutritional problems" which led inspectors to search for evidence of nutritional deficiencies.[59]

Nevertheless, some weeks later Baker announced that firm figures now indicated that 30 percent of the city's schoolchildren were undernourished and she estimated that the figure rose from forty to fifty percent in some working-class schools. An incredulous NYAICP researcher thereupon wrote Burritt that it was "hardly credible that in four years the percentage of children suffering from defective nutrition could have risen from 4 to 30 per cent without this condition being reflected in the death and morbidity rates of children of school age. It is perfectly clear that the increasing number of undernourished children in the schools is due rather to the changing standards of the Health Department than to an actual increase in the number of cases."[60]

Still, Baker and her statistics prevailed, and the city government was finally persuaded to assume complete responsibility for school lunches, and other municipalities did the same.[61] The New York City program remained restricted to schools in poor neighborhoods. Because the conviction that ignorance of nutrition was as much a scourge as poverty remained strong, domestic science teachers were put in charge of food preparation, and meals were accompanied by pamphlets and lectures on nutrition.[62] However, in 1923 the educational effort was abandoned in the face of economies to be gained through centralized food preparation and, it would seem, because of student indifference. Indeed, none of the experiments using lunch programs to teach nutrition proved effective.[63]

However, if school lunches failed to educate the working class in the ideas of the New Nutrition, they were much more successful in another direction: "Americanizing" the immigrant diet, for no concessions to non-American tastes were made.[64] Whether or not they developed a taste for chicken croquettes, salmon loafs, and scalloped dishes, which were the staples of school lunch programs,[65] thousands of immigrant children were exposed to foods vastly different from what they ate at home. Leonard Covello remembered growing up as an Italian immigrant boy in east Harlem, where he and his friends—accustomed to the substantial crusty bread of southern Italy—regarded the white bread served in their school lunch program as better fit for spitballs than for eating.[66] Nevertheless, when the authorities served the bread of the dominant culture, the message that they were the odd ones out was clear.

In other, more ethnically variegated schools, it was not so easy to resist. Another Italian immigrant, John Fante, recalled:

> At the lunch hour I huddle over my lunch pail, for my mother doesn't wrap my sandwiches in wax paper, and she makes them too large, and the lettuce leaves protrude. Worse, the bread is homemade; not bakery bread, not "American" bread. I make a great fuss because I can't have mayonnaise and other "American" things.[67]

Italians were more resistant to the pressures to Americanize their eating habits than were other immigrant groups. Yet the pressures which school lunches put on immigrant children were immense. Like Fante, the children may have remained chained to their mothers' cuisine, but they were learning an important lesson: it was the food in their homes, not on the steam tables, which was out of the main stream, and that to enter that stream they would ultimately have to learn to appreciate its food.

The growing awareness of the basics of the New Nutrition—that the quality of food was as important as the quantity—lent credibility to assertions that malnutrition was rife among the better-off.[68] The most prominent purveyor of the idea of middle-class malnutrition was Dr. William R. P. Emerson, whose competitive nutrition classes failed among the poor of New York in 1918–19.[69] Emerson's diagnosis of malnutrition relied on height/weight charts. For each 7 percent below the average weight for his height on the scale a child was deemed one year "retarded" in growth. Even 3 or 4 percent below the requisite weight was regarded as dangerous, for the child who was that far below at age seven would likely be 10 percent "below weight" at twelve and "grow to maturity with reduced vitality."[70] The other important indicators were defects which might interfere with breathing, namely inflamed tonsils and adenoids.[71]

Claiming that height/weight statistics showed 150,000 New York City school children were "stunted in their growth, retarded one to three years both in height and weight," Emerson tried to shake the middle class out of their belief that malnutrition was associated with poverty. "If poverty is the fundamental cause of malnutrition," he wrote in the *New Republic* in 1918, "how are we to account for the fact that malnutrition occurs as much among the well-to-do as among the poor?"[72] The solution, said Emerson, lay in "measured feeding," taught in nutrition classes using his method. This meant competition stimulated by measuring the amount of food the child ate and entering the child's weight on graphs against the weights of "normal" children. Children were encouraged to eat more by emphasizing that the girls would be considered beautiful and the boys athletic only if they attained "normal" weight.[73] He also recommended excising "diseased" tonsils and adenoids, "a frequent cause of malnutrition. . . . The removal of such obstructions usually means an immediate gain of several pounds, followed by a steady rise to normal [weight]." Rest was very important, and he ordered the underweight to limit attendance at school to half-days and abjure "all outside activities, especially music."[74]

After writing a series of articles on the problem for the *Women's Home Companion*" in 1919, Emerson formed a private corporation, Nutrition Clinics for Delicate Children, Inc., which ran over forty nutrition clinics from Maine to Hawaii.[75] However, his empire was short-lived. His competitive eating method found little favor among professional dietitians in the 1920s,[76] and his requirement that children spend half-days at home could not have sat well with parents or school authorities.

Still, the idea that malnutrition could afflict the well-off as much as the poor became part of nutritionists' credo. While she acknowledged that poverty was likely the single most important cause of malnutrition, Lydia Roberts, the decade's leading expert in malnutrition among children, pointed out that it was by no means the sole cause, and in the 1927 edition of her standard textbook warned that malnutrition was common among the well-off.[77] Most important, the vague rumblings of Emerson's idea that malnutrition could afflict the better-off as well as the poor helped make the middle classes receptive to the message of nutritionists more sophisticated than Emerson, who would be talking in terms of deficiencies of vitamins and other mysterious elements.

"Best for Babies" or "Preventable Infanticide"?: The Controversy Over Artificial Feeding of Infants, 1880–1930

The malnutrition scare concentrated on children, but it paralleled another great concern of the prewar era, mortality rates among infants. To many experts, extraordinarily high death rates of infants under age one seemed linked to perhaps the most revolutionary change in diet made possible by the ideas of New Nutrition, the rise of proprietary, brand-named artificial foods for infants.

Artificial feeding of babies—that is, feeding infants food other than human milk—is by no means a recent development in Western or any other culture. Wooden feeding bottles have been discovered in archaeological sites in the Nile Delta; references to artificial feeding appear in the Old Testament; and artificial feeding seems to have been quite common in ancient Rome. But a more widespread practice of mothers who either could not or did not wish to nurse their infants has been wet-nursing. The practice of employing lactating women to nurse one's children has risen and fallen in popularity through the ages and has generally been the preferred alternative of the wealthier classes. Those whose infants were not nursed made do with animals' milk, honey, butter, mashed bread, farina, chopped meat, or other substitutes.

In the nineteenth century, thanks in part to the Romantic spirit, there was a growing belief in feeding infants exclusively the food that Nature seemed to have intended for them: milk. By mid-century and after, mothers were being discouraged from feeding their children anything but milk

121

until teething signaled that they were ready for solid foods. But what kind of milk was best? Wet-nursing was declining, in part because of the disruptive effect of wet nurses (who often thought themselves more privileged than other servants) "downstairs" in large households, in part because of old fears that wet nurses transmitted moral as well as physical characteristics in their milk—fears reinforced by new "proof" that venereal diseases were also transmitted in human milk. The greatest drawback in America was the servant shortage, which meant that by the 1880s and 1890s only the wealthiest could afford to have a servant who did little else but feed a baby. Yet, not only were there increasing numbers of middle-class women, many of whom now had social, religious, and other interests outside the home to interfere with their nursing at the generally recommended two- or three-hour intervals, but there were also more married working-class women in the labor force, especially toward the end of the century, making it necessary for many of them to wean their children soon after birth in order to return to work. The stage was therefore set for vendors of various substitutes for human milk to step in.[1]

The most common substitute, of course, was cow's milk, but it presented problems. First, long before the germ theory of disease demonstrated the bacteria-coddling properties of cow's milk, it was widely regarded as a baby-killer. Europeans in the first half of the nineteenth century had taken to boiling it, but this seemed to do little to reduce the appalling infant-mortality rates associated with it. Americans rarely even boiled it. Some mid-century experts recommended suckling infants directly at the udder of a cow (it should be "known for her gentle disposition," warned one) or a goat, but this was clearly impractical, especially for city dwellers.[2] Second, as modern chemistry soon demonstrated, the composition of cow's milk was quite different from that of human milk. It was difficult for many babies to digest and produced hard, undigested curds in their stools. Thus, in the second half of the century various systems for altering cow's milk to make its chemical composition more like human milk found favor among scientists and doctors. Many of these involved the dilution of cow's milk with water and the addition of sugar or some other sweetener, but by the 1860s a growing number of doctors, scientists, and entrepreneurs realized that a new market was opening up for proprietary, brand-named infant foods.

Perhaps not surprisingly, a major step in capitalizing on the new advances in chemistry by marketing proprietary infant foods came from the scientist who laid the foundations of the New Nutrition, Baron Justus von Liebig. If indeed foods were constituted of protein, carbohydrates, and fats, could these nutrients not be combined into a replica of mother's milk? Thus, in 1867 the Baron introduced Liebig's Soluble Food for Babies in the European market. By the next year it was being manufactured and sold in London by the Liebig's Registered Concentrated Milk

Company and within a year after that it had migrated to the United States.[3]

Liebig did not challenge the prevalent notion that mother's milk was the perfect infant food. Rather, he claimed that he had succeeded in concocting a substance, at first liquid, then powdered, whose chemical make-up was virtually identical to that of mother's milk. Liebig's Food was soon followed by a host of imitators. Some contained dried milk and called only for the addition of water. Others, like Liebig's original formula, were to be added to diluted milk. Soon some doctors were proclaiming these foods to be superior to the milk of wet nurses. By the 1890s the most popular by far of the powders to be added to milk was Mellin's Food, developed in England and manufactured in Boston, whose advertisements claimed that it was "the genuine Liebig's Food." The best known of the dried-milk products was another European import, Nestlé's Milk Food, which was manufactured and distributed under license by a New York City firm.[4]

Advertisements for the various proprietary infant foods became well-nigh ubiquitous by the 1890s. The Mellin's babies, uniformly chubby, became as well known as the Gerber babies of later years. Testimonials accompanied the pictures, usually thanking Mellin's for saving apparently doomed babies' lives. "Ten days ago my little one, only two months old, was a mere skeleton," said one. "I tried every other kind until my boy was nothing but skin and bones," said another. Needless to say, both mothers reported that within days of switching to Mellin's their babies were flourishing. Most of the competitors' advertisements were variations on Mellin's theme. "After trying almost every Food on the market, without success, for our little girl, I resorted to Eskay's Food," read a letter typical of those cited by the Smith, Kline, & French Company in support of their powder. "Immediately our baby began to thrive." Nestlé's ("Best for Babies") said it was better for babies than milk, for "impure milk in hot weather is one of the chief causes of sickness among babies. Nestlé's Milk Food is the safest of all foods, as it requires in preparation the addition of water only." The American manufacturers of Ridge's Food, an English import, acknowledged that breast feeding was best of all. Alas, they said in 1882:

> The mammary glands have suffered . . . outrages at the hands of the corset-maker, the dressmaker, and the manufacturer of bosom pads, so that what is left of our mothers is in the majority of cases only an apology for the ideal which nature designed . . . In all classes and conditions of modern life, the mother's milk is most frequently neither in quantity nor quality adequate to the nourishment of the child, . . . BUT THE BANE HAS AN ANTIDOTE.[5]

A favorite promotional technique was to offer free samples by mail to the readers of middle-class magazines. Perhaps most effective with middle-class mothers, though, were the free handbooks on infant care and feeding distributed by the companies. Mellin's, with its own press, was especially active in this field. The handbooks explained the chemistry of milk and feeding in clear but relatively sophisticated language, adding an aura of science to the food they were promoting. Not only did they prove effective in convincing mothers of the efficacy of proprietary infant foods, they convinced many doctors as well.[6]

The major alternative to the powders among the processed, brand-named foods was condensed milk. In the 1870s and 1880s, many physicians recommended it for infant feeding, usually diluted at twelve-parts water to one part condensed milk, and most brands carried directions for dilution on their labels. Because it required no cool storage, was already sweetened, and (especially when overdiluted) could cost much less than fresh milk, it was often the preferred food of the few members of the lower classes who used proprietary foods in infant feeding.[7] Artificial feeding was also encouraged by the promotion of nursing bottles and nipples, whose technology was recently improved. These new devices were touted as the most modern and scientific available, making "hand feeding" much easier than in the past and preventing colic as well.[8]

Thus, by the 1890s a number of sources spread the growing impression that artificial feeding was both scientific and modern. The proprietary foods claimed to be based on the formula of one of the century's greatest scientists, or at least to have been "prepared with scientific skill in every detail." Borden's and the other condensed-milk manufacturers emphasized the modern, sanitary nature of their processing, and the nursing bottle and nipple advertisements projected an image of technological perfection. By the later 1880s and early 1890s, though, a growing number of pediatricians were looking askance at both proprietary foods and condensed milk, pointing to evidence that babies raised on them had higher mortality rates than babies who were breast-fed. Those who continued to recommend condensed milk were forced to admit that devastating results sometimes accompanied its use, but they blamed the problem on overdilution, especially among the poor, which resulted in slow starvation of the infant. In the late 1890s both proprietary foods and condensed milk were attacked (wrongly) by prominent pediatricians as prime causes of infantile scurvy and rickets. The well-known New York City professor of pediatrics, L. Emmett Holt, whose pediatrics text would soon become the Bible of twentieth-century pediatricians, warned in 1897 that even though "the feeble resistance of condensed milk babies to acute disease has long been noted by many observers," condensed milk was still widely used and recommended by many physicians. Yet during the past five or six years, he said, he had "yet to see an infant reared solely on canned condensed milk who did not exhibit the signs of rickets to a greater or lesser degree."[9]

In 1898 an American Pediatric Society investigation of what was purported to be an epidemic of infantile scurvy concluded that scurvy was most prevalent among children fed on proprietary foods and condensed milk and somewhat less common among those fed on boiled and pasteurized milk. "The farther a food is removed in character from the natural food of a child the more likely its use is to be followed by the development of scurvy," it reported. A prominent Detroit pediatrician charged that not only were proprietary foods and condensed milk the prime causes of scurvy and rickets, they also predisposed infants to infectious diseases and led them to "suffer from constipation, and its various intoxications all through infancy and childhood." In 1911 the evidence against condensed milk accumulated by Holt and others inspired the journal *Pediatrics* to condemn its use in infant feeding, citing the "sinister coincidence" between its employment and epidemics of infantile diarrhea as well as the likelihood that it brought on rickets. While acknowledging that there was "some deficiency in even the most carefully devised artificial foods for infants" and that the best infant food was mother's milk, *Pediatrics* said that because "breast feeding seems to be falling more and more into disfavor [the] most efficient substitute must be sought." No kind of condensed milk fit that bill, it concluded, and skimmed condensed milk was "distinctly injurious."[10]

Most of the pediatricians' charges were unfounded, but this is not surprising, in view of the nutritional notions of the day. More interesting is the great extent to which their attacks on proprietary foods were linked to criticism of general practitioners for recommending such foods. "The average practitioner does not care to give much time and study to infant feeding and readily accepts and prescribes formulas that the proprietary food manufacturers print on the label for him," wrote one pediatrician, reflecting a feeling common in his specialty in 1905. "In spite of the efforts of eminent pediatricians to decry them, the proprietary infant foods have been the mainstay of the general practitioners" said an important text on infant feeding in 1912.[11]

Although undoubtedly the result of genuine concern over the mishandling of the acute problem of infant feeding, the pediatricians' criticisms also contained an element of self-interest. For many years they struggled to achieve recognition as a respected specialty within the medical profession, battling those who argued that there were no such things as diseases specific to infants and children; that the so-called diseases of infancy and childhood, whose treatment pediatricians tried to monopolize, were merely adult diseases writ small and could be handled by general practitioners or the appropriate specialists. Infant feeding was recognized as involving peculiar problems, but the relatively simple rules of most systems could be easily mastered by general practitioners and even nurses and laymen. Now, however, came an exceedingly complex system of artificial feeding that pediatricians could uniquely call their own. This became a new and important weapon in their struggle to elevate the status of their specialty.

Formula, or percentage, feeding was perhaps the *reductio ad absurdum* of Liebig's notion of reproducing an exact duplicate of mother's milk. It likely owed much to the assertions of the German pediatrician P. H. Biedert that the differences between cow's milk and human milk, especially in the amount of casein, could be overcome by diluting cream with water until its percentage of protein was the same as that of mother's milk and then adding sugar to bring up the level of carbohydrates. The proportion of fat in mother's milk could be replicated by starting with cream containing whatever percentage of fat was necessary to yield the desired result after dilution.[12] In the United States, Thomas Morgan Rotch, a Boston pediatrician who had studied in Germany and taught at Harvard Medical School, took this a major step further and created a system whereby the percentages of each element could be varied to suit the needs of individual infants. He thereby elevated the process of concocting formulae to levels of pseudoscientific complexity of which even the Germans had not conceived.

According to Rotch, percentage feeding developed in the late 1880s out of his concern over the wide variety of foodstuffs—especially cereals—being used for infant feeding. Most galling to him was the widespread notion that infant feeding could be left in the hands of non-specialists, and particularly that mothers and nurses knew as well as anyone what infants should be fed. "The mothers and nurses . . . dominated the physicians," he later recalled with disgust, "and the physicians . . . took refuge with . . . the commercial venders of patent and proprietary foods innumerable." He had long felt, he said in 1892, that the endeavor should be made "to rescue this important branch of pediatrics from the pretentions of proprietary foods and the hands of ignorant nurses."[13]

At first Rotch followed the Europeans and prescribed formulae based on what was thought of as prototypical mother's milk: 3 percent fat, 6 percent sugar, and 1 percent protein. However, when his research indicated that all mother's milk was not chemically identical and that infants' digestive systems also varied, he began to alter the proportions of the various elements in search of combinations that would best suit particular infants. This was the crux of the difference between his system and those of Liebig, Biedert, and others who were content to prescribe one basic mixture for all infants, varying the contents only with an infant's age.[14]

When, in 1889, disturbing reports began to reach Rotch that his method had not been notably successful in reducing infant mortality or morbidity, he decided that the problem lay in mixing the exact formulae at home. In 1891 he managed to persuade George H. Walker, a well-to-do Boston lithographer, to fund a special laboratory to turn out formulae in sanitary scientific surroundings, responding only to the requisitions of those armed with a physician's prescription. The Walker-Gordon laboratories, as they were called, proved to be a major breakthrough for the system. The white-coated laboratory technicians with their test tubes and instruments added an attractive aura of science and efficiency to the process.[15]

Rotch's system was reinforced by a plethora of theories regarding exactly what made cow's milk indigestible and dangerous to infants. Some blamed it on the fats; others on the carbohydrates. Later some blamed sucrose, while others disagreed and pointed at lactose (milk sugar). Still others focused on inorganic salts. Formula feeding and the Walker-Gordon laboratories gave pediatricians the chance to follow any of these theories simply by filling out prescriptions for formulae. As he became more committed to the laboratory and formula system, Rotch became less committed to any one particular theory of infant feeding and recommended formula feeding even to the recalcitrants who still believed that infants could digest starch. The important thing, he said, was knowing exactly how much of the various elements were being given to babies, "so that the treatment should not be simply empirical, but should be exact." Indeed, his original attack on proprietary foods had been based, he said, not so much on their composition but on the "irregularities and changes, slight perhaps in the eyes of the makers," that might "creep in" as their makers opted for "cheaper production," making the foods more different from human milk than they had originally been.[16]

So finely tuned were the formulae supposed to be that they were to be changed only in slightest degree, usually by 0.05 percent per week. Moreover, although alterations often had to be made day by day, only one element at a time could be changed. The effect of the new system was to give pediatricians an arcane skill at a time when they were desperately searching for such things to set them apart from other physicians. By 1894 Holt was teaching percentage feeding to new pediatricians in New York City. A doctor who studied with him shortly after he was appointed Professor of Pediatrics at Columbia University in 1901 recalled that Holt "enveloped the subject with an esoteric aura. Indeed it appeared the very Eden of Pediatrics, where skill was most needed and the pediatricians reigned alone and supreme." By 1901 the craze had spread so far that there were Walker-Gordon laboratories in eighteen cities in the United States and Canada, and one had also opened in London. Doubters such as the aging dean of American pediatricians, Abraham Jacobi, who said rather cryptically, "You cannot feed babies with mathematics, you must feed them with brains," were viewed as old-fashioned, unable to see progress.[17]

Although Rotch, Holt, and most other pediatricians still affirmed that nothing was superior to mother's milk, they now directed much of their effort toward devising and promoting a method of infant feeding, labeled by Holt the "American or scientific method," that proved much more attractive than breast feeding to many mothers. Perhaps the final recognition of the system's lure came in 1908, when Mellin's Food began promoting a method of percentage feeding that appeared every bit as sophisticated as that of Rotch.[18]

The commitment of so many prominent pediatricians to one alternative to breast feeding could not help but endow artificial feeding as a whole with a modern, scientific, and American image. This was reflected in the medical training of general practitioners, who in most medical schools received very little encouragement to promote breast feeding. The modern image was also reflected in the much greater propensity of native-born mothers to employ artificial feeding than the foreign-born, regardless of class. Indications that artificial feeding of infants among the foreign-born increased with greater mastery of English by the infants' parents would seem to imply that greater exposure to American norms and advertising led immigrants of child-bearing age to regard artificial feeding as modern and American.[19]

We now know that percentage feeding was needlessly elaborate and expensive. The minute gradations in formulae contents were particularly unnecessary. The main advantage of the system was that the cleanliness of the ingredients and the surroundings in which they were produced tended to ensure that the formulae had lower bacteria levels than most concoctions fed to infants. Yet production costs put the formulae beyond the reach of all but upper-income groups. The necessity for doctors' supervision and prescriptions at a time when only those in the middle classes and above had regular access to medical advice in child rearing also helped restrict percentage feeding to upper-income groups. Percentage feeding was, therefore, primarily the plaything of Fifth Avenue and Beacon Hill physicians and their well-to-do clients. It is significant that when Holt conducted a study of various methods of artificial feeding used in the tenements of the Lower East Side of New York from 1901 to 1903, apparently none of the families surveyed reported using percentage feeding. Perhaps even more significant, Holt, one of the archpriests of the system, never suggested that it might be a suitable tool for bringing down the area's appalling infant-mortality rate.[20]

Artificial feeding expanded at a time when infant mortality was beginning to be perceived as one of the great social problems of the day. Philanthropists, social workers, physicians, and politicians in many countries began debating methods for reducing the horrifying death rates that new statistics on infant mortality revealed. "Preventable infanticide!" became a battle cry for reform. Although everything from hot weather to working mothers was blamed, the fact that the largest percentage of infant deaths were ascribed to intestinal disorders and diarrhea naturally led many people to search for solutions to the problem in the field of infant feeding and to heed the pediatricians' warnings of its importance. By 1905 a consensus seemed to be emerging, at least among public-health reformers, that much of the problem lay in the apparent increase in the popularity of artificial feeding, especially in cities. These reformers now joined pediatricians in attacking proprietary infant foods. Public-health officials combed their rudimentary statistics, proving time and again that breast-fed children survived infancy with much greater frequency than the bottle-fed.

As with the malnutrition scare, much of the onus for high infant mortality was thrust on the poor themselves. A prominent Philadelphia pediatrician accused slum dwellers of succumbing to the blandishments of the purveyors of proprietary foods and abandoning breast feeding "for mere convenience,"[21] but more commonly their ignorance was blamed. The thrust of the reformers was therefore in two major directions: first, to provide alternatives to proprietary foods and canned milk by making available fresh-milk-based formulae for those mothers who bottle-fed and, second, to educate the poor in infant hygiene, encouraging, where possible, breast feeding.

Aside from a general concentration on lowering the bacteria levels in milk, there was little that unified the reformers. One group was inspired by the discovery that bacteria were killed by high temperatures. By 1886 some doctors were suggesting scalding fresh milk to "destroy microbes" and diluting it only with boiled water. When the concept of sterilizing milk spread in the late 1880s, much of the medical profession heralded it as an advance of the greatest importance.[22] However, in the hands of late-nineteenth-century pediatricians the process was made so complex that it was not useful to the vast majority of the poor, whose children were the main sufferers from milk-borne diseases. As evidence mounted that simply boiling milk did little to reduce infant mortality and morbidity, advocates of sterilization insisted that everything that came into contact with the milk should be sterilized. They also recommended progressively longer periods of boiling. By 1898 one of the more prominent proponents of sterilization was advising that if the milk was to keep for any length of time, "a sterilization of three to six consecutive days at a high temperature for very many hours was necessary." As a result, real sterilization, as opposed to merely heating or boiling milk, was practiced mainly by the well-to-do. A further problem was that boiling cow's milk changed its taste without making it more digestible. Moreover, to boil milk seemed to make it even more chemically remote from mother's milk, thus contravening the cardinal belief that chemical identity was to be aimed at above all. By the late 1890s, then, sterilization had fallen into disfavor in America.[23]

One of the reasons for the decline of sterilization was the rise in hopes for a supply of clean raw milk. The new bacteriological methods were helping to identify dairy farmers who were successfully applying rules of sanitation to the production of raw milk, keeping it away from fecal and other matter in the barns and storing it in cool sanitary containers for transportation to the city. The prospect now opened for the identification of this clean milk, and its segregation from milk from other, less sanitary farms. The most prominent advocate of a system for certifying milk as pure was a New Jersey doctor, Henry L. Coit. His virtual obsession with the subject led to the establishment of the Medical Milk Commission in New Jersey and the delivery of the first bottle of officially certified milk in 1894. Milk reformers in many cities took up the cry for certification, either through voluntary means, such as those Coit was busily organizing, or through government regulation and legislation, which Coit opposed. By 1906, when the movement approached its zenith, thirty-six milk commissions in the United States were supervising and taking bacterial counts of the production of hundreds of dairymen. Yet they had little impact in reducing infant mortality, for certification was an expensive process, and only upper-income groups could afford it. At its peak in 1910, only between 0.5 and 1 percent of the milk sold in major American cities was certified.[24]

By that time certified milk was rapidly being overtaken by Coit's dreaded rival, pasteurized milk. Pasteurization generally referred to any method of heating milk to a temperature below its boiling point but high enough to kill many of its bacteria and then cooling it rapidly. In the 1890s, while pasteurization could only be done on a small scale, it was thought that the small milk peddlers of the large cities commonly used the technique to camouflage stale milk and prevent it from going rancid. Advocates of pasteurization of milk for infants therefore had to overcome suspicions about the process, especially among pediatricians. In 1892, however, New York philanthropist Nathan Straus began subsidizing summertime milk stations in the slums of New York City to distribute bottled pasteurized milk to mothers of infants, as well as to teach a method of home pasteurization using a contraption he had invented. Straus and his supporters argued that pasteurization was preferable to boiling or sterilization because, while the milk was heated to a level "sufficient to kill all noxious germs . . . the nourishing quality and good taste of milk are retained."[25]

Growing concern over infant mortality inspired reformers such as the Women's Municipal Leagues and settlement houses to set up milk stations in major industrial cities and to press for regulation of the milk industry. In New York City the New York Association for Improving the Condition of the Poor spawned the New York Milk Committee, which opened eight milk stations in the summer of 1908 and was running thirty-one by the summer of 1911. By 1912 milk stations existed in at least thirty of the American cities with more than fifty thousand inhabitants. In line with the philanthropic ideas of the time, milk was distributed free only to the very needy. The rest paid the prevailing rate for ordinary milk.[26]

Most milk-station milk was not pasteurized, because until about 1914 large-scale pasteurization was not possible. Neither was home pasteurization a solution for the poor. Although some settlement houses did try to teach the poor to "modify" milk at home, home pasteurization proved too complicated. Thus, the mainstays of most milk stations were certified milk and other forms of relatively expensive, clean milk. Pediatricians in clinics associated with the stations often contributed to keeping costs high by prescribing formulae tailored to individual babies. In 1910, for example, the Straus milk depots in New York City were making five different formulae, the creations of three major pediatricians. That year the Babies' Milk Fund Association of Louisville, Kentucky, reported that while it paid ten cents a quart for certified milk, which it sold at eight cents a quart, "modified" milk cost seventeen cents and had to be sold for ten cents. Their Boston counterparts were forced to sell prepared formulae at well above the prevailing retail rate for ordinary milk.[27]

The efforts of the milk stations to teach home modification of milk often failed because pediatric wisdom verging on the occult made the process unnecessarily complex. "In the absence of a nurse specially trained for the purpose it becomes necessary for the physician to give careful written and verbal instructions, and then to see personally that these are carried out," warned one of the leading doctors' manuals. "There are many nurses, both graduate and otherwise," it lamented, "whose conceptions of infant feeding and milk preparation are practically useless. Like many medical students and recent graduates, they understand more about laparotomies than they do about milk." And no wonder. The text outlined nine different techniques for modification, most of which required a keen mathematical mind and some of which even required slide rules and home pasteurization. Moreover, the unsanitary conditions that prevailed in the homes of the poor deterred those who might teach home modification. "Because of the unfavorable home conditions very little is being done and probably never should be done in the teaching of the home modification of milk," reported Boston's largest settlement house in 1911.[28]

Those who operated and subsidized the milk stations generally believed that artificial feeding of any kind was second best to breast feeding. Yet the very nature of the milk stations made them vulnerable to the charge that they were inadvertently discouraging breast feeding. Some milk stations claimed that they demanded "positive proof" that the mother either could not or should not nurse before allowing her to receive their products. However, it was virtually impossible to obtain proof of ability to lactate after a mother ceased nursing. The most common reason for not nursing given by mothers of all classes, whether at milk stations or not, was inability to produce milk, and although child-welfare workers might suspect the veracity of many of these claims, it was difficult to disprove a claim.[29]

Again the reformers were victims of the expert, yet erroneous, concepts they were trying to apply to the poor, for physicians were now unduly pessimistic about the ability of most women to nurse. Since at least the 1860s, when the specialty of pediatrics first emerged in England and Germany, there had been a strong tendency among pediatricians to underestimate the proportion of mothers who could nurse and of babies who could survive nursing.[30] Changes in the medical profession, as well as the late-nineteenth-century infatuation with psychosomatic illnesses, helped to diffuse these attitudes among the urban middle class. By the 1890s midwives and home delivery of babies had been largely displaced among the middle and upper classes by deliveries by male physicians. These physicians, perhaps afflicted by a prudishness that made it difficult to demonstrate nipple massaging and other techniques used to get mother's milk flowing, tended not to urge breast feeding. A much larger proportion of mothers than might have been expected in a reasonably well-fed middle-class population seem to have either convinced themselves or been convinced by physicians that they were incapable of nursing. Interruptions, diminutions, or apparent changes in mother's milk of the most inconsequential kind often occasioned early weaning. "Almost any abnormality in the behaviour of the infant . . . is seized upon as sufficient reason for inaugurating bottle feeding," complained a dissenting doctor in 1910. "While extremely neurotic mothers do not secrete the best of breast milk, a ridiculous number of women are excused or restrained from fufilling their maternal duties upon this and other insufficient grounds," he said. Rotch, for example, ascribed many infant maladies to inadequacies in the mother's milk. "Where continual shocks are brought to bear upon the mother in her daily life, or where her own temperament is such an undisciplined one that the milk, ordinarily good, becomes totally unfitted for her infant, [it] at times acts as a direct poison," he warned. Holt estimated that "not over 25 percent of the well to do and cultured of New York City who had earnestly and intelligently attempted to nurse had succeeded in doing so for as long as three months." (His insistence that babies should be nursed every two hours may well have played a major role in these failures.) By 1910 child-welfare conferences were even considering the idea that maternal lactation was a disappearing function in human evolution.[31]

A number of child-welfare activists were concerned that milk stations were counterproductive, worsening rather than improving the health of tenement infants by encouraging artificial feeding. Only in New York City, however, did this criticism lead to drastic action. In 1909 the New York Milk Committee, a major milk-station operator, closed its milk-modification laboratory, sold its equipment, and abandoned the distribution of modified milk in individual feeding bottles at its four milk depots because the system "placed undue emphasis on hand feeding and . . . actually discouraged feeding at the breast." (Significantly, the committee's new emphasis on encouraging breast feeding and teaching home modification of milk was severely criticized by social workers, mothers, nurses, and doctors.) In 1912 Josephine Baker warned that milk stations should concentrate more on education than on milk, and placed the encouragement of breast feeding among their most pressing future tasks, but in New York, as in other cities, milk stations continued to function for some years, performing their apparently contradictory function of encouraging breast feeding while teaching and facilitating artificial feeding.[32]

One of the ironies in the whole controversy was that while pediatricians and reformers denounced the supposed epidemic of artificial feeding among the poor, the practice was much more widespread among upper- than lower-income groups. In his 1901–1902 survey of tenement district artificial-feeding habits, Holt, who expected to discover ammunition to use against Mellin's and Nestlé's, was surprised at the difficulty his researchers encountered in finding a large enough number of artificially fed infants to study. While every street of the Lower East Side neighborhood studied seemed awash in children, the researchers had a difficult time finding more than half a dozen bottle-fed children per block.[33] The rarity of artificial feeding among the poor was confirmed by a series of studies of infant mortality in various cities undertaken from 1910 to 1915 by the newly created United States Children's Bureau. Most showed that "as the income increased, maternal nursing decreased."[34]

The urban poor of America were relatively resistant to the attractions of artificial feeding because of the high proportion of immigrants among them. The foreign-born, regardless of economic status, tended to feed their babies artificially at significantly lower rates than the native-born. In Montclair, New Jersey, for example, whereas 34.3 percent of the native-born white mothers weaned their babies by age three months, only 8.4 percent of the foreign-born did. On each rung of the economic ladder a higher proportion of immigrants nursed.[35]

Yet despite the relatively small proportion of artificially fed infants, the foreign-born urban poor still suffered appalling infant-mortality rates. Although the Children's Bureau studies demonstrated that artificially fed children of all classes had higher mortality rates (usually from three to five times greater) than their breast-fed counterparts, they were unable to pinpoint artificial feeding itself as the crucial variable. Rather, the most striking correlations in the studies were almost always between declining fathers' incomes and rising infant mortality. In the elliptical words of the Montclair study, "it would seem . . . that the disadvantages of a low income were sufficient to offset the greater prevalence of breast feeding among the babies of the poorer families."[36]

Like so many other Progressives, few of the opponents of proprietary and canned infant foods could see beyond their crusade to the wider problem of urban poverty with which it was intimately connected. Artificial feeding was connected with high infant mortality, but more because of the living and working conditions of the poor than because of the particular methods of feeding used. This is not to say that the obvious connection with poverty was not recognized at all.[37] However, even those who saw the connection and tried to understand the conditions of slum life usually managed to avoid attacking the roots of the problem.[38]

The milk-station movement peaked in about 1912–14. Within six years the depots were rapidly disappearing from urban America. They were put out of business not by concern over their promotion of artificial feeding but by commercial pasteurization. Despite opposition from proponents of home pasteurization and other systems, the "holding method," which allowed commercial pasteurization on a very large scale, spread rapidly through the large cities of America in the 1910s. New machines for rapid heating and cooling of milk enabled pasteurized milk to be produced in great quantities and sold at competitive prices. Because the process involved a sizable capital investment in new equipment and returnable bottles, it drove out of business the small milk peddlers and storeowners whose overripe product and unhygienic cans and dippers had contributed to the problem. The rapid expansion of a clean, affordable milk supply was a further blow to breast feeding, more than counteracting the simultaneous campaign of national and municipal child-welfare officials to encourage breast feeding, especially among the poor.[39]

The apparent drop in infant mortality that followed the introduction of large-scale pasteurization in many of the nation's large cities also played a major role in ending the hocus-pocus surrounding formula feeding. Pediatricians, their successful drive for recognition now crowned by newly constructed children's hospitals in a number of cities, abandoned percentage feeding in droves. By 1921 most pediatricians were suggesting that pasteurized cow's milk diluted with water and with some sugar added was safe and digestible for most infants. The recent discovery of vitamins enabled them to dispel the fear of infantile scurvy, always overblown anyway, by recommending small amounts of orange juice as well. This helped open the floodgates for the introduction of other non-milk foods at progressively earlier stages. By the end of the 1920s, as in the mid-eighteenth century, infants were being fed mashed and pureed fruits, vegetables, cereals, and even meat products by the age of six months.[40] A declining reliance on milk in the first twelve months of life helped weaken the mystique of breast feeding as well, for its dwindling number of advocates were no longer talking of babies' sole source of alimentation.

Meanwhile, the manufacturers of proprietary infant foods worked out a mutually beneficial arrangement with pediatricians and general practitioners. Many physicians had rejected Mellin's and its competitors because the proprietary foods, with the directions for preparing formulae on their labels, obviated the need for the medical supervision of infant feeding. As Rima D. Apple has written, "Such a situation could be physically unheal-

thy for the infant and economically harmful to the physician."
Increasingly, then, after 1912 most infant-food companies began marketing products requiring detailed instructions from physicians regarding
their preparation. Promotional campaigns were directed primarily at the
medical profession, the extravagant claims in the lay media replaced by a
judicious mix of appeals to medical science and physicians' self-interest.[41]
Led by the Pet Milk Company, whose "Research Division" assiduously
cultivated doctors, nurses, and hospitals, canned milk companies followed
suit.[42] With proprietary infant foods now reinforcing rather than undermining physicians' status and income, medical opposition practically
vanished.

By the late 1920s, the opponents of artificial feeding seemed soundly
defeated, their positions crumbling in the face of increasing artificial feeding and declining infant mortality rates. Many were forced into the stance
they would maintain into the 1960s: a posture that found its expression in
organizations such as the La Leche League, which emphasized psychological factors such as the "bonding" that occurred between mother and
suckled child. But in fact the widespread notion, among advocates of both
breast feeding and artificial feeding, that it was pasteurized milk that
reduced infant mortality to very low levels in the period from 1910 to
1930 was not as well grounded as it might have seemed. Rather, Robert
Morse Woodbury's 1924 statistical analysis of infant mortality in the first
seven cities studied by the Children's Bureau demonstrated that high
infant morality was most directly correlated with low income of the
fathers. This was connected, of course, with a number of intermediate
factors, such as neonatal care, housing and sanitary conditions, and the
mother's employment status, as well as the method of feeding. But the
analysis still indicated "that artificial feeding was fraught with greater dangers to the baby's health in the lower earnings groups." Significantly, this
was true of the breast-fed too, for there was a similar gap in mortality rates
between breast-fed children of the various earnings groups.[43] The most
ambitious attempt in subsequent years to link declining infant mortality
and pasteurization showed only the most general correlations between the
two and failed to establish a direct causal link.[44]

In fact, no one has yet been able to explain this century's decline in
infant mortality in a manner convincing to most of the other experts in the
field. The matter remains as controversial today as it was in the early years
of the century, when advocates of the various types of feeding and methods of improving child welfare flayed each other with their scanty statistics. If a consensus is emerging, however, it seems to be leading to a
"standard of living" explanation in which nutrition plays a major role. This
sees infant feeding in more or less the way that Woodbury did in 1924, as
one of a number of intermediate factors whose effects are directly linked
to real incomes.[45] Among other things, low incomes lead to poor maternal

nutrition and poorly nourished mothers have smaller babies than well-nourished ones. In the words of a 1982 editorial in the *Journal of the American Medical Association,* "put simply, poorer mothers have smaller babies, and smaller babies are at higher risk of early death.[46] In a way, this explanation represents a return to one of the earliest studies of infant mortality in the United States, undertaken in New York City in 1894 by Henry Dwight Chapin, one of the pioneers in the field, who concluded that inadequate income was the chief cause of infant mortality.[47] Studies of infant mortality in the Third World which indicate that a "synergistic" relationship exists between malnutrition and susceptibility to disease supports the conclusion that this century's decline in infant mortality was at least as closely linked to improved nutrition as it was to pasteurization.[48]

As for why nutrition improved, if in 1930 pollsters had asked adult Americans what had been the most important factors in improving their eating habits, it is likely that a large proportion of middle-class Americans, would have cited their experience during World War I.

CHAPTER 11

"Food Will Win the War"

It is no wonder that middle-class Americans thought World War I marked a watershed in their attitudes toward food. The massive food conservation program directed by Herbert Hoover seemed to have had an extraordinary impact on food habits and ideas. Thanks to Hoover's United States Food Administration, said a 1930 article in the *Saturday Evening Post,* "Americans began to look seriously into the question of what and how much they were eating. Lots of people discovered for the first time that they could eat less and feel no worse—frequently much better."[1]

Even though a number of forces were already encouraging Americans to reduce and simplify their food intake well before the United States entered the war in April 1917, there was some merit to these claims. However, they must be qualified by a consideration ignored by Hoover's admirers: the marked differences in the war's impact on the different classes, for the influence of the USFA was restricted mainly to the middle and upper middle class.

This was not its original intention, for the Food Administration (FA) was conceived amidst the food crisis of the winter of 1916–17. By March 1917, American entry into the war seemed imminent, and even if it could be avoided the continued fighting in Europe promised to bring even more disruption to the food production and distribution system. The Wilson Administration drafted a measure designed to allow it to assert some kind of control over the food supply in order to prevent hoarding, shortages,

inflation, and recurring food riots. In April, shortly after the official decla-
ration of war, this bill, the Lever Bill, began to wend its way through a
fractious Congress. It provided for the creation of an agency to license and
regulate food producers and distributors, intervene into the market to
purchase and distribute foodstuffs, and, as a last resort, fix farm prices and
impose rationing.

There seemed little question as to who would be appointed to head the
new body, for Hoover had already carved out a formidable reputation for
himself in overseeing the distribution of the millions of dollars' worth of
foodstuffs sent by Americans to neutral Belgium. A Quaker in origin and
an engineer by profession, Hoover's success in running the voluntary
organization from a makeshift London office reinforced his faith in the
principles of voluntary cooperation and lean, efficient administration.[2]

For some three months, while the legislation was pummeled in Congress, the FA functioned as a voluntary committee, but this enabled Hoover to concentrate on mounting the campaign for voluntary restriction of
food consumption that would become the centerpiece of the FA's strategy. The FA would persuade, not force, Americans to cut down on their
consumption of white wheat flour and meat, as well as sugar and butter.

The talented crew, many of them volunteers, whom Hoover recruited
included a number of home economists and reformers who were influenced by the ideas of the New Nutrition. Thus, while the FA occasionally
issued calls for general reductions in food consumption,[3] its strategy in
promoting measures such as "wheatless and "meatless" days rested on the
bedrock concept of Atwater and his followers: substitution. If Americans
could be taught about the interchangeability of proteins, fats, and carbohydrates, they could be persuaded to get their proteins from beans and
pulses rather than meat, their carbohydrates from corn meal, oats, and
grains other than wheat, and their fats from lard and vegetable oils. If they
could learn to fill their bellies on fruits and vegetables too perishable to
send to Europe, then soldiers and civilians overseas could be supplied,
pressures on domestic prices could be eased, and there would be no need
for rationing.[4] When combined with a drive to reduce "waste," the thrust
was strikingly similar to the New Nutritionist effort to teach economical
cooking. The home economists and reformers had been preparing the
appropriate lessons for years. All that was necessary were some minor
adjustments to accommodate the new value placed on perishable
vegetables.

If it took its message from the home economists, the FA borrowed its
tactics from an incongruous combination of the prohibition movement
and the fledgling advertising industry. From the former it took the idea of
the "pledge," mounting campaigns to induce housewives to sign cards
pledging to obey the rules set out by the Food Administrator.[5] It also sent
out orators to arouse enthusiasm from the pulpits and women's clubs of
the nation.

From the advertising industry the FA learned the importance of slogans, brand names, and visual propaganda.[6] It also developed a keen appreciation for the susceptibility of the nation's press to the lure of the "canned" article: free material which could be altered slightly by a tenuous local angle to help propaganda masquerade as news. Women's magazines and women's page editors signed up enthusiastically for its offer to supply them with one article per week and sent in requests for tailor-written articles.[7] Even political journals such as the *New Republic, Nation,* and *Independent,* could not resist FA pieces written especially for them.[8]

While the FA benefited from the expertise of home economists and food reformers, the home economists in turn profited from their association with the new agency. Ray Wilbur, president of Stanford University and head of the FA's Food Conservation Division, set up a special Home Economics section in his division staffed by "trained specialists." A director of home economics was appointed for each state, and Wilbur encouraged the heads of the home economics departments of state universities to assume these posts. Coming to work in Washington would "bring home economics into its own more than anything else," he told the home economists.[9]

The home economists used their talents to devise recipes and menus which would employ substitutes for wheat, beef, butter, and sugar.[10] The American Home Economics Association set up an Emergency Committee to turn out war recipes for the press, write pamphlets for women's clubs, and create course outlines for home economics courses in the schools.[11]

The FA was particularly supportive of the scientific approach to food. Hoover told home economics graduates to devote themselves to "issues that demand the rarest talent and the highest scientific training," and "pursue studies dealing especially with food . . . reinforced by courses in chemistry, physiology and economics."[12] This faith in science echoed down the FA line. Introducing a pamphlet popularizing the New Nutrition, Ida Tarbell, the ex-"muckraking" journalist employed by the agency, wrote that solving the food problem required scientific knowledge. "To learn to do every common thing in the most scientific manner is one of our high duties at the moment," she wrote, and was also "a contribution to peace."[13]

The FA home economists turned out an impressive array of material. They prepared a textbook for upper-level school children explaining the principles of the New Nutrition—one of the first such texts to reflect the growing awareness of the nutritional value of fruits and vegetables.[14] The Collegiate section prepared outlines for three different college courses on food, sending them out in weekly installments during the spring semester of 1918 before publishing them in textbook form as *Food and the War.*[15]

Other home economists and cooking instructors recycled old messages to meet the new demands of war. The cooking teacher Ida C. Bailey Allen, a former *Good Housekeeping* columnist and cookbook author now employed as a lecturer by the FA, rearranged many of her old recipes into *Mrs. Allen's Book of Wheat Substitutes, Mrs. Allen's Book of Meat Substitutes,* and *Mrs. Allen's Book of Sugar Substitutes.*[16] Perhaps the most ambitious of the menu-planning aids was a book by Thetta Quay Frank called *Daily Menus for War Service.* This *tour de force* not only provided detailed menus using only poultry, fish, lamb, and other non-essential foods three meals a day for each day of the year, it also noted the calories per portion for each dish and gave three different menus for each day, in ascending order of expense![17]

The FA was not the only agency to employ home economists. The federal Department of Agriculture was supposed to carry on its normal duties during the war and avoid bloating its bureaucracy, but Dr. Alfred True had been steadily expanding the role of home economics within it before entry into the war. The war provided an opportunity to attempt a massive national nutrition survey which it dubbed the War Emergency Food Survey. The department's newly created Office of Home Economics sent home economists into hundreds of homes, asking inhabitants to record their daily consumption of foodstuffs in minute detail. The amounts and costs of the protein, carbohydrates, fats, and various minerals in their diets were then calculated and the results sent to Washington.[18]

The home economists in the FA and the Agriculture Department worked well together, particularly in ensuring that the food conservation program did not fall into the hands of amateurs. Although the Women's Committees of the Council of National Defense—comprising many thousands of women chomping at the bit for a greater role in the war effort— wanted to play a more central role in planning and carrying out the program, they were shunted aside by the professionals and relegated to distributing pledge cards and encouraging the planting of Liberty Gardens.[19]

The Women's Committees were not particularly effective in their first appointed task. The first pledge card campaign, in July 1917, in which they played a central role, was a disaster. However, after intensive reorganization by the FA, which assembled a network of nearly half a million workers in its state organizations, a second campaign in late October managed to sign up nearly half of the nation's estimated 24 million families. When women canvassers failed, they were followed by Boy Scouts, schoolchildren, and finally, in some cases, the police.[20]

The rather impressive degree of success was based very much on the FA's ability to rally the key middle-class institutions and organizations to its cause. Protestant churches, women's clubs, chambers of commerce, schools, colleges and universities, Boy Scouts, fraternal organizations, men's clubs: all played important roles in producing social pressure to promise, as the second pledge card did, to have one wheatless day a week, one wheatless meal a day, one meatless day a week, and one meatless meal each day and then to hang cards attesting to their oath ("the service tag of American women") in their windows.

Although consuming food prepared from many of the home economists' recipes (particularly those for leaden breads using wheat substitutes) may well have involved a form of sacrifice, this rationing was perhaps the least onerous ever undertaken by a modern nation at war. "Meatless," for example, usually only meant beefless and porkless. Thus, when the Chicago, Milwaukee and St. Paul Railway devised a special breakfast menu for "Meatless Tuesdays" it hardly imposed undue hardship on its passengers. It included fresh fruit and juices, dry and hot cereals, fried, stewed or broiled oysters, grilled whitefish, broiled mackerel, half a grilled spring chicken, shredded chicken on toast, crabmeat au gratin, various kinds of eggs, broiled squab, omelettes, including one with fresh oysters, French toast with maple or corn syrup, and other choice items.[21]

While the lessons of the New Nutrition formed an integral part of the push for substitution and economical cooking, the overall campaign rested on appeals to patriotism rather than good health and economy. "Recipes for Menus that Serve Your Country" was the title of a typical FA women's magazine article.[22] "Lick the plate and lick the Kaiser," was a favorite FA slogan.[23] Hoover himself was wary of appeals to good health and referred to malnutrition only in reference to Europe, and then mainly to rally support for continued shipments of food to Europe after the Armistice to head off what FA propaganda called "the red scourge of revolution."[24] Hoover's reluctance to emphasize good health seems to have stemmed from a morbid fear of food faddists. When the Lever Bill was being debated in Congress he told President Wilson that a clause giving him the power to force millers to mix wheat flour with other grains was expendable because it would be difficult to enforce and yet bring pressure on him to do so from "the large number of misguided faddists in the country."[25]

In the postwar era, when disillusion with the patriotic war was rife, some took a rather jaundiced view of the FA's patriotic message and its effects. In 1931, a food lover wrote that "the decline in American dining began . . . when the Food Administration set out to change the eating habits of the nation." It turned the nation's hotels and restaurants into "experimental stations" and "caused a scaling down of portions and the use of substitutes in cooking." While some hotels and restaurants were initially alarmed, when they discovered that "the Food Administration permitted them, in the name of patriotism, to serve reduced portions without any corresponding reduction in prices, they became reconciled to the situation." As for the public, "it got used to skimpy helpings and has stayed used to them." The result was "a general deterioration from which we have never recovered."[26]

Nevertheless, one of the few conclusions which could be drawn from the Department of Agriculture's wartime food survey was that, while it likely did reconcile middle-class Americans to smaller portions of meat and other items, the war also saw them, and the better-off farmers, eating more fresh fruits and vegetables and drinking more milk.[27] Exactly how much of this was due to the FA's efforts is, of course, impossible to assess, but the impact of a campaign of persuasion which enlisted so many millions of individuals cannot be minimized.

While patriotic eating may have stirred the middle and upper classes, it had less impact on those on lower rungs of the socio-economic ladder. The vast majority of American families who did not take the pledge rested firmly in this category. FA administrators noted ruefully that five million of the country's twenty million heads of families were foreign-born and tended to ascribe working-class indifference to their campaign to "disloyal inclinations."[28] Touring the Midwest in December 1917, Ray Wilbur wrote Hoover that there were "some bad German spots where no cards were signed." Cincinnati was "one of the most difficult cities in America— a mixture of Germany, Africa, Italy and America."[29]

The FA tried to win the immigrant groups over by establishing a Vernacular Press Division to send out literature to the foreign language press and by making special appeals to particular immigrant groups. "You Came Here Seeking Freedom. You Must Now Help to Preserve It—Waste Nothing" said a Yiddish poster portraying immigrants gazing at the Statue of Liberty.[30]

The Vernacular Press division was not unaware of the difficult task ahead of it. Soon after its creation it sent one of its staffers to study immigrant food habits. In September 1917, it asked Jane Addams and other social workers to tell of "the staple foods and dishes of the various races," asking Addams for sample recipes and food combinations so that it could have "full information on the food found in the homes of Italians, Jews, Poles, Syrians, Greeks, Austrians, and the different Slavic peoples."[31] It secured an endorsement from W. E. B. Dubois, head of the National Association for the Advancement of Colored People, and circulated his statement to the Negro press that "Americans and colored Americans in particular eat too much."[32]

But the FA effort among blacks and immigrants was almost wholly ineffective. Although it had a small (segregated) Negro press division which prepared some special publications for blacks, it had little in the way of special articles for the Negro press. In September 1918, realizing that blacks had been almost completely ignored and untouched, the FA urged state Food Administrators to appoint black chairmen who would form "Colored Food Clubs," but little came of this.[33]

More effort was devoted to immigrant groups, but to little avail. Jane Addams was enlisted as a speaker, but spoke mainly to middle-class women's groups and businessmen.[34] The Vernacular Press division was hampered by a shortage of translators. While many immigrant papers were happy to receive its free copy few would translate it themselves.[35]

Some in the agency were plagued by doubts about the appropriateness of its conservation message to those already hard-pressed economically.

The Vernacular Press section refused to circulate an FA article entitled "We Can Fight Back with Our Teeth" because it centered around a call for reduced consumption of meat. "Practically all" readers of the foreign-language press "eat very little meat now," said its head, because "they can't afford to eat much meat." Therefore, they would likely resent such gratuitous advice.[36] The Food Administrator in Louisiana wrote that poor Italians in his state could not "be impressed by pleas to conserve a little bread, butter, milk, and fat, because [they are] forced to economize on these items all the time."[37]

Some FA material was irrelevant because ethnic groups were already carrying out its prescriptions for their own reasons. The editor of a Lithuanian paper in Boston thanked the FA for its bulletins on conserving white wheat flour but pointed out that "in conservation of wheat Lithuanians perhaps excel every nation in America" because the Lithuanian workingmen despised white bread. They called it "straw bread," and ate only rye bread.[38] When an FA home economist held a series of home preservation demonstrations in a Boston settlement house in the summer of 1917, the board of directors noted that "the audience was able to give the teacher instructions."[39]

Sometimes material translated for the foreign-born might better have been left alone. When the pledge card was translated into Yiddish, not only was it full of incorrect words and translations but it had the oath-taker promise to try to eat shellfish, a serious violation of the Orthodox dietary laws which most Yiddish-speakers followed. An FA circular to synagogues asked them to urge their congregants to forego the usual dishes of beef, mutton (which Jews never ate), and pork![40] Even Regina Mermelstein, the FA's resident expert on Jewish folkways, made some noteworthy gaffes. She told an interviewer from the Jewish press that "the duty of the Jewish woman does not stop with putting a few pennies in the charity box every Friday night" when she should have known that Orthodox Jews do not handle money on the Sabbath. Moreover, she warned that "the fact that she fasts on your [*sic*] Kippur and other holy days does not mean absolution from sin."[41]

The FA had a particularly hard time gaining voluntary compliance with its regulations from the smaller food distribution concerns not subjected to direct controls, and most ethnic food dealers and restaurateurs were in this bracket. The calls for meatless and wheatless days were ignored by most ethnic restaurants, something of no little significance to the FA. The frustrated director of the FA's Hotel and Restaurant Division complained that his greatest problem was securing compliance from "alien hotel and restaurant proprietors. . . . We found out from the police that there were 18,900 eating places in New York City and out of this number only 8,000 were English-speaking."[42]

Immigrants aside, the FA had difficulty reaching working-class institutions in general. There seems to have been no effort to work through labor unions, even though Samuel Gompers and the top leadership of the American Federation of Labor lobbied hard for passage of the Lever Bill.[43] The organization of the first pledge card campaign in Florida was typical of those in many states. Lead by the head of the Women's Committee of the Florida Council of National Defense, who also headed the state's Federation of Women's Clubs, it sent the cards out to the Women's Christian Temperance Union, the Daughters of the American Revolution, the Colonial Dames, the Equal Suffrage League, the Florida Federation of Women's Clubs, and, to reach farm women, to the Home Demonstration Agents, whose canning clubs normally comprised the better-off white farmers' wives.[44] Ida Tarbell gave an indication of the class background of most FA supporters when she ascribed the problems encountered in the first campaign to the fact that it took place during the summer, when most of the women who would have supported it were off on vacation.[45]

When the FA did come into contact with workers, it had difficulty adjusting its message to their needs or interests. Its Speakers Bureau was composed of articulate people from the upper echelons, and included people such as the employee of the American Bankers Association who, assigned to address a group of Alabama miners on food conservation, instead warned them that their union was pro-German and that if they dared to strike they would be shipped to the front and replaced by British miners.[46] The six men "from various walks of life" chosen by the FA to tour the front and report back to the nation on the need for conservation were a Buffalo lawyer, the field secretary of the National Chamber of Commerce, the ex-football coach at Cornell, a Swedish Lutheran pastor, a prominent New York banker, and a lawyer-businessman from Orange, New Jersey.[47]

The greatest obstacles to changing working-class eating habits, however, were higher wages and more hours of work. Not surprisingly, the FA found its propaganda particularly ineffective in communities where working-class wages had risen sharply during the war.[48] Rare was the workingman's family, whether native-born or immigrant, which could be persuaded not to spend at least part of the new gains on more and better food, particularly meat. C. F. Langworthy concluded that meat consumption "among the more well-to-do" declined during the war as they learned that "with less meat than they had been accustomed to their daily fare could be attractive and adequate for the needs of their body." However, he pointed out, "since persons of small means commonly consider a generous use of meat a mark of good living," many workers whose incomes rose during the war seem to have spent more on more and better cuts of meat.[49] The same applied to the rural poor. In the rural Southeast, when the war brought higher incomes to black farm laborers and sharecroppers they quickly abandoned dry salt pork in favor of the fancier, meatier cuts of cured pork.[50]

In the spring of 1918, with evidence accumulating that the working classes were not responding to the FA's admonitions and were increasing rather than decreasing their consumption of beef and pork, Hoover himself confessed to being baffled over what could be done to dissuade them. At an FA staff meeting in March 1918, he ascribed "these curious developments," which caused 1917 beef consumption to actually rise by 11 percent over "prewar normal" to the "increasing prosperity of the industrial classes." This brought about a rise in their standard of living "while on the other hand the well-to-do classes are actually reducing their food consumption." Hoover admitted he knew of no "radical" or voluntary action which could affect working-class beef consumption: "With the increase in wages in the industrial centers the natural tendency was to lay on the porterhouse steaks and I rather sympathize with that attitude from a personal point of view but from a national point of view it is hard on us."[51]

If one had to choose a government institution which had a significant impact on the eating habits of the "other half," it would have to be the War Department. Until the late nineteenth century, there were no standard or even suggested recipes for the Army or Navy. Messing was adapted to different local situations and cooks were untrained and often inexperienced. ("God sends the food, the Devil sends the cooks," was an old Navy saying). When an Army manual for cooks was developed in 1896, the emphasis was on cooking what soldiers were thought to like. There was no evidence of the new nutritional ideas; admonitions about cleanliness constituted the only health-related information. Although most of the recipes were resolutely "American," there was a separate section with "Spanish" recipes which included variations on Mexican dishes such as tamales, tortillas, stuffed chiles, and frijoles con queso. It even called for grinding chiles in a *metate,* the traditional Mexican stone grinder.[52]

By 1916, when a new manual was issued, the military obviously abided by the maxim which still guides the nutrition of military people throughout the world: that the last thing the men want is anything "different." The idiosyncratic "Spanish" section was gone and the recipes were almost uniformly "American." Now, one section explained the bases of the New Nutrition and cooks were mandated to strive for a proper "balance" among proteins, carbohydrates, and fats. With the exception of those for emergency conditions in the field, most of the recipes could have come from any contemporary middle-class woman's magazine or, worse, home economist's lab.[53] Meanwhile, 386 home economists who specialized in nutrition, now calling themselves "dietitians," were recruited by the War

Department and assigned to supervise the menus of all army hospitals, at home and overseas.[54]

The service experience must have had a particularly great impact on thousands of young men of two major origins: immigrants and rural folk from areas such as the southern and southwestern "hog 'n hominy" belt. For the latter, the change from a cured pork and cornmeal diet to a beef, potatoes, white bread, and milk must have been as profound as that experienced by many immigrants and their children. They must have suffered from spice deprivation as well,[55] but they were also, unwittingly, playing important roles in the process of the nationalizing of American food tastes.

Ironically, if the FA campaigns failed to change working-class eating habits, they did have some effect on middle-class attitudes toward the food of at least one immigrant group, the Italians. Italy's new status as one of the nation's major Allies helped alleviate the disdain with which its food was regarded by the prewar elite. Articles on "spaghetti, food of our ally," appeared in women's magazines which had previously ignored the existence of a thriving pasta industry in basements, storefronts, and small factories throughout the nation. Also, while other immigrant groups indulged in veritable orgies of beef and pork consumption when they could afford it, Italians increased their meat consumption but still retained their attachment to many of their meat-stretching dishes. They thereby provided some readily available meatless or meat-conserving recipes which were easy to adapt to the American household, particularly since the fear of tomatoes had long since dissipated. The rising popularity of pasta and tomato sauce during the the 1920s helped make Italian food (or at least an Americanized version of it) the first immigrant food to gain widespread acceptance in America.[56]

To say that the FA's impact was felt mainly by the middle and upper classes is not to minimize its importance. As a consumer advertising specialist noted in the mid-1920s, the wartime campaigns to "Save the sugars, save the fats, save the wheat" taught millions of people for the first time that there was a difference between potatoes and tomatoes, that there were things called calories, that some foods were similar to each other and others were not. These would be important concepts that the advertising industry of the 1920s would exploit.[57] But the postwar era would see the confluence of even more powerful forces, making use of the ideas of the New Nutrition as well as those of the Newer, vitamin-based, Nutrition, to complete a revolution in eating habits whose depth and extent could hardly have been dreamed of by Ellen Richards and the first generation of New Nutritionists.

CHAPTER 12

The Newer Nutrition,
1915–1930

The housewives who assiduously practiced the Food Administration's
rules for substitution represented a victory for the ideas of the New
Nutrition. Yet even as they were finally learning that beans and meat were
nutritionally equivalent, the discovery of vitamins was revolutionizing scientific concepts of food and redirecting ideas about nutrition.

Atwater, Richards, and most New Nutritionists had concentrated on
the "practical economy" of food, arguing that people could maintain good
health while spending less on food. Home economists used these ideas to
appeal to middle-class women concerned not about health but about the
burdens of housework. Dr. Harvey Wiley and the pure food advocates of
the Progressive era had aroused nationwide concern over food and health,
but their thrust was a negative one: to protect consumers from illness
caused by unscrupulous adulterers of food. Chittenden, Fletcher, and
their faddist supporters had gone half a step further, lowering the estimates of the amount of food required to "fuel the human machine" and
promising positive improvements in health and longevity as well. The
discovery of vitamins now shifted the ground decisively toward good
health.

At the heart of what the American pioneer in the field, Elmer
McCollum, called "the Newer Knowledge of Nutrition" was a great de-
parture from prevailing ideas regarding the causes of illness and disease.
The vast majority of health professionals of the time and most of the

faddists were mesmerized by the discovery of bacteria and the germ theory of disease, which saw illness as the result of the ingestion of foreign agents into the organism. Their cures for ailments normally involved abstaining from certain foods and/or cutting down on total food intake. The thrust of the scientists who discovered vitamins was in the opposite direction, for they showed that illness could result from the *absence* of certain elements. Moreover, they could support these claims with striking evidence, visible and understandable by all, from their laboratories.

One key to it all was the rat. Human nutrition studies had always revolved, quite naturally it seemed, around human beings, dogs, or other large mammals. Yet the Liebig-Voit-Atwater approach had produced puzzling results when scientists mixed together the optimum amounts of proteins, carbohydrates, fats, and inorganic salts into artificial foods. As in the case of artificial infant foods, feeding these foods to large mammals often resulted in sickness or death. When Elmer McCollum and others at Yale began to experiment on rats in 1908, their shorter life cycle enabled scientists to perform a large number of experiments to confirm that there were indeed, as some suspected, other unknown elements in food essential for life and health, substances which in 1912 were labeled "vitamines" by the European chemist Casimir Funk.

In 1911, Funk isolated a water-soluble nutrient, later called Vitamin B, and the next year McCollum identified a fat-soluble vitamin, which he labeled Vitamin A. Most important, McCollum demonstrated that the absence of Vitamin A led to severe deterioration of vision and stunted growth in rats. In 1916 he proved that there was a direct link between the absence of Vitamin B and beri-beri.

From then on research and discovery accelerated rapidly. Nutritional scientists abandoned True and Langworthy amidst their expensive respiratory calorimeters and nutrition surveys, re-equipped their labs with rats, and began the searching for other hidden nutrients and the ailments they prevented. It had long been suspected that scurvy was caused by a dietary deficiency and, although the deficient item was not actually isolated until 1928, by the early 1920s it was known to exist in citrus fruits and potatoes and was labeled Vitamin C. McCollum and others had induced and controlled rickets with diet among rats for a number of years before McCollum finally isolated the "accessory factor" and called it Vitamin D in 1922. The following ten years saw other discoveries, both of new vitamins and of the importance of various minerals and trace elements. All of this bred a growing awareness in the importance of what McCollum labeled "protective foods."[1]

Two characteristics of the early years of vitamin and mineral research made the new tack a boon to the food industries. First, although a number of vitamins were isolated from 1915 to 1930, methods for synthesizing most of them were not discovered until later. Thus, they could not be ingested in the form of inoffensive little pills. They had to be eaten in foodstuffs. Second, practical methods for measuring the amounts of vitamins in foods did not begin to emerge until the early 1930s, making it impossible to recommend how much of any particular kind of food should be eaten. The "Newer Nutrition" was thus made to order for the extravagant claims of food advertisers.

In 1914, scientists such as Henry C. Sherman and Lafayette B. Mendel alerted the public to the fact that there were mysterious food factors about which little was known, but they could do little but recommend "physiological liberality in diet."[2] In 1918 McCollum declared that "milk and the leaves of plants are to be regarded as protective foods and never omitted from the diet." He also recommended that these foods supplement a basic diet of seed products, tubers, roots, and meats, but was vague regarding how much of each was required.[3] The realization that milk contained vitamin A and that whole grain cereals and many vegetables contained vitamin B fit in well with the United States Food Administration's goals and Food Administration materials sent to colleges and high schools in late 1918 included information on these vitamins; but again, it was impossible to specify quantities.[4]

On the surface, the rapidity with which interest in vitamins overtook the middle class during the 1920s might seem rather curious. After all, the specific diseases which they cured, the so-called dietary-deficiency diseases, were not exactly rampant, certainly not among the classes who became vitamin-conscious. Beri-beri and scurvy, caused by deficiencies of vitamins B_1 and C, were almost unknown in America. Rickets, caused by insufficient exposure to sunlight and/or lack of vitamin D, was more widespread, but was still concentrated among the urban poor. By the mid-1920s it was apparent to Dr. Joseph Goldberger and others aware of his studies that pellagra was related to the corn meal diet of the Southern poor and its deficiency in vitamin B_3, niacin, but because of the opposition of politically powerful people intent on preserving the cotton economy it was not officially recognized as a vitamin-deficiency disease until the 1930s.[5]

But middle-class concern over vitamins and minerals really had little to do with deficiency diseases per se. Rather, what struck home were indications that the newly discovered substances affected health, longevity, and growth. "Food for Health's Sake" was the title of a 1924 book by Lucy Gillett, an Atwater-Teacher's College product who, although employed by the New York Association for Improving the Condition of the Poor, aimed her popularization of the Newer Nutrition at the middle class. In an introduction to the book Henry Sherman assured readers that eating "protective foods" would not only head off deficiency diseases but would "also promote a higher degree of positive health." A core chapter was entitled "Increase the Length of Your Life."[6] "How Long Do You Want to Live?"

was the title of a typical article popularizing the Newer Nutrition in a 1922 issue of *Collier's* magazine. Learning the lessons propounded by McCollum and the Newer Nutrition would lead to good health and longer life, it assured readers.[7]

Indications that vitamins promoted human physical growth proved equally compelling. During the past thirty years or so, middle-class American families had become increasingly child-centered. The abolition of child labor and the enforcement of compulsory education laws reinforced this trend among the lower classes, lengthening the stage of childhood and placing more emphasis on the mother-child relationship.[8] Concern for the health of children led to the formation of a number of child health and protection leagues and in 1914 the federal government had created a special Children's Bureau, headed by Julia Lathrop, who twenty years earlier had established a New England Kitchen in Hull House.

As the child-oriented nature of the malnutrition scare of those years would indicate, much of the concern over children was directed toward their physical growth and feeding. Ample weight, height, and robustness of appearance were regarded as signs of health among children of all classes. Mothers prided themselves in their children exceeding the weight-age and height-age charts, which now festooned schools and doctors' offices, as much as earlier generations found satisfaction in their children's moral attainments.

Fortuitously, one of the first vitamins discovered, vitamin A, visibly affected the growth of rodents. Widely reproduced photographs of McCollum's mice, which showed the striking contrast between the fat and healthy white mice fed on adequate diets of the vitamin and their deprived siblings, made an extraordinary impact on mothers. McCollum's statements that milk contained the crucial vitamin made mothers of young children regard it as a magic potion. This was reinforced by the municipal health authorities' clean milk campaigns, the Children's Bureau's studies of infant mortality, and its pamphlets on child-rearing in the post-infancy years, all of which portrayed milk as a miracle food for infants and children.[9]

The Newer Nutrition also appeared just as the food industries were entering a stage where manipulation and control of the market was becoming not only possible but necessary. During the nineteenth century, the ups and downs of food production had affected mainly farmers, who had little control over market forces. As we have seen, the late-nineteenth-century trend toward concentration into large units centered in industries "downstream" from the farm: in areas such as meat packing, flour milling, sugar processing, and biscuit baking. The production and marketing of the items which the Newer Nutrition would declare all-important to human health—milk, cheese, vegetables, and fruits—remained the province of many small producers and distributors.

By 1915, however, this was rapidly changing. Improvements in production processes and transportation, along with infusions of capital to finance new forms of organization, led to the rise of large growers who banded together to promote their products, abetted by state departments of agriculture. In industry after industry large new organizations arose. Advances in distribution, occasioned by better roads, trucks, and automobiles, played major roles. So did continuing improvements in the technology of large-scale manufacturing and packaging of foods. Inspired in part by the much-discussed success of the FA in persuading consumers to change their food habits, the large new organizations were ready to devote their resources to massive advertising campaigns to create consumer loyalty toward their nationally distributed brand names.

Among food processors, the prewar trend toward concentration and growth in some of the food industries paled before the spurt of organization and consolidation of the 1920s. The era of the great individual entrepreneurs faded quite rapidly. H. J. Heinz, so concerned over the morals of his white-smocked female employees, passed from the scene, replaced by his business-school-educated sons, more concerned about competition from Campbell's. The newer age belonged to the anonymous giant corporation, organized and capitalized by Wall Street magnates whose closest encounters with food in its raw state were likely with the apple orchards near their summer homes.

Perhaps the transition to the corporate age was best symbolized by the marriage, in the early part of the decade, of the daughter of C. W. Post to Wall Street financier Edward F. Hutton. Ex-cowboy Post had risen to the top in the breakfast food scramble because of his genius for promotion and a substantial measure of blind luck. Hutton, the new kind of businessman, took control of the Postum Company and used the latest techniques of financial wizardry to organize the capital necessary to expand it. He brought in managers schooled in the latest Taylorite dictums to reorganize the corporation and multiplied the effectiveness of its sales force by diversifying into other food areas. In less than four years, from 1925 to 1929, Postum acquired fourteen other food companies, including the Jell-O Company, whose sales comprised half the total of the new parent's. By that time, Hutton had turned Post's operation into an immense conglomerate called General Foods.

Similarly, the J. P. Morgan company, which had concentrated on heavy industry before the war, moved its faceless financial men into food in the 1920s. It acquired control of the Chase and Sanborn coffee company and Royal Baking Powder and built another impressive food conglomerate, Standard Brands, Inc., around them.[10] By the end of the decade the amounts of capital invested in the food processing industries had made them the largest of American manufacturing industries, surpassing even such giants as iron and steel and textiles in terms of capital investment.[11]

Capital investment in the manufacturing segment of the food industry more than tripled from 1914 to 1929, and almost quadrupled in the modern processing sectors such as canning.[12]

The battle among these giants for the consumer's dollar was made particularly fearsome by some commonly accepted ideas regarding food expenditures. Most important was the knowledge that the market itself was limited: Americans had enough to eat and could not be persuaded to eat more food. This meant that any increase in the consumption of one food commodity would have to be at the expense of others; the advertiser's version of the rule of substitution.[13] As a result producers of the same commodities formed trade associations to promote the virtues of their products. Flour millers joined an "Eat More Wheat Campaign," California's citrus growers extolled the heathful qualities of their Sunkist fruits, while the state's raisin growers adopted the Sun Maid label and the very successful slogan "Had Your Iron Today?" Southern rice growers claimed the kind of rice grown in their region was better than all others. Even the pasta manufacturers joined together in the National Macaroni Institute, published a trade journal (the *Macaroni Journal*), and tried to stimulate consumption by touting pasta's nutritious qualities. They campaigned to have Friday proclaimed national "Macaroni Day," and fretted that the fad for spaghetti-eating contests "disparages the product."[14] In some cases, shrewd advertising campaigns were able to introduce completely new foods to American tables. Asparagus, for example, was practically unknown in the United States until the 1920s, when the Asparagus Section of the Canners League of California invested in a substantial promotional campaign.[15]

As canning and other forms of processing boomed, pressure on processors to come up with catchy brand names and promotional gimmicks to differentiate their products from those processed in essentially the same fashion increased. The Washburn-Crosby flour milling company changed its name to General Mills and created a food service department which could communicate directly with housewives through the medium of a fictional character, Betty Crocker, who answered their letters and sent them recipes. This was so successful that Crocker was given a face for the print media and a voice for a weekly radio program.[16]

The struggles for market share soon made food and beverage manufacturers the decade's second largest purchasers of newspaper advertising space.[17] Desperate for anything that could help differentiate foods and brands, advertisers turned to the Newer Nutrition for weaponry. Invisible, unmeasurable, and tasteless, obviously important but with little knowledge of exactly why, vitamins and minerals were an advertiser's dream. One could claim virtually anything for them and almost everything was. At first, advertisers were surprisingly negligent of the potential of the Newer Nutrition. In the first years after the war many continued to mine the New Nutrition. Quaker Oats advertised itself as an inexpensive source of calories, much more economical than veal or halibut. California walnut growers said their "vital food" possessed "important heat and energy producing qualities," while their raisin and prune-producing colleagues touted their products as sources of energy-producing sugar.[18]

By 1920 and 1921, however, the message of the Newer Nutrition, with its promises of growth and health, was coming to the fore. Predictably, breakfast cereal manufacturers were among the leaders. Post's Grape-Nuts asked, "Are you bringing up your children properly?" It pointed out, "It is possible to give children all the food they can possibly eat—and still their little bodies can be under-nourished." Luckily, Grape-Nuts was there to save them, for it contained *"iron, calcium, phosphorus,* and *other mineral elements* that are taken right up as vital food by the millions of cells in the body."[19]

Fleischmann's Yeast rapidly became one of the decade's most shameless purveyors of half-truths and falsehoods regarding vitamins. Hard hit by the decline in home-baked bread in the 1920s, it turned to advertising yeast cakes as a health food. Eating its yeast, "the richest known source of water-soluble vitamin," headed off "the two constant dangers—not having our body tissues built up and not ridding the body of poisonous waste matter." Millions of Americans were now spreading Fleischmann's yeast on crackers or bread, it said, and mixing it with water, fruit juice, and milk. Two to three cakes a day (later increased to four) was the recommended dosage, to be taken at home and in the office ("Eat it at your desk. Ask for it at noon-time in your lunch place"). An added benefit was that it also cleared up skin disorders, and corrected run-down conditions, indigestion, and constipation.[20]

Other manufacturers tiptoed along the borderline of dangerous misinformation. Morton's Salt became "health salt," bringing "new health and vigor to countless thousands of youngsters.[21] Welch's Grape Juice, which consisted mainly of enormous amounts of sugars, advertised itself as "Rich in Health Values," containing vitamins, mineral salts, and "the laxative properties you cannot do without."[22] Even manufacturers of chocolate bars touted their products as vitamin-packed.[23]

Sunkist lemons exploited one of Elmer McCollum's less fortunate "discoveries": that there must be a balance between acid-forming and alkaline-forming foods in the diet. Its advertisements warned against "acidosis" caused by "eating freely of such good and necessary foods as cereals, bread, fish, eggs, and meats—all of which are of the *acid-forming* type—without sufficient fruit, vegetables, and milk (alkaline reaction foods) to balance them." There was a "seeming paradox": that although called "acid fruits," citrus fruits created an alkaline reaction in the body. An accompanying cartoon showed the president of a company lamenting the failure of one of his underlings to "get ahead." Despite his apparent intelligence

and diligence, he somehow lacked "punch." The manager had a ready
diagnosis and the remedy: "Doctors call it Acidosis. Oranges and lemons
would do him a world of good—as they have for me."[24] The campaign
found ready support among nutritionists and home economists in colleges
and universities as well as in the Bureau of Home Economics in Washington, who, convinced by anything McCollum said, helped create a
national vogue for oranges, grapefruits, and lemons. Further ammunition
for the campaign was provided by the "discovery" that orange juice was
nature's remedy for tooth decay.[25]

The milk industry demonstrated that, in the hands of the new commercial forces using the latest promotional techniques, the Newer Nutrition
could be a major force in shaping food habits. There, a number of powerful interests managed to use conclusions derived from McCollum's photographs of fat and scrawny mice to have milk, previously regarded as
necessary for infants but merely a refreshing beverage for children and
adults, come to be seen as an essential drink for all.

The process of concentration of control over milk distribution accelerated in the 1920s. Giant holding companies such as National Dairy Products (Sealtest) and Borden's used exchanges of stock, leverage, pyramid-
ing, and the other new devices of the corporate finance markets to come
to dominate milk distribution in most major cities.[26] In one week alone,
Borden's purchased fifty-two concerns.[27]

The giant milk distributors formed a national organization to inform the
public of milk's nutritional value, inundating the schools with posters,
pamphlets, and lesson outlines. Pictures of healthy children sipping their
daily quart of milk (the recommended dose) smiled from the newspapers
and magazines of the nation.[28] In New York, Pennsylvania, and the midwestern states, powerful Dairymen's Leagues joined with milk distributors
to encourage state departments of agriculture to study and propogate the
good word about milk's healthful properties.

Fast-growing companies specializing in additives that they claimed made
milk more palatable to children also helped. Thompson's "Double Malt-
ed" milk promised to make "Little Milk Rebels" who wouldn't touch the
"most important single food for a child" change their tune.[29] According to
Walter Baker and Company, doctors prescribed cocoa to get children "to
take good milk regularly" and 80 percent of childrens' doctors interviewed
gave their own children Baker's Cocoa (which also contained "indispensable food elements in excellent proportions").[30] Cocomalt played
unabashedly on the new child-centeredness:

> So many things you do for them, . . . which will count most in the years to
> come. . . . So many little garments to be mended . . . so many childish faults
> to overcome . . . so many difficulties to be smoothed away. . . . How you
> work and plan for them, those children of yours—how *much* you try to do!
> But most of all you think about safeguarding their health. . . . Like most

modern mothers you know a great deal about the essential elements of the well-balanced diet. You know how valuable a food is milk.[31]

Baker's was not to be outdone in exploiting the child health vogue: the American Child Health Association had just pointed out that "average health is not enough to aim at for children." "Optimal Health . . . the highest physical ideal of childhood" must now be the goal. "Nurses, domestic science teachers, women's magazine editors, and home demonstration agents" all seemed to prefer Baker's Cocoa as a ladder to reach this new level.[32]

Advertisements such as these, along with a tremendous amount of propaganda in the schools, helped milk producers and distributors reverse the trend toward reduced per capita consumption of milk which seemed to prevail after 1909. It may or may not be coincidental that a bottom was reached in 1914, 1915, and 1916, just as milk's miraculous properties were being discovered. After that, consumption of milk and milk products rose steadily, reaching a new high of over 800 pounds per capita in 1925.[33]

One argument for eating "protective foods" generally ignored by advertisers was that many of the original nutrients had been lost in processing. McCollum made this point a number of times during the 1920s, particularly with regard to white flour and sugar. White flour was the most important energy food in the American diet, he wrote, yet "it is notably deficient in more dietary factors than any other food entering into the diet, except sugars, starches, and fats which are sold in the pure state." While there could be no objection to eating "certain quantities" of white flour and white sugar, he said it was particularly necessary that they be supplemented by sufficient quantities of milk, eggs, leafy vegetables, and meats.[34] "The American public has been educated to like white bread and white flour by skillful advertising," he said.[35]

Shortly after writing this condemnation, McCollum signed on as a nutrition consultant to General Mills and became a spokesman for the virtues of white flour. In the early 1930s he lent his name to advertisements emphasizing the "wholesomeness" of white wheat flour and (along with fellow vitamin-scientist Lafayette Mendel) joined a group of Hollywood stars organized by "Betty Crocker" to testify to the importance of white bread in maintaining healthy diets. He then appeared before a congressional committee to condemn "the pernicious teachings of food faddists who have sought to make people afraid of white-flour bread."[36]

McCollum's support of the flour manufacturers was typical of the larger nexus which developed between nutritional science and food processors and producers. In the prewar era the New Nutritionists looked to government, rather than to business, to support nutrition research, seeking aid from businessmen only in their roles as philanthropists. The governments, universities, and foundations they worked for were all at one remove, at least, from the food businesses. They used school systems, governments, and women's organizations to propogate their ideas and expected little in this regard from the food businesses. The atmosphere of the 1920s was much different. In place of suspicion, the rise of big business now engendered admiration, and the growth of the food industries provided new opportunities for employment and funding for research.

Home economists no longer depended only on schools or government for jobs. Food processors now hired hundreds to develop recipes using their products, demonstrate them, and give testimonials to their nutritive value. The membership and orientation of the American Home Economics Association came to reflect this. In 1924 it created a Home Economics in Business Department which specialized in making available to home economists in the schools the "educational material" produced by home economists in food corporations. Its scholarly journal, the *Journal of Home Economics,* became an important vehicle for food advertisers, and in 1926 it opened its convention floor to commercial exhibits and invited "*Journal* advertisers and other desirable manufacturers" to participate. By the end of the decade, over 30 percent of the organization's budget came from the food and appliance advertisements in its journal.[37]

Whether or not they worked directly for food corporations, the home economists' message was influenced by the newly ascendant business civilization. This was reflected in its shifting emphasis from the importance of production to the importance of consumption. Whereas prewar home economists concerned themselves primarily with the production of materials in the home, postwar specialists saw the modern world as one where efficient business methods had finally brought most production processes out of the home. Therefore their prime consideration was to train women in consumption, rather than production. "Most of us are becoming more and more convinced that a principal function of home economics instruction is to train for the wise selection of and utilization of household goods," said an editorial in the *Journal of Home Economics*. The field was becoming "the science of ultimate consumption."[38]

Much of the material sent out to the schools by food firms' home economists emphasized two interrelated themes: the nutritive values of the foods being promoted and possibilities they presented for attractive presentation. Eye appeal was regarded as important because so much of the struggle to have people eat what was good for them, rather than what they liked, involved persuading people to eat things such as canned spinach, whose taste was not widely appreciated. Home economists in the schools were provided with an enormous amount of free literature and graphic material for teaching about the new and old nutrients. As a result, millions of schoolgirls (and many schoolboys subjected to classes in "Health") learned of the importance of the iron in spinach (these were the pre-Popeye years), the calcium in milk, the existence of vitamins, and so on. Those who missed the lessons in elementary school imbibed it in high school, as the proportion of teen-agers attending secondary schools expanded rapidly.

Here and there offbeat events signified the rising status of home economics. In the mid-1920s, the National Committee on Prisons and Prison Labor demanded that home economics be taught in women's prisons and reformatories. As a result of its efforts, no one was declared eligible for parole from the Indiana Girls School in Indianapolis until she had passed a domestic science course.[39]

As their status rose in a society concerned mainly with what William Leuchtenburg called the "perils of prosperity," home economists, nutritional scientists, and dietitians lost much of their prewar interest in the poor. In the early 1920s, the malnutrition scares disappeared more rapidly than they had begun. In part, this was the result of the new social and political attitude of the time, which became one of celebration, rather than criticism, of the economy's achievements. However, while not more relevant to the rich than to the poor, the message of the Newer Nutrition, with its focus on health rather than on economy, also played a role.

While home economists and nutritionists evinced a new enthusiasm for the health benefits of milk, fruits, vegetables, and other "protective foods," they displayed little flexibility when it came to adopting new ways of cooking and spicing. The cooking they taught remained resolutely Anglo-Saxon in origin, reflecting none of the ethnic mosaic that America had become. Although interest in specialized programs for changing ethnic diets declined, particularly after the Immigration Act of 1924 effectively cut off immigration from southern and eastern Europe, home economics teaching remained an integral part of the "Americanization" process. "To the average nutritionist," said Lydia Roberts, "the only adequate diet is the conventional American one, and any diet that departs from this is regarded as hopelessly faulty."[40]

Among the more absurd examples of the persistence of the earlier tradition of teaching "Americanization through Homemaking" was a course in southern California designed to teach Mexican-American girls "both homemaking and citizenship." Its director warned that malnourishment not only led Mexicans into lives of thievery but it also contributed to revolutionary tendencies. It was therefore necessary to teach them the basics of the New and Newer Nutritions in the Anglo-Saxon cooking manner. A prime objective was to convince them to abandon the traditional Mexican sauces (whose tomatoes and chiles provided vitamins and whose nuts and cheese provided protein, calcium, and vitamins), in favor of only two sauces: White Sauce, consisting of flour, butter and milk, and Hard Sauce, mainly sugar and butter.[41]

Other Americanizers, however, became attuned to the needs of corpo-

rate America. Winifred Gibbs, who before the war taught home economists to Americanize immigrant diets, now became a freelance endorser
and, billing herself a "Consulting Home Economist," tried to adapt home
economics themes to the needs of food processors.[42] Whereas before the
war she had devised schemes to convince Italian immigrants to abandon
their pasta-centered diets, in the 1920s she told macaroni manufacturers
how the Newer Nutrition demonstrated the economy and healthfulness of
their product.[43]

Mutually beneficial relationships developed between the food industries and "pure" nutritional researchers, such as McCollum, and helped
establish the path for future American nutritional research. The discoveries of the first vitamins led to a frantic search for other vitamins and their
relationship to disease, particularly cancer. This, of course, was due mainly
to the nature of the discoveries themselves, and the new scientific frontiers they seemed to open. However, by the late 1920s, business interests
were also a factor because studies which indicated that processing
deprived certain foods of vitamins and minerals led to the desire to learn
how to add these nutrients to foods. Food manufacturers therefore funded
research into how processed foods could be reinvigorated, as it were, by
adding nutrients. Moreover, the discovery that iron was important to
human health and the widespread belief that copper was healthful as well
led the producers of other minerals, such as manganese, phosphate,
nickel, and iodine to fund research into the beneficial properties of their
products.[44]

The University of Wisconsin set the pace for this kind of research. The
university's biochemists built a powerful research empire, mainly by having food companies fund graduate students in return for studies of the
(they hoped healthful) properties of their foods. Wisconsin granted 140
Ph.D.s in biochemistry between the wars, far more than any other university, and helped bias nutritional research in the United States toward the
commercial needs of the food industries. Typically, when Wisconsin biochemists working for the milk industry developed a process for infusing
pasteurized milk with vitamin D through irradiation, an elaborate scheme
was concocted to prevent the process from falling into the hands of the
rival oleo-margarine industry.[45]

The postwar era saw a great increase in the number and circulation of
women's magazines. Unlike the prewar era, advertising and the revenue
from it now played an all-important role in them, and much of it came
from food processors. Not only did this discourage hints that certain kinds
of processing might rob foods of nutrients, it led to a tendency to portray
the food industries as bringing more nutritious food to the people. "There
is an extraordinary ferment of activity among progressive food men, a
sensitiveness to new needs, a desire to live up to the newer knowledge of

Nutrition," said a typical *Ladies Home Journal* article on the wonders of modern food processing.[46]

Food, nutrition, and health were popular themes in these magazines, and they and the women's sections of newspapers had stables of experts whose articles explored the mysteries of the Newer Nutrition, suitably packaged to avoid offending food advertisers. Although American physicians, oriented toward curing rather than preventing illness, knew little about nutrition, a woman's magazine was not complete unless it had at least one M.D. dispensing advice on diet. Due to McCollum's readable *Newer Knowledge of Nutrition,* the doctors were able to write as if they were on the cutting edge of science and emphasize the importance of vitamins and minerals to good health. "The physicians in their practice, dietitians in their kitchens, chemists in their laboratories and manufacturers in their factories, all are constantly learning more about food," said a typical physician summarizing McCollum's ideas.[47]

The bow to the nutritional contribution of food manufacturers was typical. Even prewar pure food crusader Dr. Harvey Wiley, who became the health columnist of *Good Housekeeping* magazine, the largest-circulation women's magazine of the decade, accommodated himself to their new supremacy. At first, the emerging discoveries of the Newer Nutrition fed his suspicions of processed foods by indicating that processing robbed foods of vitamins. At the end of World War I, he declared himself optimistic about the future of the American diet because the wartime lesson that the "wholesome" foods were those which were "simple and as near to nature as possible" would inaugurate a new era of simple cooking and less processing.[48] Alas for Wiley, within a few years his magazine had worked out tie-ins with its advertisers whereby their products were given the "Good Housekeeping Seal of Approval," attesting to the endorsement of their claims by experts on its staff. This meant that Wiley's *imprimatur* was soon being given to Jell-O and all sorts of other foods of dubious nutritional value. "You may safely rely on those articles of food which are advertised in GOOD HOUSEKEEPING," he assured readers in 1928. "Only those foods which have been fully investigated and found to be worthy are admitted to GOOD HOUSEKEEPING advertising columns." These included Fleischmann's and similar distorters of scientific evidence, and products such as Cream of Wheat, which tried to turn its lack of nutrients and fiber to advantage by proclaiming that its digestibility was the result of containing "none of the harsh, indigestible parts of the grain."[49]

The commercial media and their advertisers were not the only ones promoting the Newer Nutrition. Many public and other private forces had important roles as well. Pamphlets and circulars on nutrition were churned out by the U.S. Public Health Service, state agricultural and health departments, and boards of education. American Red Cross chapters in twenty-three states hired nutritionists to give courses in nutrition and food selection;[50] private charities hired dietitians to teach the poor; the National Catholic Welfare Conference even published its own book on food and nutrition.[51]

By the time of the Great Depression, the basic ideas of the Newer Nutrition—that vitamins and minerals were essential to stimulating growth, protecting good health, and even prolonging life—prevailed in middle-class America. To a great extent, the rapid dissemination of these ideas was due to a remarkable confluence of interests which made these ideas useful to businesses struggling to sell food. These commercial forces managed to shape the message to suit their own needs, enlisting the aid of many of the most influential groups in America: the media, the educational systems, and the scientific establishment. Clearly, their efforts had an enormous effect on the American diet. However, they would have had much less impact had important social changes not made Americans particularly receptive to these new concepts. It is to these changes which we now turn.

CHAPTER 13

A Revolution
of Declining Expectations

The crisis in the middle-class kitchen occasioned by the servant shortage, the scientific approach to food and eating purveyed by middle-class food reformers and home economists, and the wartime food conservation campaign were all important factors in changing the way Americans ate, and prepared the middle classes for the messages of both the New and Newer Nutrition in the 1920s.

However, changes in the female labor force, women's role in the family, and relations between the sexes also spurred dietary change. It was not so much the steady increase in the number of women working outside the home as the shifts in the kinds of jobs they held which made a difference. From 1910 to 1930 the service industries expanded and the steady march of bureaucratization created thousands of new, white-collar jobs for women, particularly native-born white women. While the number of women in the manufacturing industries increased only slightly in the 1910s and 1920s, those in the clerical service and professional service categories rose spectacularly. By 1929 the "office girl" had overtaken the "factory girl" as the number of females in clerical jobs alone passed the total of those in manufacturing and moved into second place among the Census Bureau categories.[1]

Although there was little change over the two decades in the proportion of female workers in the top category, "domestic and personal service" (about one-third of the total), there was a dramatic decline in the propor-

161

tion of those who "lived in." By 1920, almost one-half of the domestic servants were living in their own home, a substantial increase from 1900, when only one-third did, and the ensuing ten years saw the acceleration of this process, particularly outside the South.[2] By the mid-1920s, the "servant crisis" was being solved much in the way Edward Bellamy had forecast: with the disappearance of the live-in servant from the middle-class home and her replacement by the "cleaning woman."[3]

The virtual disappearance of the live-in servant from middle-class homes affected and reflected changed eating habits. While "cleaning women" may have taken over the house cleaning, laundering, and even child-care duties of the ex-live-in servants, food preparation was usually a casualty of the new arrangements. This was by no means accidental, for the prewar complaints about servants had centered, not on their cleaning, child care, or other abilities but on their incompetence with food. The fact is that the postwar middle class solved the servant problem by lowering its expectations regarding servants, particularly with regard to food. Significantly, the declining expectations regarding food were not accompanied by a lowering of other household standards, which continued to rise, as did standards of personal cleanliness and dress. In part this was because new household technology, including cleaner gas and electric stoves, made higher standards of cleanliness attainable in the 1920s.[4]

Middle-class interest in cooking did decline. It is interesting that while the 1920s were, in the words of one historian of women, "a period of rising expectations with regard to standard of living, an increased emphasis on consumption, and a new definition of economic need"[5] this did not seem to apply to their kitchens and dining rooms. Sumptuous dinner parties no longer held center stage in middle-class socializing, replaced, in part, by bridge, mah-jongg, dancing, and other parties. When the middle class did entertain at dinner, guests' expectations were markedly lower than in the prewar era, for it was understood that meals were prepared by otherwise busy women with no "help" in the kitchen. Needless to say, Middletown's competitive dinner clubs became lost in memories of prewar days.

The traditional role of food-sharing in reinforcing family solidarity and establishing lines of authority also declined in the face of competing loyalties to peer groups and, most important, to the new leisure activities. To "eat and run" became acceptable family behavior, as did family members eating at different times to accommodate their other social obligations. "It's getting so that a fellow has to make a date with his family to see them," said one middle-class Muncie father.[6] While this kind of sporadic, *a cappela* eating was ill-suited to the services of a live-in cook, housewives, who wanted to get on with their own leisure activities, could deal with this by using canned, processed, and prepared foods. However, despite advertisers claims to the contrary, it was generally recognized that this involved reduced expectations regarding the quality of food.

Contemporary observers often remarked on the decline in attention paid to cooking by middle-class women and read various meanings into it. One social scientist who noted the shrinking size of kitchens in new housing and the abandonment of real kitchens in apartment buildings in favor of tiny "kitchenettes" saw these as the result of an inevitable movement of the family's productive functions outside the home.[7] Others thought improved technology, in the form of better stoves, electric appliances, canned goods, and other prepared foods had so reduced the amount of time and effort which needed be devoted to food preparation that women could spend less time in the kitchen and yet produce essentially the same results as before. This idea was particularly popular in women's magazines which promoted the new products. "Every day sees some ingenious new wrinkle devised to lessen labor," enthused a typical article on the "Grocery Revolution" in the *Ladies Home Journal.* "You don't have to clean up tea grounds; tea comes in individual bags, made possible by new packaging machinery . . . You don't have to prepare the morning grapefruit any more; if you wish you can get all the meat of the grapefruit in cans or glass containers ready for the hurried commuter's breakfast. . . . Ten years ago every woman made her own mayonnaise. Now almost every woman buys it in a jar. There are few things except soft-boiled eggs that you can't buy almost ready to eat today.[8]

But paeans such as this neglected the fact that grapefruit in the can was cooked, not fresh, the sweet "mayonnaise" in the jar bore little resemblance to the real thing and readiness to accept canned and other prepared foods normally represented a conscious lowering of culinary standards. Housewives themselves recognized this. A 1926 Department of Commerce survey showed an overwhelming preference among consumers for fresh rather than canned goods in terms of flavor. Over half of those surveyed also believed that fresh products had higher food values. There was 100 percent agreement, however, that canned goods were more convenient.[9] Clearly, behind the soaring sales of canned and other prepared foods in the 1920s were millions of individual decisions to sacrifice taste, and even nutrition, in order to lessen preparation time.

More perceptive observers thus saw the diminution in the time devoted to food as linked to broader changes in family life. The Lynds thought that cooking occupied a much less important place in the life of the middle class of Muncie, Indiana, in the 1920s than in the 1890s, that preparation was much less elaborate and more rushed, to allow more time for proliferating social activities outside the home. "I only ate seven meals at home all last week," said one father, "and three of those were on Sunday." The lure of the automobile on pleasant days often curtailed the evening meals which were taken at home into informal "bites."[10]

Christine Frederick, a contemporary home economist and marketing consultant, also thought the decline in time, effort, and interest devoted to middle-class cooking was the result of competing activities. In the nineteenth century, grandmother cooked to pass the time, she wrote. She did not have such things as radio and movies to compete for her attention. Frederick recalled that even with six black servants at her disposal her own mother spent hours in the kitchen, hovering over her fruit cakes and other specialties. Now, she pointed out, not only did the servants have outside jobs, so did the daughters who had previously stayed home to help. There was more interest in cooking and cooking lessons in small towns than in larger cities, said Frederick, because there was less competition from other leisure activities.[11] Those promoting canned and processed foods recognized this early on. In 1919, *Good Housekeeping* advised that canned goods were particularly useful in the summer because "every housewife finds the summer months busy with social and other activities which require more of her time."[12]

The increased emphasis on leisure activities was also part of a larger, more subtle change in the nature of middle-class marriage. The social segregation of the sexes was breaking down as companionate marriage became the universal middle-class ideal. Increasingly during the previous hundred-odd years the idea that happily married couples must be chums who share a variety of outside interests and mutual sexual attraction challenged older conceptions which saw husband and wife as playing separate but complementary roles in marriage's all-important function: the raising of a family. Ideally, husbands and wives now constituted "a couple" who participated jointly in leisure-time activities: listening to records and the radio, going to the movies, for automobile rides, and to "parties," where they danced and even drank together in the company of other couples. Frank G. Shattuck made a fortune out of the middle-class loss of interest in cooking by promoting his chain of Schrafft's restaurants as places where one could get the "home cooking" which mothers no longer had the inclination to cook. "When I talk about the pies mother used to make, it means something that is really excellent. Mothers today do not make such pies. They aren't particularly interested in pies. Their time is taken up with other things—movies, bridge parties, automobile rides. A young man contemplating marriage no longer asks whether a girl is a good cook; he wants to know whether she is a good sport."[13]

"From the Nursery to the Bedroom" is the label that one writer has given to the decade's increased emphasis on wives as sexual partners. However, given the era's high expectations regarding motherhood, "From the Kitchen to the Bedroom" would be more apt. As with so many of the phenomena we associate with the 1920s, the idea that mutual sexual attraction was important in marriage became well established even before the war. So was an appreciation for slimmer bodies. Concern regarding the physical fitness of American women rose in the late nineteenth century, when physicians and educators began to take more seriously feminist critiques of the dire physical effects of chain-mail corsetry and shut-in pallor. Consequently, women were encouraged to take mild physical exercise such as bicycling, tennis, and swimming, particularly outdoors. Since it was virtually impossible to indulge in such activities in the voluminous clothes of the time, lighter and simpler fashions that allowed more physical movement became acceptable. Also, as upper- and middle-class women went out more to shop and socialize the bulky long dresses which swept up dirt and manure from sidewalks and roads became intolerable. The increased number of women working in offices and stores after 1910 also demanded less burdensome attire, and fashion moved away from the heavyweight materials and constricting corsetry of the past. By the 1910s, they had freed themselves from the most burdensome of the clothes, although prewar shop and office girls were still expected to dress demurely in long black dresses with white shirtwaists and black ties. By 1920, even these restrictions had broken down and the ladies' ready-to-wear clothing industry began to take off, specializing in relatively simple, colorful clothing and undergarments for the growing middle- and working-class market. Although "girdles" were still used, these relatively inexpensive clothes generally followed the natural lines of the uncorseted body.

At the same time, the conceptions of what were the natural lines of an ideal body changed dramatically. The large-bosomed, massive-hipped "voluptuous" woman of the Lillian Russell type was challenged after the turn of the century by less robust but more athletic-looking ideals such as the drawings of the "Gibson Girl": amply but not massively endowed upstairs, slim-hipped, with a small waist which seemed to owe much more to one of nature's miracles than to the high technology of corsetry. After the war, she was replaced by more nymph-like ideals, bordering on the boyish, whose most extreme version was the "Flapper." The ever-shortening skirt lengths of the period drew attention to the shape and thickness of legs, thighs, and even buttocks, parts of the anatomy that prewar women had been able to hide from critical view.

Had these new styles merely affected single girls on the marriage market, the effect on food habits would have been negligible. In earlier times it was not unheard-of for women to starve themselves until marriage and then abandon all concern over bulging bodies as they enjoyed the pleasures of the family, the table, and the sweet shop. But the heightened sexual expectations of middle-class marriage meant that married women now had to engage in a two-front battle against aging (for youthfulness in women was still regarded as sexually attractive) and weight.

The new ideal of slimness affected men as well. Gold watch-chains surmounting gigantic bellies were now signs of age and decrepitude in a society fond of youthful zest for life's pleasures. Gaunt figures such as F. Scott Fitzgerald and the slender Rudolph Valentino now became the male ideals. It is almost inconceivable that after 1920 a man of William Howard

Taft's enormous girth could have been elected to the presidency. (Indeed, since 1913, when the cadaverous Woodrow Wilson replaced Taft, a fat man has not been able to make it to the White House.)[14]

Changing sexual ideals were complimented by new attitudes toward weight and health. Despite the prewar efforts of Chittenden, Fletcher, Kellogg (none of whom was exactly slender) and the activities of Hoover's Food Administration, the old idea that ample weight was a sign of good health had been remarkably resilient. By 1918, however, the idea that being overweight was unhealthy had caught up with the traditional idea that being underweight denoted poor health. This was evident in the still-flourishing world of patent remedies and quack medical literature. Whereas most of the remedies of the previous era had been directed toward curing skinny people, the years from 1917 to 1920 saw overweight and underweight reach a kind of balance in public concern. One author reflected this by offering two different advice books, one entitled *Eat and Grow Fat,* the other called *Eat and Grow Slender.*[15] An advertisement which assured readers of *Good Housekeeping* in 1919 that they could have a "good figure" by subscribing to Susana Cockroft's program reflected the same ambivalence, for Cockroft claimed to have reduced the weight of forty thousand women and raised the weight of forty thousand others.[16]

In her 1919 book, *Diet and Health with Key to the Calories,* the California doctor and woman's magazine writer Lulu Hunt Peters offered advice on both losing and gaining weight. In 1922, however, her emphasis was almost wholly on how to lose weight.[17] By 1923, there was no doubt as to which way the tide was flowing. There was now "a flood of advertised methods of reducing," said an article in the *Woman's Home Companion.* "With the revolution in clothes has come a revolution in our attitude toward avoirdupois," it said. "Once fat was an asset: now it's a liability, both physical and esthetic."[18]

"Dieting" and "calories" now became middle-class obsessions, particularly among females. One writer linked the death of the women's club movement to married women's new mania for losing weight. The women of the day wanted above all to grow slender, he wrote in 1923, an obsession which had drawn them to the tennis court, golf links, and swimming pool rather than to club meetings.[19] "The word "calorie" is as familiar as the word "food" and is heard in conversation at the luncheon table even though socially it should be taboo," said one of the less trendy cookbooks in 1928. Yet even this book began with suggestions regarding sensible dieting.[20]

Concern over excess weight combined with other social forces to drastically reduce the quantity and elaborateness of middle-class food. The result was a victory for the kind of menus and dishes that still form the core of American eating habits: breakfasts built around citrus fruit, dried cereal or eggs and toast, light lunches, usually involving a sandwich of some sort, and dinners consisting of roast or broiled meats with a potato and vegetable garnish and a simple dessert. (The sweet tooth could not be forgone.) Gone were the old concerns about mixing various foods together in the same dish, as Americans discovered the magic of "one-dish dinners" which were sometimes bland versions of European peasant dishes they had so recently despised. "The One-piece Dinner, ladies, is like the One-piece dress," enthused one book on the topic, for they both saved time and motions while the dinner conserved flavor and vitamins. Among the more inventive suggestions was Shepherd's Pie with Marshmallow Crust, a dish which not only combined meat, potatoes, and vegetables, but also included dessert![21]

The great age of the main course salad (fruit, vegetable, or both) now dawned. Encouraged by advertisers, women's magazines and women's pages, and spurred on by the desire for more leisure time, millions of housewives now thought that, armed only with a can opener, some Jell-O, and a bottle of mayonnaise they could create wondrously healthy and easy meals for the family. "In the old days a salad meant a few leaves of indifferent lettuce sprinkled with sugar and vinegar," wrote an enthusiastic Christine Fredericks. "Today, salads are not only used as side courses, but are demanded as a complete meal dish. On every side we hear that vitality, vim, vitamines [sic] and vegetables go hand in hand. Instead of paying $2 a bottle for Dr. Whoosis Bitters for rheumatism or taking Dumb's Kidney Pills for backache, we prefer to buy our blood purifiers at the vegetable stand and the salad counter."[22]

Home economists were particular admirers of these efficient methods of preparing healthy foods, adding admonitions regarding the importance of eye appeal in convincing men and children to eat what was good for them. The result was a vogue for "dainty"-looking composed salads, with multi-colored layers, surrounded by contrasting colored objects and topped off with eye-catching swirls of bottled mayonnaise. The well-known Kansas newspaper editor William Allen White grumbled that the domestic science taught in schools and colleges had hardly helped American cooking at all, "making our cooking decorative, inept, and given to fruit salads, boiled mayonnaise, paper frills, and striped ice cream."[23] Later in the decade, even Frederick, herself a home economist, reacted against the decorative overkill. While restaurants did improve their salads over the course of the decade, she wrote in 1928, they were often "too elaborately concocted, too heavily loaded with mayonnaise, too full of feminine frills. I want food, flavored food and not millinery!"[24]

One of the chores of turn-of-the-century housewives had been planning weekly menus and ensuring that the necessary materials were at hand. Now, the amount of foresight and planning devoted to cooking diminished and cookbooks catered, not only to those who had not planned but to those who had not shopped as well. "Emergency" substitutes for ingre-

dients which themselves were substitutes for the real thing abounded.
Perhaps the *reductio ad absurdum* of this was a recipe for "Emergency
Cream of Tomato Soup" for use when a can of that already *sine qua non* of
"emergency" foods was not available: one cup of diluted thin cream or
condensed milk to which three tablespoons of catsup were added.[25]

Prohibition also had an impact on middle-class cooking. By making
cooking with wine taboo in public and expensive in private it helped
eliminate the French style of cooking's tenuous foothold in the prewar
middle-class kitchen. The recipes for French dishes which survived in
middle-class cookbooks became charades of their former selves: wineless
"Chicken Bordelaise," and Chicken Marengo which was merely chicken in
tomato sauce.[26] A Teachers' College instructor even published a book
entitled *French Home Cooking,* which managed to avoid mentioning wine in
any context, not even to note omitting it in many dishes where it would
normally be considered indispensable.[27] Perhaps the saddest case was that
of the French chef who, after twenty years in the kitchens of wealthy
Americans, finally produced a French cookbook for American kitchens,
only to have Prohibition take effect before it could be published. Likely
consumed by despair, he seems to have simply gone through the manuscript glumly striking out "wine" wherever it appeared and substituting
the word "broth."[28]

Not all the middle class was enamored of canned and prepared foods or
chicken in tomato sauce masquerading as French cuisine. There is some
evidence that as one ascended the educational ladder the lessons of the
Newer Nutrition were applied with more dedication and more serious
concern for freshness of fruits and vegetables. Perhaps the pinnacle in this
respect was represented by twelve "professional" or "well-educated" families, nine of whom were headed by professors, surveyed in Berkeley,
California, in 1927. The surveyors (home economists, of course) concluded that "this group with some dietetical knowledge approached more
closely to the standards of an adequate, balanced diet than any other
American group studied. . . . The Berkeley diet emphasized fresh vegetables and fruits, especially the leafy and citrus varieties, milk products, and
eggs, in contrast to the average urban diet which substituted the cheaper
cereals and potatoes and spent relatively more for meat. The extraordinary
amount of fresh fruits and vegetables were especially noteworthy. Beef
and lamb were the common meats used and the amount of pork consumed
was low compared to the amount reported in other studies. Canned soup,
fish, vegetables, and canned and dried fruit were the only types of prepared food used to any appreciable extent and of these items only the last
was of real importance in the diet. The meals served were charac-
teristically American and simple, the dinner limited to two courses."[29]
Clearly, although tofu, alfalfa sprouts, and wheat germ are absent, and the

red meat might add a jarring note, it was not a diet which would be utterly condemned in Berkeley today.

Like their present-day counterparts in the Bay Area, this small group of Berkeley families were obviously very nutrition-conscious. More significant, however, was a statistic that emerged from a study of larger group of "professional" families in Berkeley that same year: that they spent only 16 percent of their income on food. Indeed, in dollars, the average Berkeley family spent considerably less on food than a sample of 819 New York City families of the same class surveyed seven years earlier, in 1920, even though the New Yorkers' incomes averaged less than half that of the Californians.[30] It would seem that for these well-off Californians food was simply not an important item of expenditure or concern, and simple, relatively light meals had become the norm for them as well.

The trend toward lighter, simpler fare was also evident in public occasions, which saw the virtual demise of the grand old multi-tiered banquet menu. The contrast between the prewar banquets and the one given in 1927 by the Mayor of Boston to honor Charles Lindbergh for his heroic transatlantic flight could hardly have been greater. The Lone Eagle was treated to fruit cocktail, filet of sole with tartare sauce, roast chicken with potatoes and peas, lettuce salad with Roquefort dressing, ice cream, cake and coffee.[31] How fitting it was that the all-American hero should be served what (without the fish course) had become the all-American dinner! This roast or broiled chicken dinner with french fries and canned peas which countless hapless politicians, convention-goers, and travelers faced in countless dining halls in America over the next five decades became the standard in the early years of the decade. The Menu Collection of the New York Public Library also contains a menu for the Franklin Bicentennial Dinner of the New York Club of Printing House Craftsmen in January 1923. The broiled chicken, french fries, and canned green peas dinner could be enshrined as a classic. Not only does it contain that mainstay of the next thirty years, Mock Turtle Soup, but it also begins with a grapefruit half (garnished, one presumes with a red marischino cherry). Only the presence of pineapple salad (the popularity of pineapple verged on a craze in 1923) dims its luster as a perfect prototype.[32]

Some simple menus became virtual national dinners for home entertaining as well, surviving, with remarkably few changes, to become familiar to almost any middle-class person who ever entertained at dinner or was invited to one during the next fifty years. How often have Americans eaten virtual replicas of the Dinner for Six in a 1927 middle-class cookbook: shrimp cocktail, vegetable soup, roast beef, Yorkshire pudding, roast potatoes, stuffed tomatoes, string beans, and Peach Selma![33]

Nation-wide forces were at work in fashioning the new way of cooking and eating. The women's magazines from which so many of the recipes derived were national magazines, and much of the editorial content of the women's pages of the dailies was wire-service copy, produced in a few major centers. The millions of free recipe pamphlets emitted by the giant food processors were distributed nationally, encouraging the housewife in Arkansas to cook her Armour ham or use her Del Monte canned pineapple in the same way as her counterpart in Vermont. Betty Crocker did not teach shortcuts in making hominy grits and Kraft did not encourage the use of New Mexico chiles with its cheese dishes. The result was the further nationalizing of American eating habits and the strengthening of the food tastes of British origin which had always rested at the core of middle-class food habits. The surviving local and regional culinary traditions were being pushed in the same direction as the cooking of the first generation of European immigrants: to the ritual "Sunday" (or less frequent) family dinner and the occasional festive event.

The nationalization of food habits was reflected in restaurant fare as well, and regional cuisine was given short shrift in this booming industry. "I have eaten in Florence, Alabama, in Logan, Utah, in Mansfield, Ohio, and Penobscot, Maine," wrote Christine Frederick in a restaurateurs' trade journal in 1928. "Is there any difference in the meals served in one locality from another? No. The customer will always sit down to the same old steak, or canned beans, bottled catsup, French fried or Adam and Eve on a raft. Where, I ask you, is the sweet potato pone of Maryland for a slice of which General Lee would walk a mile? Where is the genuine clam chowder of New England? Gone, or rapidly disappearing under . . . an absolutely false effort of the restaurateur to standardize his food."[34]

In early 1931, a restaurant trade journal tried to be more positive, constructing a profile of what was now the national cuisine by polling 115 food specialists on the question "What do guests mean when they say American Cookery?" Although the magazine tried to put the best face on it, for those who preferred prewar food habits or who relished zesty regional cooking, the composite response to the survey which it constructed must have been rather depressing: "American cooking is simplified cooking—cooking that brings out the original flavor of foods and does not alter flavor with rich sauces and seasonings. It is food served with limited amounts of garnishing and fancy trimmings. American cooking includes the use of many vegetables and fruits and is always a well balanced dietetic combination of foods."[35]

Of course, regional cooking traditions did not vanish. Indeed, after the editorial, "What Is an American Dinner?," which commented on protests from proponents of various regional cuisines over the supposedly typical American dinner served to David Lloyd George at the Waldorf hotel, the *Nation* commissioned a number of them to write of a "home dinner typical of their section of the country."[36] The results were generally as varied as they were mouth-watering. H. L. Mencken, an avid gourmand, wrote of Chesapeake Bay oysters, terrapin Maryland style, and roast wild duck. A New Englander extolled broiled scrod or codfish tongues for breakfast, doughnuts and coffee, "boiled dinners," and fish chowder, as well as a meal of baked beans, spare ribs, potatoes, biscuits, pumpkin and apple pies, Indian pudding, and tea. A Tennessee correspondent contributed a menu for a succulent fried chicken dinner, with boiled ham, sweet potatoes, butter beans, okra, tomatoes, hot biscuits, and a big bowl of gravy on the side. The *Nation* man in New Orleans described two kinds of meals: the first (of the kind served "in the home of a prominent Creole family" by a "sepia-toned old Senegambian" who "yassahs and 'scuses-me's in the best tradition") was very much the New Orleans adaptation of French cuisine: oysters, consommé or crayfish bisque, *pâté de foie gras, filet mignon bordelaise* or mallard and stuffed eggplant or veal roast and candied yams, watercress salad, and so on. A simpler "mother's" meal revolved around what was in season, and comprised an impressive list, including some local specialties such as gumbo, corn fritters, red beans, and cow peas, but most of it is not particularly distinctive to Louisiana. The Alabama contributor got much more to the heart of traditional Southern cooking, also presenting two menus: one of typical dinner of a black field or furnace hand and a white mill hand or mountaineer, which he said would be about the same. It consisted of sow-belly (fat pork), turnip greens, and pot liquor (the water in which the greens are cooked), string beans, snap beans, boiled onions or another in-season vegetable, corn pone, and coffee with "long sweetening" or molasses. The second menu, for more prosperous families, white and black, would have been a fried-chicken dinner not dissimilar from the one suggested for Tennessee. Other contributors put in a word for roast pork and sauerkraut from Pennsylvania and the *tortillas, frijoles,* and *chiles* of New Mexico.

But even amidst the praise for local specialties, it was clear that regional cooking was fast disappearing. Kansas newspaper editor William Allen White pointed out that there was indeed such a thing as American cooking. Although "American cooking is in general bad—both public and private," he wrote, "in every town and village there is at least one righteous woman who can cook." American cooking was seasonal, he said: fried or broiled spring chicken was accompanied first by strawberry shortcake, then by corn on the cob, blackberry cobbler, or green apple dumpling. "When young chickens become passé, turkey appears with its trimming; and then pie—pumpkin pie, apple pie, or mince pie . . . and the glacé sweet potato, the parsnip, and the rutabaga." However, said White, these were company dinners. The "most American of our dishes" was the beefsteak. "It is one of the things which may be found in American homes served better than in public. . . . No other nation knows it—this big, thick, rare, four-pound T-bone steak. . . . It is not regional. It is as accessible in Seattle as in Palm Beach. A good beefsteak is the same on every American table."

Even some of the authors extolling regional cooking conceded that these culinary traditions were verging on extinction. Mencken's Maryland dinners "are now only dreams," he lamented. "Prohibition has extinguished them, save in the homes of profiteers. Even the profiteers, alas, can't bring back the past. The Chesapeake Bay oyster has been going downhill for a dozen years past, canvas-back ducks have become extremely scarce, and genuine diamond-back terrapins are almost unobtainable. The Marylander today eats the common fodder of the republic. Like all other Americans, he has been ironed out."

E. E. Miller said his ideal Tennessee dinner was "a farm dinner, of course, since city dinners, like cities themselves, trend away from the individual and towards standardization."[37] Yet even as this was being written, in 1923, it was being overtaken by events, for by the end of the decade even this ancient line between rural and urban diets was becoming blurred, and so were many of the old distinctions between the diets of the middle and the working class.

CHAPTER 14

Workers and Farmers During the "Prosperity Decade"

When Edward Atkinson, disappointed by workers' failure to listen to reason and eat economically, declared man an essentially "imitative" animal, he was shifting to a cultural, rather than material, explanation of food habits. This idea that food habits were the products of social and cultural forces rather than material ones based on rational economic and ecological grounds was echoed later by anthropologists. In the 1940s Margaret Mead emphasized the complex interrelationship between food habits and social distinctions, family relationships, and tradition.[1] In the 1960s and 1970s, Claude Lévi-Strauss's "structuralist" analyses of the food habits of primitive tribes, which found deep-rooted universal meanings in various methods of cooking and eating, excited American anthropologists. Some, like Mary Douglas, a transplanted Englishwoman, also emphasized the cultural significance and origins of food habits. Then they met a spirited challenge from Columbia University anthropologist Marvin Harris, who asserted the primacy of "material" factors. He emphasized the essentially rational economic and ecological origins of even such apparently irrational food habits as Aztec cannibalism, Jewish dietary laws, and the supremacy of beef in America.[2]

The story of the transformation of the American middle-class diet could provide evidence to support both approaches. On the one hand, the emergence of the new food habits would have been inconceivable without the post-1870 changes in "material" areas such as the production, trans-

173

portation, processing, financing and marketing of food. Yet non-material (Harris somewhat misleadingly labels them "idealist") considerations such as conspicuous consumption, class emulation, a love affair with science and technology, health fads, patriotism, and fashion were also of great importance.

The limitations of a one-sided emphasis on either factor are exemplified in the attempt by Harris and Eric B. Ross to ascribe the American love affair with beef to the circumstances surrounding the rise of the large-scale beef-production industry after 1870. By concentrating mainly on the role of the cattle companies and the packers in promoting the consumption of beef over pork they downplay the high status of beef earlier in the century, even when pork was the most commonly eaten meat. They also neglect the historically high status of beef in the British and other European cultures whose food habits form the core of American ones.[3]

On the other hand, to search for the kind of "meaning" of American food habits which the Lévi-Strauss and Douglas approach looks for is to search for wills-o'-the-wisp. As Douglas herself points out, Lévi-Strauss's generalizations are essentially unprovable, and as Harris has pointed out, so are hers.[4]

Part of the problem seems to lie in the thicket created by the Marxist concept of "material" forces and the imbroglio over "structure" and "superstructure" into which this concept almost inevitably leads. When one tries to classify factors such as the "servant shortage" (an economic problem created by cultural aspirations) or vitamin-consciousness (rational concerns fostered by irrational advertising) as either material or mental/cultural the concepts themselves begin to seem very fragile. Nevertheless, when it comes to analyzing the changes which occurred in the diets of workers and farmers in the years after about 1915, the concepts are of some use, for here the importance of unalloyed material forces is evident. This in turn raises the question of whether the twentieth-century homogenization of American eating habits was the product of the increasing hegemony of middle-class ideas and values among the other classes or was simply the result of workers and farmers responding to the new culinary opportunities which economic and ecological changes were creating for them.

The answer would seem to be that both forces were at work, but that the latter, economic considerations were of greater importance in influencing workers' diets than those of the middle class. There is some irony in this, for the frustrated Atkinson, Richards, and Abel had ultimately labeled working-class food choices as essentially irrational and thought that only the middle class could be swayed by sound economics and reason. Yet while the middle class was not particularly moved by the strictly economic appeals of the New Nutrition and instead responded readily to irrational considerations of "pride," fashion, and patriotism, new economic equations were stimulating changes in workers' diets.

Wage differentials between skilled and unskilled workers remained wide in the years during and after the war, but the great gap between the living standards of the two main components of the working class, the immigrant unskilled and the native- or northern European-born skilled, narrowed. Immigration was effectively cut off by the war and, after a brief spurt in 1919–20, by Congress. Although cheap labor continued to migrate to the industrial centers from the South, Canada, and Mexico, the pressure for jobs at the bottom which had helped keep the wages of the unskilled low was thereby considerably relieved. From 1914 until 1929, then, the real wages of American workers improved significantly. After little or no increase from 1890 to 1914, from 1914 to 1926 the purchasing power of a week's work by the average worker grew by 20 percent.[5] This was partly the result of relatively cheaper food. While food prices did double from 1916 to mid-1920, they plummeted in the fall of 1920 and leveled off at about 35 percent higher than in 1916. They then fluctuated at about that level for the rest of the decade while wages caught up and then moved ahead.[6]

To some extent workers took advantage of the improved ratio of wages to food prices by spending more on non-food items, but food continued to be of prime importance in workers' expenditures, taking up almost 40 percent of the average worker's family's budgets.[7] The most important changes took place in how the food dollar was allocated and what it bought, for the cost of key items in the worker's budget such as flour, potatoes, and some meats declined substantially or stabilized at a relatively low level. This freed income for more fruits and vegetables, whose prices remained about the same.[8] In 1914, typical families in Chicago's stockyard district (many of whom were immigrants from Eastern Europe) spent a very large proportion of their total family budget, over 25 percent, on baked goods (including flour) and meat. Only 2 percent went for fruit and 4 percent was spent on vegetables, mostly potatoes and cabbage.[9] New York City workers surveyed that same year followed a similar pattern. In 1928, fourteen years later, when New York City workers were again surveyed, marked changes were evident. Although meat consumption remained at the same high level in terms of quantity, a much smaller proportion of the budget was devoted to it and a much larger part went for milk, cheese, fruits, and vegetables. They did eat less flour and cereals, however, and as income increased, the tendency to eat more meat and less grain became more pronounced.[10]

Can the increase in workers' consumption of the "protective" foods which evidently took place be ascribed to their greater affordability or to the impact of the new food ideas which were sweeping the middle classes? An either/or answer seems out of the question. In noting that working-class diets in Muncie became much more varied in the 1920s, particularly with regard to fruits and vegetables, the Lynds credited both factors. First, they said, the increased availability of fresh fruits and vegetables over the winter was eliminating the old distinction between "winter" and "summer" diets. Second, the new ideas on nutrition, spread through home economics courses and women's magazines, were affecting all classes.[11] These cultural influences were part of a nationwide pattern, for now working-class girls were attending the high schools where home economic training was concentrated, and their mothers were reading the women's magazines which before the war had been the exclusive preserve of the middle and upper-middle classes.[12] Mass circulation newspapers with women's pages purveying the latest ideas on nutrition and child-rearing now cultivated a readership among increasingly literate working-class women.

Immigration restriction also spurred the spread of the new ideas by helping to "Americanize" ethnic eating habits. The immigrant communities were now bereft of the infusions of newcomers from the old countries who helped preserve the old ways and were therefore more susceptible to pressures to fit in with the dominant culture around them. Many of these influences came through the children, now growing to maturity amidst home economics courses, school lunch programs, women's magazines, and movies: all of which bred self-consciousness, if not shame, about their old-country food habits.

Also, having put in their years slaving over monstrous stew pots and rolling out dough on kitchen tables, putting up innumerable Mason jars every August and September, many immigrant housewives began to succumb to the lure of Corn Flakes, canned goods, and other prepared "American" foods. Bottled ketchup, mustard, mayonnaise, and even pickles became common in their homes. Jell-O became a favorite dessert, often mixed with canned fruits. Quickly broiled steaks and chops replaced the slow-cooked *gulyashen, cholents,* and pork and cabbage dishes or the rolled and stuffed dough dishes at dinner tables. Crusty dark breads gave way to soft white bread from chain bakeries and sandwiches made from them became lunchtime favorites. Like regional American cooking, old-country cooking was increasingly relegated to Sunday dinners, holidays, and family festivities, to serve as a reminder of common origins and a common past.

Yet by no means did the working classes wholly adopt the new middle-class food habits. For example, working-class people tended to be avid movie-goers who apparently responded positively to the sexual ideals purveyed by the films. Whether it was Theda Bara's slinky, dark, vamp look or Mary Pickford's perky blonde innocence, or the Mediterranean exoticism of Rudolph Valentino, 1920s screen idols normally had figures as slim and boyish as the "flapper" who emerged earlier in the decade as the middle-class ideal. Yet, while they may have admired the same skinny actors and actresses, the working class was not yet secure enough about its food supply to succumb to middle-class calorie-counting and dieting.

These practices were relatively rare among working-class women and practically unheard-of among working-class men. There were few dietary surveys of working-class people during the 1920s, for business civilization was little interested in them, but the 1928 New York City survey indicated that the quantity of food they consumed actually increased, by about two pounds per man per day, over their counterparts' in 1914.[13]

The fact that the majority of working-class Americans seem to have eaten more and better quality food during the 1920s did not mean the end of nutritional deficiencies. As one moved down the working-class income ladder, consumption of "protective" foods and meat protein declined and that of highly refined white bread and starches rose.[14] At least in part as result of this, health problems rose in inverse proportion to income.[15] Moreover, while workers and their families ate more fruits and vegetables, they also ate much more sugar and sweets, likely more than compensating for the drop-off in alcohol consumption which followed Prohibition.[16] As a result, obesity became a working-class problem and helped make hypertension, diabetes, and other related ailments more common among that class than among those above them. It was likely in the 1920s that the traditional cartoon images of the fat bloated rich man and the emaciated worker came to portray, as they do today, quite the reverse of the corporeal norm.

That the working class was not prepared to be as complacent as the middle class about the quantity of its food is understandable. For many workers the "Prosperity Decade" was a time of recurring hardship. At least one in ten workers was unemployed at any given time during the decade, and for a number of years the unemployment rate exceeded 13 percent.[17] With no unemployment insurance to fall back on, bouts of joblessness brought the kind of major cutbacks in family food budgets which discouraged complacency regarding food once the hard patch was traversed. An unemployed Muncie family reported that they had five dollars a week to keep a family of five going. Although they had two children, this meant that they had bought no fresh milk for over a year, using only canned milk. They ate beans and potatoes twice a day and spent only two dollars a week on meat.[18] The long months spent eating mainly bread and potatoes and stretching bits of bony meat into stews did little to undermine atavistic dreams of beefsteak and roast-beef dinners.

Meanwhile, the social problem that would persist for the rest of the century was already emerging: a seemingly permanent urban underclass who shared little in the economic advances of the rest of society. Hundreds of thousands of blacks had been migrating from the rural South to the cities of the industrial North and Midwest. Isolated from white middle-class culture in ghettoes, most had neither the means nor incentive to change their food habits. Like first-generation immigrants from Europe, they tried to preserve old methods of cooking while taking advantage of previously out-of-reach foods. (Some even shunned the gas outlets built into their apartments and persisted in cooking on wood or coal-burning stoves.)[19] But this often meant they altered the salt pork and corn meal diet of the rural South to the northern cities in an unhealthy way, consuming more refined white flour, sweets, and highly processed foods while neglecting milk, fresh vegetables, and other "protective" foods. Many families arrived in the North with mothers as single parents, and many others became single-parent families under the pressure of ghetto life, forcing a high proportion of mothers into jobs as laundresses, domestics, and chambermaids. As a result, although food played an important role in solidifying black mothers' bonds with their children, they had little time for their own kitchens and often fed their families on dried breakfast cereals, sweet snacks, and other nutritionally deficient foods. The resulting nostalgia about the home-cooked meals of the South did little to combat infant mortality rates which were twice that of urban whites.[20]

Inadequate, indeed, unhealthy diets were not uncommon in rural America either. The "three M's" diet persisted in many parts of the rural South and outbreaks of pellagra plagued the region. Although its connection with deficiencies of milk and others forms of the B vitamins was becoming apparent, tenants and sharecroppers tied to the production of cash crops still found it impossible to diversify and improve their diets. Dr. Joseph Golberger, the man whose research ultimately pinpointed the economic and social origins of the disease, called "King Cotton" the thief who robbed thousands of southerners of their health by keeping vital food crops from being grown and maintaining a stranglehold on the region's economy. This earned him the hatred of a Southern political and economic establishment unwilling to undermine the traditional cotton economy merely for the sake of improving the health of the rural poor.[21]

In Appalachia, thousands of mountain people were thin, not because of current fashion but because of their difficulties in wresting anything of commercial value out of their impoverished land. Studies of Appalachian diets in Tennesee, Georgia, and Kentucky in 1901 and 1904 indicated that the fall and winter diets of the large majority were based on about one pound of flour and cornmeal per person per day together with three to four ounces of fat, mainly lard and salt pork. Lean meat, eggs, fish, milk, and vegetables, with the exception of potatoes, were consumed only sparingly.[22] A 1921 study of farmers in the mountains of Kentucky showed little change. Corn bread and salt pork were still the basics, supplemented by biscuits made of white wheat flour. Worse, much of the corn bread was now made of refined or "bolted" meal, deprived of much of its nutritional value. Luckily, buttermilk was used in making bread, and some fruit— mostly wild blackberries—was consumed during the summer months. Mothers also nursed their children for prolonged periods (up to two years) and, ignorant of expert opinion of the day, supplemented nursing with adult foods from the table. However, parental ignorance was no help for older children. Although many of the mothers showed great concern for the health of their children they did not appreciate the importance of diet and nutrition in their upbringing. While they knew what they cooked, many were unaware of what their children ate. "I put the food on the table; I don't pay no 'tention to what nobody eats," was a frequent response to investigators' questions.[23]

Appalachian families in Kentucky and Virginia studied in 1930 were still locked in the "summer" and "winter" diet syndrome. They ate adequate quantities of fruits and vegetables during the summer but did not can or preserve them for the winter, when they reverted to the basic pork and refined cereals diet, supplemented by small quantities of potatoes, beans, and bits of dried fruit. While some families used milk generously, others hardly consumed it at all. As a result, signs of calcium and other deficiencies were everywhere apparent. "Many observers have been impressed by the premature appearance of old age among people of the mountains, by the poor condition of their teeth, and by their lack of energy and initiative," the study commented. There was a crying need for programs to spread nutritional knowledge and encourage the home production and conservation of the vegetables, meat, milk, and eggs which were so lacking in the diets, it concluded.[24] Clearly, the New and Newer Nutritions had little impact on Appalachia.

Many grain farmers of the central states may have known more about the new nutritional ideas, but when repeated droughts caused their topsoil to blow away and much of the ex-Great American Desert return to its former state they were left with little land on which to grow vegetables and no money to buy them. In Texas and California, rural Mexican-Americans struggling as day laborers on Anglo-owned farms lived on largely meatless diets based on corn tortillas and beans, flavored with some chiles or tomatoes. Because they ate little meat, eggs, milk or other dairy products, their diets were deficient in those amino acids not supplied by beans, as well as in vitamins, calcium, and minerals. Moreover, the processing of the corn for *masa,* which involves soaking it in lime, removes important nutrients as well and, when Mexican-Americans' incomes rose slightly, they tended to abandon corn tortillas in favor of white bread or tortillas made of even more nutritionally deficient white flour.[25]

The Mexican-American diets shone in comparison with those of most Native Americans, particularly those in the West, where the remaining Native American population was concentrated in government-run reserves. Essentially carnivorous people who had lived by hunting, by the 1920s they were in as desperate straits as the buffalo herds upon which many had depended. A 1927 study of nutrition on a Sioux reservation in South Dakota revealed some appalling conditions. The staple food was "grease bread," which, as the name implies, was white-flour bread or biscuit dough fried in fat. Potatoes and beans were the only vegetables in widespread use and, although there was some consumption of squash and canned tomatoes, green vegetables and fruits were almost totally absent from the diets, as were milk, eggs, butter, and cheese. For meat, although young dogs were sometimes eaten, the Native Americans were dependent on a monthly government ration of beef. While the 25 to 40 pounds per month allotted to each head of family on the ration roll sounded fairly generous, the issue day each month attracted many relatives and friends not on the ration roll. They would stay for a week or two until the beef ration was consumed, often leaving families to live on bread and coffee for the rest of the month.

To nutritionists, the results of the unbalanced Sioux diet were visible. One nutritionist estimated that "40 percent of the adult women, 27 percent of the men, and 11 percent of the children would be termed distinctly fat, while 21 percent of the women, 25 percent of the men, and 27 percent of the children were extremely thin. . . . Even a casual observer could not fail to note the prevalence of decayed teeth, bow legs, and sore eyes and blindness among these families. Even more striking were the infant and child mortality rates. One-third of the children reported born were dead before the age of two and almost one-half had died before seven years of age.[26]

Obviously, the new ideas about nutrition and the new trends in eating were quite unknown, irrelevant, or impractical to those on the lower reaches of the rural scale. However, as one moved higher on the rural socio-economic scale, the ideas had more effect, at least to the extent of reinforcing what seems to be most peoples' natural tendency: to diversify their diets when the opportunity presents itself.

We now tend to associate poor farms with self-sufficiency and wealthier farms with the production of a few cash crops and the purchase of most food items in stores. However, this was not quite the case during the first two decades of this century, for, as we have seen, a large number of tenant farmers and sharecroppers tended to be tied to cash crops and were painfully dependent on store-bought foods. On the other hand, many of the better-off farmers tended to be quite self-sufficient in food. Most of the farmers surveyed by the Department of Agriculture from 1917 to 1919, who were generally among the better-off, produced the vast bulk of the food they consumed: practically all of their bread, butter, pork, lard, sausage, salt pork, milk, corn meal, bacon, canned (or otherwise preserved) fruits and vegetables, popcorn, and eggs. Tropical and citrus fruits were purchased in town, along with sugar, salt, and flour. (They also bought considerable supplies of Post Toasties, Wheat Puffs, and other prepared breakfast foods.)[27]

Increased federal funding for home economics work after 1915 helped expose the better-off farmers and their families to the lessons of the New and Newer Nutrition through a variety of sources. The proliferation of automobiles and trucks and the improvement in roads encouraged the consolidation of school districts and the creation of school bus systems which brought more rural students into expanded high schools in towns.[28] The home economics courses in these schools, which sometimes taught canning, drying, and otherwise preserving foods, were much more relevant to the daily lives of these students than they were to their urban counterparts, and one can assume that their nutritional messages had an impact as well.

At the same time, home economists funded by the federal Department of Agriculture and state agricultural extension services (also aided by the new mobility made possible by the automobile) went into rural America from state universities and colleges, lecturing, demonstrating, and organizing farmers' families into clubs where they were taught how to grow and utilize the foods which were thought to be nutritionally important. By 1929 over three-quarters of a million farm boys and girls were enrolled in 4-H Clubs, while 3,787 county organizations fostered the "demonstration work" in which the home economists specialized.[29]

The collapse of cotton, wheat, and other farm commodity prices after the wartime and postwar boom also encouraged farmers to break away from their dependence on one or two cash crops and diversify. Agricultural extension workers encouraged this for health as well as economic reasons, for they believed that single-crop farms bred dietary deficiencies. "Teach them to produce for sale and consumption will result," was a common saying among southern agricultural extension workers, and those farmers who did manage to diversify into other cash crops did have better diets. In November 1927, the typical day's fare of a family in Mississippi's brown loam cotton and corn belt who had diversified into truck gardening left little to be desired: breakfast was fried eggs, flour muffins with butter and molasses, coffee and milk. For dinner they ate roast pork with baked sweet potatoes and cabbage, cornbread, and custard pie. Supper was spaghetti and tomato sauce, fried sweet potatoes, biscuits and butter, fig preserves, and milk.[30] That year, county agents noted changes in the kind of meals served at farm community gatherings. "Salads of succulent vegetables and fruits were fast becoming the rule rather than the exception. Many covered dishes contained hot buttered or creamed vegetables which formerly contained starchy foods or pie. Milk was served to children . . . and fewer kinds of desserts were in evidence."[31]

Milk, especially for children, was now becoming commonplace throughout rural America, for one of the most common ways to diversify was to buy some milk cows. This was particularly important in the southern and border states, for it allowed many farmers in areas traditionally dependent on the nutritionally deficient "three M's" diet to escape its worst consequences. By 1930, only 10 percent of the rural population of South Carolina had no cows and purchased no milk. While few of the 47 percent who had only one cow had provisions for a family milk supply during periods when the cow was dry, at least they had fresh milk for a good part of the year, a substantial improvement over the situation in the 1880s and 1890s.[32] Ninety-four percent of the farmers in two cotton-growing areas of Mississippi surveyed in 1927 had their own milk cows.[33] All but twenty-nine of the 1,331 farm families surveyed in Kansas, Kentucky, Missouri, and Ohio surveyed in 1922–24 had milk cows, and not one of the 1,331 purchased any milk or cream during the year.[34] The idea that milk was a miracle food seems to have had as great an impact among farmers as in the cities. Of 895 farm families surveyed in New Hampshire in the early 1930s the 73 percent who owned cows drank an impressive average of almost one quart of milk per capita a day.[35]

Farmers were also affected by the mania for citrus and other "protective" fruits. As transportation improved, and better-off farmers became more reliant on store-bought foods, sacks of citrus foods became commonplace in the Model-Ts and pick-up trucks returning from shopping trips to town. Farm families surveyed in Kansas, Kentucky, Ohio, and Missouri consumed an average of over 100 pounds of lemons, oranges, grapefruits, and bananas per year. The influence of nutritional ideas of urban origin on these food choices was apparent, for those living closer to towns and cities generally bought more of these and other "protective" foods than farmers in more remote areas.[36]

Although farmers now had better access to town and village merchants who sold canned and prepared foods, home canning of vegetables seems to have expanded, rather than contracted after 1917. Home economists taught and encouraged it during the war, and the subsequent boom in canning for the urban market provided many farms in fruit and vegetable growing areas with local canneries where they could take their own produce for canning. A survey of Maryland farm families toward the end of the 1920s showed that almost half prepared all the canned goods they used themselves, while many others brought their corn, beans, and tomatoes to local commercial canneries for processing.[37]

By the end of the decade, then, the new nutritional opportunities and ideas had changed the diets of most of the nation's workers and farmers. The American diet was becoming more homogeneous, more like the emerging diet of the still-expanding middle class. Beneath the surface, stark departures from the norm remained, but these were regarded as exceptional cases and were ignored, for the most part, by a society more determined to celebrate the successes of business civilization than to probe its failures.

CHAPTER 15

The Old (Restaurant) Order Changeth

In a 1931 article on "What's the Matter with American Food," journalist Julian Street wrote that gastronomes might differ on the exact year in which the "Golden Age of eating in the United States" began, for it was difficult to pinpoint exactly when in the 1890s French cuisine achieved its ascendancy in America. However, "lovers of good food" were sure about the date on which it came to an end: "The art of noble dining, they will tell you, was assassinated under legal process on January 16, 1920, the day on which the prohibition laws became effective."

While they would not have agreed with Street's gloomy assessment of the quality of American food, most Americans would have agreed that Prohibition did indeed have a major impact on their eating habits. And understandably so, for its gastronomic repercussions were felt primarily where eating is most visible: in restaurants. Yet, although its effect was sudden and highly visible, it was only one of a number of forces which transformed eating out in America during the 1920s.

Street explained the economic basis of what he regarded as a gastronomic holocaust. It was not just that it was impossible to cook most of the finer French dishes, and even some American dishes, without wine, he said (a recent dish of sherryless Lobster Newburg tasted like "wet newspaper") or to enjoy them without appropriate accompanying wines. The economics of the hotel and restaurant industry were also responsible, he said. The great prewar hotels and restaurants relied on their bars for most of their profits, charging modestly for rooms and serving generous portions of food made with first-class ingredients at or below cost to attract customers who would also order high-margin wines and spirits. Deprived of this income, many fine hotels and restaurants were forced to close. The opulent Knickerbocker and Holland House hotels were no more. Delmonico's, Mouquin's, Churchill's, and Sherry's restaurants, the latter "the most elegant eating place New York has ever known," closed their doors. Those that did not close down were forced to economize in their kitchens, turning to second-rate materials and smaller portions.[1]

The culinary disaster was by no means confined to New York City. Throughout the nation, hotels and restaurants which had painfully built up a clientele for the elegant cuisine of *fin-de-siècle* Paris were devastated by legislation aimed, not at them, but at the grubby saloons and their "free lunches." Even famed Locke-Ober's in Boston, considered by many to be that city's, if not the nation's, finest restaurant, managed to hang on only by closing down and selling off the Locke part, which had housed its spectacular mahogany-lined bar-café, and scaling down its menu and operations.[2]

Closing or scaling down both amounted to the same thing: abandoning French cooking. Within two years of Prohibition, most of the French chefs who had flocked to New York, Chicago, San Francisco, and the other major cities in the prewar days were on the streets, looking for nonexistent jobs, or at the steamship offices, booking their passage home.[3] Among those who stayed were those who continued to cook in the urban mansions and Newport "cottages" of the very rich. Even there, however, the demand for French chefs slackened. The huge Fifth Avenue mansions of the trend-setting New York elite, with their gigantic dining halls, ballrooms, reception rooms, and kitchens, were being pulled down to make way for more profitable buildings. The East Side apartments and town houses where they moved, while by no means pokey, were not up to entertaining on the scale of the prewar Astors and Vanderbilts. Their Long Island and Westchester estates were too isolated for more than the occasional giant affair. The prewar solution for those with housing problems, renting Delmonico's or Louis Sherry's, would not do, for even had they not closed, wine and champagne would have to be served surreptitiously. Better to retain an aging French chef, entertain on a somewhat less lavish scale at more modest dinner parties, where alcohol could be served, out of the glare of the prewar public spotlight. Of course the chef's *equipe* of *sous-chefs* trained in the European style would have to go, replaced on special occasions by American "temporaries," and the height of the gastronomic mountains he would be expected to climb would consequently diminish.

With the culinary achievements of New York's private chefs and elite restaurants no longer glittering across the nation, the new rich of the rest of the country ignored or even deplored French cuisine. Here and there,

notably in San Francisco and New Orleans, islands of Francophilia survived in the dining rooms and restaurants of the older upper class, but for
the most part those who hied to the French tradition in the rest of the
country felt adrift in the rising tide of culinary Babbitry. Without New
York's French beacon to follow, pressed in on all sides by newly rich
stockbrokers, bankers, and real estate speculators, those who managed to
retain the old French tastes seemed like relics of a previous age and ceased
to provide a convincing culinary example to follow.

But there was much more to the gastronomic side of Prohibition than
the undermining of French cooking. While it helped to destroy the higher
echelon of the restaurant industry, it also helped spur a tremendous
expansion in the levels below, particularly among those catering to the
middle and lower-middle classes of both sexes. In the ten years after 1919
the number of restaurants in the country tripled and many of them became
much bigger businesses than Lorenzo Delmonico or Louis Sherry could
ever have imagined possible.[4] Much of this was the result of cultivating a
middle-class, lower-middle-class, and particularly a female market to
which these purveyors of fine French food never deigned to cater.

While the economics of the prewar bar-restaurant industry may have
provided some bargains for restaurant-goers, it was mainly males who
could take advantage of them. Of course working-class saloons, with their
"free lunches," were strictly male preserves, but restaurants on the higher
levels also catered to a primarily male clientele. All-male bar-cafés with
carved mahogany bars, ornate mirrors, brass spittoons, and cigar-smoke
atmosphere were an integral part of even the highest class pre-Prohibition
restaurants. Large paintings of naked women were de rigueur as centerpieces for their decor.[5] Even the restaurant sides of high-class establishments such as Locke-Ober's and Delmonico's were mainly male preserves
where the whiskey, wine, and brandy flowed all too freely for Victorian
feminine tastes. They maintained small private dining rooms, not simply
for discrete assignations but as places where the more decorous of women
could feel comfortable. This close association of restaurants at all levels
with alcohol gave the pre-Prohibition restaurant industry the stigma of
being, in the words of an industry magazine, "the tail-end of the liquor
business."[6]

The proliferation of a new lower-middle class of male and female office
and shop employees after the turn of the century created a burgeoning
market which neither the old saloons nor the higher-class restaurants
could tap. Short lunch hours and expanding cities made going home for
lunch impossible. Hot lunches were regarded as a necessity and lunch pails
were too working-class. As a result, new kinds of restaurants tried to fill
the growing gap in the middle.

Lunch counters, which served hot meals quickly, were set up in railway
stations in 1884, before the introduction of the dining car, but they were

slow to spread and initially remained confined to the largest cities. In the 1890s, a Swedish entrepreneur opened a smorgasbord restaurant in Chicago which he christened with a Spanish name, "cafeteria." But he too was slightly ahead of the market.[7] By the early 1900s, however, swelling numbers of office workers stimulated the establishment of many restaurants, most full-service, but some self-service, catering almost exclusively to this clientele. A Chicago restaurant magazine reported in 1904 that

> innumerable restaurants of the hurly-burly kind invite the mobs from offices for the noon-hour lunch. An army of waiters resists the invasion, and there is strenuous action for a space. The all-important consideration is economy of time, and the business of a meal is transacted with barbarous brevity—by a sort of short-hand system of jabs and slashes, punctuated by swallowing. Of this class many are known as cafeterias, or, in the parlance of the impolite, 'grab joints,' where heaven helps those who help themselves. Men and women hugging roast beef to their bosoms and balancing a toppling armful of dishes rush to and fro, on a perilous and exciting exploration for seats.[8]

In New York City, large parts of downtown Manhattan boasted "table d'hôte" restaurants serving set hot meals at fixed prices. These simple establishments catered not just to the lower-middle-class lunch-hour trade but to the dinner trade as well, offering clerks and shopkeepers who lived alone or with friends in small flats or rooming houses four and five course meals, with beer or wine, for thirty-five to fifty cents.[9]

The pure-food scare led entrepreneurs to create restaurant chains which emphasized cleanliness and high quality ingredients. New steel utensils, enameled table tops, mass-produced tiles, and electric lights allowed them to achieve a sparkling-clean, hygienic look. After two failures with full-service restaurants, the Greek immigrant John Raklios realized that what Americans now wanted was cleanliness and the appearance of quality and built a chain of nineteen "luncheonettes" in Chicago on these principles. He advertised that he dealt only with the major meat packers, displayed only Heinz and other high quality condiments, and employed only whites as waiters and waitresses. ("Colored help take care of the dishwashing," he said.)[10] By 1922 another Chicagoan, John R. Thompson, built a chain of 103 restaurants on the principles of absolute cleanliness (symbolized by his white-enameled nameplate on each window), no frills, modest prices, and fast turnover, squeezing his white-collar worker clientele into tiny tables for one or two hardly larger than a napkin.[11] Child's in New York followed suit, but added a more elegant decor.

But before Prohibition these restaurants met stiff competition for the masculine trade from the saloon's "free lunch" (they were rarely actually free, but charged only a nominal price, usually a nickel or so) and the "businessman's lunch," four- or five-course meals served by alcohol-purveying establishments for as little as thirty cents.[12] By destroying these competitors, Prohibition opened the way for a great expansion in restaurants catering to the lunch-hour trade. It even provided the space to expand. The closing of the saloons and *café*-bars left many of them available at reasonable rents for easy conversion to restaurants. Stools could be nailed into the floor by the carved wooden bars; soda, ice cream, and syrup dispensing machines could replace the bottles arrayed in front of the mirrors; the naked ladies could come down from the walls, replaced by coats of gleaming white paint, and a mixed clientele could be lured to the new "luncheonette" and/or "soda fountain." Even the elegant Palmer House hotel in Chicago converted its renowned ornate mirrored bar into a luncheonette, with bottles of fruit syrup, chocolate, and soft drinks arrayed behind the soda jerks who replaced a generation of deft bartenders.[13]

While Prohibition brought women into ex-saloons which had previously been off-limits to them, it also encouraged men to frequent "tea rooms." Those which had been in business before the war were generally run by ladies for ladies, and served as respectable alternatives to conventional restaurants. Lacking the space and resources to produce a wide variety of substantial dishes, they tended to offer not, as one might expect, the lightest of fare but set luncheons and dinners of three or four courses with substantial items such as roast beef or roast lamb as the main course.[14] Prohibition made them acceptable for men, particularly when out shopping or otherwise socializing with their wives. As tastes changed, they turned to lighter fare such as salads, sandwiches, chicken pies, and cakes, all served in the "dainty" manner and atmosphere so prized by the home economists of the day. Indeed, some were set up by home economists determined to put their knowledge to profitable use. Two women who transformed an old warehouse on Beekman Place in New York City into a tea room were University of Minnesota home economists who had been sent to the city by the federal Department of Labor to investigate the wartime food situation.[15]

In the first few years after Prohibition, particularly as their bills of fare shrank, the future looked rosy for tea rooms. From coast to coast, women rushed out to rent store fronts, buy old homes, or even convert their living rooms or stables to tea rooms furnished in the accepted frilly style. Miss Ida L. Frese, New York City's "dean of tea room women," even established one on the ground floor of the monstrous ex-Vanderbilt mansion on Fifth Avenue, employing 100 women who served 1800 people a day there and at her two other tea rooms.[16] One optimist even started a trade journal, *Tea Room Management*.

However, tea rooms were soon abandoned for establishments which offered faster service and lower prices. Foremost among these was the self-service cafeteria, which had swept California even before the war.[17] Its attraction to investors centered in its labor-saving economies. It was not just the obvious savings in table service which mattered but the additional savings achieved by simplifying food preparation as well. The steel steam table allowed a number of dishes to be prepared in bulk and to be served all day by unskilled labor, much of it cheap, female labor. Dishes such as macaroni and cheese and "Spaghetti Italienne," whether prepared from dried and canned ingredients or simply poured onto the steam table from a can, could be prepared by anyone. They could sit on a steam table all day, and bring profit margins of up to 500 percent. What remained at the end of the day could be mixed with leftover ham and other meats into what the industry called "workovers" and sold as other dishes the next day. The salad, bread, and dessert counters also utilized canned and prepared foods to the fullest extent and did not even require servers.[18]

The cafeterias' cleanliness, convenience, speed, and respectable atmosphere helped attract a large share of the growing shop and office girl market. This was no insignificant achievement, for by mid-decade it was estimated that close to 60 percent of restaurant patrons were women.[19] By the end of 1923, the Waldorf chain in the East comprised 112 branches doing almost $14 million in annual sales. Not only had it already gone public but soon its share price rose so high that the stock was split two-for-one.[20]

In a burst of construction activity, cafeterias broke away from the sterilized hygienic mold and adopted the Mesopotamian, Egyptian, and other exotic decor being featured in the new movie palaces. Messrs. Horn and Hardardt carved a handsome niche for themselves with a fifty-year-old system of Swedish origin which they had imported to Philadelphia before the war.[21] Their gleaming nickel-plated Automats required only that the patrons pump coins into slots beside the food of their choice, visible behind sparkling little windows. They seemed to embody the ultimate in hygiene and American labor-saving genius, for no human hands could be seen touching the food and, if they had enough nickels, patrons did not even have to confront a cashier.

By the mid-1920s, however, cafeterias were beginning to give way to luncheon restaurants featuring even lighter fare. In part, this was related to the new ideas regarding food and nutrition. The pre-1920s Automats had not been notably successful until steam tables were added to provide the hot food thought essential for a proper meal.[22] However, as the New Nutrition, with its emphasis on physiological economy, was superseded by the Newer Nutrition, the mystique of the hot lunch began to fade and sandwiches, composed salads, and other cold dishes became popular luncheon fare.

The invention of the electric toaster was a boon to places serving sandwiches. "Luncheonettes," where practically all the food preparation was done in front of the customer, now swept the nation. "It was not until a few years ago," said a bemused restaurant trade journal, "that the toast sandwich came into general popularity in restaurants and hotels, with the exception, of course, of the time-honored club sandwich." Yet many businesses now thrived, it said, on selling little more than sandwiches, beverages, and desserts.[23] A Milwaukee hotel, discouraged at seeing the working girls it hoped to attract to its new cafeteria walk five extra blocks to a sandwich shop, closed the cafeteria and replaced it with a sandwich shop.[24]

Drug stores soon invaded the light lunch market, setting up their own soda fountains, which served not only ice cream and syrup-based beverages, with their high mark-ups, but coffee, cakes, canned soups, and sandwiches as well. By 1929 it was estimated that 61 percent of all drug-store sales took place at the soda fountain and that 67 percent of this was in food sales.[25]

Although fast service at economical prices were major attractions of the light lunch restaurants, the restaurants also encouraged patronage by conforming to the new dietetic ideas. The chain restaurants that survived and prospered were those which adapted their menus to lighter, more calorie-conscious tastes. Many printed calorie-counts on their menus and featured special low-calorie salads. The Childs' chain enjoyed immense success by catering to health-consciousness. "Watch your step: Go Vegetable-Wise," was the slogan on its menus. These listed the number of "protein calories" as well as total calories beside each dish. "Items rich in vitamins" were marked with a capital "V" and those in which vitamins were merely present were noted with a lower-case "v." As concern over adequate roughage in diets rose, Childs placed bowls of free "Sanatorium Cooked Bran" on every table at breakfast time.[26]

One of the problems with calorie-consciousness was that the fattening dishes were normally the most profitable for restaurants. One way in which restaurateurs coped with this was to try to extol the nutritional value of vegetable soups, which were also high margin items, and particularly canned condensed soups, which were the highest-profit items of all. In 1929, canned soup which cost three cents a serving sold for 15 to 20 cents a serving in restaurants.[27]

This ability to adapt to the new eating habits of the day helped make establishments specializing in light lunches and snacks booming sectors of the industry by the end of the decade. A survey of new restaurant installations in 1929 showed 48 percent devoted to lunch rooms, 26 percent to coffee and sandwich shops, and only 8 percent to cafeterias.[28]

Full service restaurants accounted for only 11 percent of expansion plans, but this was partly because, like cafeterias, they had expanded earlier in the decade. Although surreptitious bottles were not unknown in many of them, in general Prohibition helped make restaurant-going a respectable diversion for middle-class women by removing the unsavory alcoholic aspect to dining out. The heightened importance placed on couples socializing outside the home encouraged this as well. Now, for the first time, middle-class housewives could look forward to regular relief from the burdens of meal preparation by "going out" for dinner.

But what did "going out for dinner" mean? It was certainly distinct from the bourgeois European idea of "dining out," with its gastronomic connotations and expectation that chefs will turn out a cuisine superior to that found at home. Rather, it provided relief for servantless housewives from the burdens of food preparation, opportunities to socialize, and, at times, a certain kind of titillation. The titillation came, not from trying new and different foods but from new and exotic locales. It was a commonplace in the restaurant industry that the nature and quality of the food in a restaurant took a back seat to its decor. The successful restaurateurs were usually those who came up with a gimmick of some kind unrelated to the quality of the food itself. When Gus Mann opened his famous seafood restaurant in Chicago in 1923 it was an instant success, not because his oysters and clams were fresher or better prepared than those of his competitors but because he thought of the then-novel idea of decorating it with portholes, fish nets, and a fake wheelhouse. The waitresses dressed as sailors, each with a pack of cigarettes jauntily protruding from her breast pocket, were a great hit.[29]

Throughout the country restaurateurs joined the battle for ever more exotic decor. In California, W. C. Lape created the "Barkies" chain of sandwich shops, which featured a gigantic puppy holding the "Barkies" sign in its teeth as storefronts and required patrons to enter a doorway between its two enormous paws.[30] Tile was imported from Italy to construct "Italian Villages," "Venetian Grottos," and "Roman Gardens." Plazas were torn up in Spain to furnish "Spanish Haciendas" in the Midwest, and the architects of movie houses were hired to design Mayan-style restaurants in North Carolina. Yet the food in these places normally remained stolidly American, and bore no relationship at all to the decor. One entered Omar Khayyam's tent to face the usual comfortable choice between steak and roast chicken, French fries or mashed potatoes, and salad or canned peas. The only exceptions of any significance were the occasional upwardly mobile "chop suey" house, which might invest in a few plaster dragons to go with food that would be regarded with blank incomprehension in China, and Italian restaurants, which developed a muted Americanized version of their cuisine. Although spaghetti and tomato sauce did achieve a considerable degree of popularity, it was Italian decor and atmosphere which drew in patrons. The owner of an Italian restaurant near Times Square, who advertised himself as "Luigino . . . the best known chef in America," specialized in familiar steaks, chops, and seafood.[31] Although "Venetian Gardens" sprouted across America, few served anything approximating the food found in Italy or in Italian-American homes. "Most of the Italian restaurants in New York are run by Italians, serve alleged Italian delicacies, and yet [with some exceptions] they number scarcely a single Italian among their patrons," wrote a restaurant reviewer in 1930.[32] So popular was Italian decor that when someone opened a restaurant called the Guernsey Plaza, which specialized in Guernsey milk and dietetic dishes, in Providence, Rhode Island, he insisted on decorating it as an Italian village.[33]

Traditional hotel dining rooms and higher-class restaurants tried to survive by adapting to the new currents. Some scrapped their elegant dining rooms completely and revamped them into cafeterias.[34] When, shortly after Prohibition came into effect, the waiters at the North American Restaurant—one of Chicago's most elegant and opulent—struck for higher wages and a closed shop, the management fired them all, set up some steam tables, and within ten hours had converted the pillared, mirrored, wood-paneled, and silk-tasseled palace with its semi-private banquettes into a self-service cafeteria.[35]

Some took the exotic decor route. The Hotel Miami, in Dayton, Ohio, adopted a King Tut's tomb motif for its lunch menu, which featured items such as ham and cheese sandwiches.[36] Others tried to trade on health and weight-consciousness, hiring dietitians to plan and supervise their menus. The Kahler chain of midwestern hotels appointed a home economist/dietitian as the corporation's superintendent of dietetics to create calorie-counted recipes for use in all its restaurants and cafeterias.[37] The maitre d'hotel at the Netherland Plaza Hotel in Cincinnati wrote a pamphlet on "a way to grow thin with plenty to eat" for distribution to diningroom patrons.[38] The Dessert hotel chain of the Pacific Northwest one-upped the rest. Not only did it feature the usual calorie-counted menu but its dietitian had scales installed in each of its restaurants and provided a register wherein regular customers could keep running tabs on their weights.[39]

The most common tactic, however, was to abandon the gigantic old menus, with their vast array of French or American dishes, and replace them with less extensive but more straightforward "American" ones. While restaurant industry leaders recognized that the appeal of the new establishments lay in their fast service, informality, and moderate prices, they thought that serving food which appealed to new, lighter tastes was crucial to success. As a result, there was a wholesale revision in traditional hotel and restaurant menus. A 1924 analysis of the great changes undergone by hotel and restaurant menus over only the past five years said the most significant of these were: first, a recognition of the rise of calorie-consciousness, exemplified by calorie-counting menus which "capitalized on and furthered the growing public interest in scientific eating"; second, they reflected the great increases in vegetable consumption, particularly by men; and third, "the menu with unpronounceable French names in giving way to the Americanized menu."[40] The next year, a survey by J. O.

Dahl, the magazine's food editor, indicated that meat consumption in restaurants dropped by about half in the past five years, while orders for dairy products, fruit, vegetables, cereals, and nuts soared. Milk was the item which experienced the greatest increase in consumption, and fully 25 percent of all beverage orders called for milk, usually in individual bottles. White bread was rarely served any more with meals, having been replaced by whole wheat, graham, or rye breads, or crusty rolls.[41]

The new food habits meant either getting rid of French cooking or, at least, in the words of *Hotel Management* magazine, "raising the delicate question of how to list European dishes." The consensus in the industry was that, unlike their prewar predecessors, the new middle class was not impressed by French names on the menu. If anything, they were simply confused. As early as 1919 tests demonstrated that labeling the same dish in English would bring more orders for it than retaining its French name.[42]

Ultimately, however, changes in nomenclature did not suffice. French cooking itself had to go. Many hotel and restaurant kitchens turned into battlegrounds as managers tried to force classically trained chefs to abandon French cuisine. In early 1931, Dahl surveyed hotel and restaurant managers regarding the effects of the past decade's rising demand for simpler "American" food. The composite answer to the question "How long since you noticed a demand for simpler dishes?" was "Ten years ago." Ninety-one percent of the respondents thought the demand for these dishes was still on the increase, yet 45 percent thought their chefs unwilling to change their cuisine to meet this need. Another 23 percent thought the chefs would change only with constant prodding from managers and only 32 percent thought their chefs would change unassisted.[43]

As a result, many French chefs were fired. The manager of a thousand-room hotel in New York City wrote that "after spending nine months trying to educate a foreign chef to simplify his cooking, to omit in many instances rich sauces, gravies and seasoning, and in addition, to make his menus intelligible to the average hotel patron who is not a connoisseur of food, we decided we could make no material headway with him and made a change." "The French chef, to my mind, is not very willing to change his cuisine," wrote a Chicago restaurant manager explaining why he would no longer employ one. "They are quite set in their ways and feel the French way is the correct way."[44]

The skilled chefs were also undermined by the new economics of the restaurant kitchen. For a time, during and shortly after the war, people in the industry hoped that these highly paid male chefs would be replaced by cheaper, female classically trained chefs. However, the simplification and Americanization of menus made this unnecessary. Now that it merely involved roasting, broiling, the heating of canned foods, and other simple operations, most food preparation could be accomplished by unskilled, barely trained, cheap, male labor.[45]

To save their jobs, some chefs adapted to the new ways. "Many of the older chefs and especially those of the old school were quite resentful," wrote the manager of a large restaurant chain of its conversion to the new simpler American cooking. However, they were "beginning to realize the wonderful possibilities in the simpler dishes, not only in pleasing the guests but from the standpoint of food percentage" [that is, profit margin]. "Our present chef, who is a native of France, plans very few French dishes," wrote a satisfied West Coast manager.[46]

As Dahl, who enjoyed French food, ruefully pointed out some months earlier, the decade had thus seen the "nouveau comfortable" undermine what good cooking there remained in American hotels and restaurants after the devastating blow of Prohibition. What had been a budding tradition of fine cooking and dining had been virtually snuffed out. French food had become "a negligible factor in American commercial kitchens," he declared. By his estimate, no more than 2 percent of the country's hotels, restaurants, and private clubs retained classical menus.[47] Perhaps the most telling symbol of what transpired over the course of the decade was the identity of the featured speaker at the National Restaurant Association's 1929 convention: the teetotalling vegetarian John Harvey Kellogg, most of whose ideas had been anathema to the American restaurant industry just ten years before.[48]

CHAPTER 16

Too Rich and *Too Thin?*

Perhaps nothing symbolizes the change in American attitudes toward food between 1896 and 1928 better than the slogans of the winning presidential candidates in each of those years. William McKinley rode to victory by promising workingmen "the full dinner pail." Herbert Hoover promised them "a chicken in every pot." Quality had replaced quantity as the prime consideration.[1]

This was reflected in what Americans actually ate. The American of 1928 ate less in terms of quantity (about 5 percent fewer calories per capita), but consumed more of a wider variety of nutrients than the American of 1890. He ate much more fruit, especially citrus fruits, and vegetables, particularly green ones, considerably more milk and cheese, and less cereals, particularly flour, potatoes, corn meal, and sweet potatoes. Even beef consumption fell precipitously, from 72.4 pounds per capita in 1899 to 55.3 pounds in 1930.[2]

The effect of the changing diet was literally visible. Any number of studies recorded surges in height from the 1890s onward. Upper-middle-class Boston schoolboys of 1926 averaged three inches taller than their class counterparts of 1876.[3] Recruits into the armed forces in 1943, particularly those born after 1913, were considerably taller than those of 1917.[4] In 1930, the daughters of alumnae of a number of private women's colleges averaged over one inch taller than their mothers and, interestingly, were nevertheless slimmer-hipped.[5] The growth in stature of the generations born between 1906 and 1931 was more rapid than that of any other period for which comparable data exist.[6] Moreover, the data for both Boston schoolboys and army recruits seem to indicate that the greatest surge in height occurred for those born after about 1915, the time that the new modes of eating were taking hold. "There can be no question," said an analysis of the recruiting data, "but that these very favorable findings with regard to stature reflect the improvement in general health and nutritional conditions over recent decades."[7]

Mortality statistics also seem to reflect a kind of nutritional revolution. The direction of mortality rates in the two or three decades after the Civil War is unclear. Some demographers hypothesize that there was a steady advance in life expectancy while others see stasis or decline. Nevertheless, there is solid evidence for steady improvements from the 1890s on.[8] Some have ascribed this to improved medical techniques and others have credited sanitary and public health measures. However, the improvement was as marked in rural as in urban areas, yet modern medicine, sanitation, and public health had little impact on rural America before the 1920s. This would seem to point to improved nutrition as the most important factor.[9]

A large percentage of the twentieth-century increase in life expectancy at birth has come as a result of a great decline in infant mortality rates. As we have seen, improved infant mortality rates appear to be closely linked to better nutrition. The decline was particularly marked after about 1915, the very period when the diets of a large number of Americans seem to have improved.[10]

Infant mortality statistics also indicate that for forty or so years after 1915 significant differences in nutrition still divided the classes, for while the improvement was generally across the board, babies born into the lower income levels still died at rates about 50 percent higher than those on the middle and upper reaches. However, by mid-century, once one emerged from the lower third of income levels, the correlation between rising income and lower infant mortality rates ceased.[11] This would indicate that a kind of nutritional equality reigned among the upper two-thirds of society: that those differences in nutrition which existed among the upper two-thirds had little to do with economic status.[12]

The revolution in vitality owed much to social and economic changes which made Americans receptive to revolutionary new ideas about food. It is therefore puzzling that the Great Depression and World War II did not seem to bring equally significant changes. At the very least, one would expect that the economic hardship of the former and the fear of shortages in the latter would have led to a revival of the economic thrust of the New Nutrition, for Atwater's old lessons on the substitution of cheaper foods for scarce and expensive foods would seem to have been more relevant than ever. But this was not quite the case. Although various government agencies did strive to spread the message among the deprived during the New Deal, and women's magazines often ran articles on economizing on food, crucial support from the food processors, whose advertising and promotion now played keyed roles in disseminating nutritional information, was missing. Indeed, the food industries hardly adjusted their messages at all. Pasta manufacturers did not tout their products' high-protein, low-cost advantage over bread; bean canners did not try to convince consumers to substitute beans for meat; breakfast cereal manufacturers did not, as they had in earlier years, cite scientific studies showing their products were more economical sources of energy or nutrients than other foods.

There would seem to be a number of reasons for this apparent indifference to food economies on the part of processors and public agencies at a time of economic collapse. In the first place, while the Depression brought bread lines, soup kitchens, hoboes begging for food at middle-class doors, and thousands of hungry families in devastated parts of rural America, starvation was unheard-of. Persistent hunger was more common, but it was localized, affecting mainly marginalized populations who played a small role in politics or the marketplace. After the initial dislocation, when local and private relief agencies were bankrupted, enough federal and state resources seem to have been mobilized to provide enough relief and/or jobs to head off serious threats to the nutrition of most of the poor and unemployed, particularly in the cities. In any event, there is no indication, in mortality or other statistics, of an overall deterioration in the health of the nation.

Falling food prices seem to have helped. Studies of low-income families in five northern industrial cities during the tough spring of 1933, when the nation's economy was in ruins, presented a bleak but by no means horrendous picture. Those whose incomes were over three dollars per person per week (not a handsome amount) consumed an average of over 3,000 calories per adult male per day. Those with incomes of two to three dollars per person per week still averaged 2,800 calories per adult male per day while only those on the very bottom, the relatively small proportion living on less than two dollars per person, lived near the margin of hunger, averaging 2,470 calories per day.[13] Even in southern mill-towns, where the Depression brought a reversion to the core "three M's" diet, the poorer workers still ate better than their counterparts of twenty years earlier. While they did cut back on meat, fowl, fish, and fresh fruit, they still ate adequate amounts of vegetables, fresh and canned. A comparison of the diets of families in a large number of South Carolina mill-villages in 1933 with surveys done in 1916 showed a greatly increased use of "protective" foods and few cases of the bane of the corn-meal diet, pellagra.[14]

This does not mean that the Depression did not scar Americans. Whether hungry or not, economic hardship was ever-present in most Americans' minds: they either experienced it, feared it, or were concerned about others living through it. But unlike the food crises which used to rack the pre-industrial world, this one took place among food surpluses, not shortages. The newspapers carried pictures of protesting farmers pouring cans of milk on midwestern roads, told of the slaughter of thousands of piglets in a New Deal attempt to reduce pork supplies, and reported that coffee had been burned as fuel in Brazilian railroad engines. But while the awful paradox of food being destroyed while people waited in bread lines was often remarked upon, this led inevitably to the question of how to get the food onto the plates of the needy without undermining the capitalist system. Government agencies therefore concentrated on what seemed to be the problems of overproduction and underconsumption. In this context, whether consumers would make the most intelligent and economical food choices possible did not rank of the first importance. This attitude was shared by food processors, who saw, correctly, that those who could afford to have choices among the foods they bought would not be swayed by the old appeals to the economic dicta of the New Nutrition. Also, since most food profits now arose from food processing and packaging, it ill behooved major advertisers to raise the question of the economies of their product. After all, for the canners of spaghetti or beans to suggest that their products made economical substitutes for others would raise the question of the actual cost of the spaghetti or beans in the can.

The food processors thus continued on their 1920s tacks, emphasizing health, convenience, and, paradoxically during "hard times," slimness. "Health and Freshness Comes in Cans," said the Continental Can company, because "the cooking is done in the sealed can—to retain the vitamins." "But the sun doesn't always shine," warned Pet Milk alongside a picture of a beautiful child playing in the sun. Sunshine should be supplemented with cans of Pet Milk, which was irradiated with ultra-violet rays to "create an extra supply of precious Vitamin D" and prevent rickets.[15] Fleischmann's Yeast continued its dubious campaign to promote its yeast cakes as health food, claiming to have developed "an entirely new 'strain' of yeast . . . much stronger, quicker-acting." "The new yeast amazes doctors," said Dr. R. E. Lee, the "prominent Director of Fleischmann Health Research," for it "corrected constipation, indigestion, and related skin problems far faster." It was also "rich in hormone-like substances" and thanks to "newly-added Vitamin A," it combated colds too.[16] Quaker Oats adopted the vitamin B campaign too, claiming that its oatmeal, in which "Wise Old Mother Nature" stores "the magical yeast-vitamin (B)," curbed nervousness, constipation and stimulated children's appetites, while one penny's worth of it contained as much vitamin B as three cakes of yeast.[17] (Finally, in 1938 the Federal Trade Commission stepped in, and forced Standard Brands, Fleischmann's parent, to agree to stop making such claims, as well as to cease advertising that its yeast prevented tooth decay, kept the intestinal canal healthy, cured "fallen stomach," and would not make one fat.[18])

In line with the era's drive to get women out of the job market and back into the home, the food industries emphasized the importance of food in ensuring a happy marriage. If its advertisements are to be believed, Chase and Sanborn's coffee alone saved many a marriage. The cartoons in its advertisements pictured a number of irritable husbands yelling at their wives because drinking "stale," that is, "undated" coffee had frayed their nerves to the breaking point. While Chase and Sanborn's "dated" coffee restored their happy homes, other cartoon husbands were placated by canned hams. "Peg, you're positively brilliant," said one as he ate the Swift's ham his wife had cleverly contrived to reheat after baking it the day before.[19] When another housewife, "Sue," heeded her father's advice that "the best insurance for a happy marriage is to know how to bake" and joined the Pillsbury Cookery Club, her husband proclaimed himself "the luckiest man in the world" upon tasting the toothsome results.[20]

As in the previous decade, housework was not to diminish wives' sexual allure, and advertisers promised that beauty, youthfulness, and vigor need not be sacrificed to the demands for food that would please husbands, family, and friends. "Entertaining is grand fun," Campbell's Soups assured women, "when the hostess looks her very best . . . fresh . . . radiant . . . no little tell-tale lines of fatigue on her face." The slim and beautiful cartoon hostess serving canned soup in the ad's elegant dinner party (men in white tie and tails, women bare-shouldered) apparently owed her radiance to "letting the skilled Campbell's chefs strike the first note."[21]

Although New Deal agencies provided a temporary refuge for some home economists not enamored with the food processing and household appliance industries, for the most part the links between home economics (including the branches now calling themselves "nutritionists" or "dietitians") and the food industries strengthened. By the late 1930s, it was no longer just the innovative industry leaders who employed full-time home economists to promote their goods, they were practically de rigueur for all. National Dairy Products had not one but two diet kitchens (one for its Sealtest brand name, the other for Kraft), which together turned out over 10 million recipe booklets a year.[22]

Appliance companies employed home economists to demonstrate their products; gas and electrical power companies hired them to extoll the wonders of their sources of energy. Both donated appliances to schools, where the home economics field continued to expand. By 1938, almost nine-tenths of the junior and senior high school girls in the country were enrolled in classes dealing with food and nutrition. Now that working-class children attended school more regularly and left later, the messages had a greater impact on the lower reaches of the socio-economic order, particularly when students berated their uneducated parents for not serving proper meals. In the mid-1930s anthropologists in San Francisco discovered that peasant immigrants from Tuscany, conscious of the poor diets and stunted growth they had left behind in Italy, took to heart the nutritional lessons their children brought home from school and spoke the language of calories and vitamins.[23] By the 1960s, lessons in nutrition were being given earlier (as they had been originally) and were integral parts of the curricula of many of the nation's elementary schools. There were even recurring attempts to use school lunches as instructional tools.[24]

Home economists continued to expand their role in the schools, while continuing their ceaseless struggle against the "cooking and sewing teacher" label. ("First, a home economist is not a cook!" wrote an outraged professor of the subject in 1973 when the *New York Times*'s food critic charged that they ignored the taste of food. "We in the field have for many years been fighting the image of 'cooking' and 'sewing.' "[25]) In this battle, the scientific cachet of nutritional science continued to be an invaluable weapon, and professionals remained as disdainful of "fancy cooking" (now mislabeled "gourmet cooking") as Ellen Richards, Helen Campbell, and the other founders had been.

Home economists and dietitians played much more important roles in the feeding of the armed forces during World War II than they had in the previous war, particularly as nutritionists and dietitians in hospitals or on large bases. As in World War I, those on the home front cooperated as well, but now many of them did so from their kitchens in the food industry. Like the home economists at National Dairy Products' Kraft and Sealtest kitchens, who produced a breezy little booklet, "Cheese Recipes for Servicemen," for free distribution among army cooks, they could serve the Flag and Mammon at the same time.[26]

As in the World War I, the food of the armed forces acted as a homogenizing, nationalizing influence, and, in line with American tradition, fighting men were thought of as carnivores of the first order. "He's the greatest meat eater in the world," proclaimed Armour and Company, pointing out that the U.S. Navy ration mandated one pound of meat per man per day. A typical Navy day began with prunes, corn flakes, and one-fifth of a pound of bacon with fried scrapple; lunch brought cream-of-tomato soup, half a pound of pot roast of beef with potatoes and spinach, followed by chocolate cake, while the geometrical compartments of the dinner trays brought half a pound of grilled hamburger, with spaghetti, salad, and pudding. Even allowing for disappearances of food on the way from the suppliers to the mess, a not-unheard-of occurrence, Armour was probably not far off the mark when it claimed that "not one man in ten ate as nourishing, well-balanced meals at home as he gets in the Navy today."[27]

The problem of feeding those in the service, and on the home front, according to the latest scientific principles brought to the fore the embarrassing fact that there was still little agreement on what these principles were. While the Newer Nutrition now reigned supreme, and it was becoming possible to accurately measure the amounts of vitamins and other nutrients in foods, there was nothing approaching a consensus on how much of these nutrients were necessary to maintain human health. For example, estimates of requirements for ascorbic acid—vitamin C— ranged from 10 to more than 100 milligrams per day and those for vitamin A ranged from 1,000 to 10,000 international units daily.[28] There was not even agreement on what the nation's nutritional goals should be: adequate health or "optimum" health, the minimum necessary to head off deficiency diseases or enough to promote better health and greater longevity?

Initially, the Roosevelt Administration tackled the problem in much the same way FDR had put together New Deal economic legislation: by putting opposing factions in a room together and telling them to come up with a compromise. At a special nutrition conference called by the President in early 1940, three female nutrition experts on the newly created Food and Nutrition Board of the National Research Council were given one evening in which to come up with a complete set of nutritional standards! After over a year of jockeying, the Food and Nutrition Board finally approved a set of standards, but it managed to obtain support for them only by framing them in terms of recommended, rather than required, allowances. Opposition was also muted by the unstated understanding that, in the many cases where there were divergent views on requirements, its recommendations leaned toward the high rather than the low side. (After all, it was difficult, in wartime, to protest too much about the troops or war workers being oversupplied with nutrients.) Thus, for example, while the protein and calorie requirements were high enough to have a decidedly old-fashioned ring (70 grams of protein and 3000 calories per day for a seventy-kilo male), they could hardly be attacked for being insufficient.

The allowances were modified in 1944 and a number of times thereafter, but the understanding (by nutritionists, if not the general public) that they were not minimum daily requirements allowed them to be kept on the high side. In 1958, Lydia Roberts, who headed the original committee, acknowledged this, but said that "the allowances can continue to be used, as they were meant to be, as *goals at which to aim* in providing for the nutritional needs of groups of people." By this time, however, the Food and Drug Administration, charged with regulating the promotion and sale of special diet foods and vitamins, had begun to recommend minimum daily requirements of the major vitamins and minerals. These would soon supplant the NRC's recommended allowances as benchmarks for health professionals, consumers, and the food industry.[29]

Meanwhile, wartime planners anticipated that the feeding of those on the home front would present the same kind of problems in changing food habits that Hoover's Food Administration had faced. Whereas Hoover turned to advertising men and home economists, however, the New Dealers turned to social scientists, particularly anthropologists. In December 1940, a year before the United States entered the war, a Committee on Food Habits, headed by anthropologist Margaret Mead, was established under the wing of the National Research Council to recommend ways in which national food habits could be altered in the face of the expected wartime shortages. As it turned out, the crisis was not as severe as anticipated and shortages were dealt with in ways which were anathema to Hoover: rationing and price controls. This was fortunate for the committee, for it never came near to formulating a program for changing food habits. Instead, its studies emphasized the complex connections between food habits and other aspects of culture, highlighting the difficulties faced by those who sought to deliberately change eating habits.[30]

One reason for the social scientists' pessimism about the possibilities for changing food habits through persuasion was that they were practically mesmerized by studies of the food habits of poor, rural Americans which emphasized the essentially irrational, uneconomic basis for their food choices and preferences. One, a study of "Riverbottom" people in the Ohio River Valley in southern Illinois, reported that the actual taste of food played little role in the food preferences of the fishermen, sharecroppers, and tenant farmers at the low end of the socio-economic scale. Although their food likes and dislikes were very strong, they derived more from status considerations than concerns about taste or economy. They rejected "nigger foods" such as muskrat and greens and fish (fishermen were the lowest-status occupational group) and aspired to urban food: oysters, canned salmon, hamburgers, celery, and canned chili, which the investigators thought they could not afford.[31] Another study, of poor farmers in the Southeast in 1940 and 1941, revealed a preference for processed, "urban" foods over cheaper, often more nutritious, home-grown ones. Canned hams were preferred to country hams, and beef and canned salmon were high-status items. Their own culinary tradition and foods were denigrated as "old-timey," "country," and "nigger." The anthropologists concluded that for them, the artificial-looking, lightly colored, packaged brand-name foods of the city connoted purity, prestige, science and being a part of the wider, more sophisticated urban-centered culture. Their conclusions echoed Edward Atkinson: the only way nutrition education could improve the eating habits of these people, they wrote, would be if "the overfed middle class and the 'beautiful' people would themselves hasten to choose the protein and iron-rich foods. If they do, these will be the prestige foods sought after by the malnourished as symbols of vertical mobility."[32]

Enamored as they seem to have been with highly processed foods, the poor Georgia farmers (a number of whose wives were readers of *Women's Home Companion*) had an accurate sense of where the urban diet was heading over the next thirty or so years. American food processing became more complex and the wizardry of food chemists rivaled the ancient dreams of alchemists, turning the pedestrian contents of their beakers into substances that looked and tasted like sugar, bacon, cream, and other delights. Most American consumers were impressed by these achievements, and until well into the 1960s they showed little concern for the methods and ingredients which food processors employed to turn out a host of new products. In an age in which, as in the 1920s, the achievements of American business seemed apparent to all, there was little inclination to question the products of the food business, which seemed to be making life easier for the housewife with each new chemical breakthrough. Much as canned goods had done earlier in the century, most of the new products that carved niches for themselves on supermarket shelves did so by appealing to "convenience," rather than superior taste or status. This was understandable, for harried postwar housewives seemed to be more pressed for time-saving and labor-saving devices than ever before. The millions of new households of the postwar "baby boom" were often presided over by mothers in deadly earnest about maintaining the highest standards of child-rearing and housekeeping. Like their grandmothers in the years before World War I, they visited each others' houses with eyes aglint, looking for signs of laxity in the corners of linoleum floors, mentally comparing the quality of coffee and cakes with those of the neighbors. After a wartime interlude in which work outside the home became acceptable, married women were again expected to find fulfillment in their wife-mother role. "At first I found it hard to believe that being a woman is something in itself," wrote one housewife, explaining to *Good Housekeeping* readers how she quit working and found happiness in housework. "I had always felt that a woman had to do something more than manage a household to prove her worth. Later, when I understood the role better, it took on unexpected glamor."[33]

Despite some similarities, the back-to-home atmosphere did not really represent a recrudescence of turn-of-the-century ways, for the housewife was still expected to be the glamorous sexual and social partner who had arrived in the 1920s. Food was still a way to get a man (Wesson Oil thoughtfully provided a recipe for "Man-Winning Tomato Salad" in the same issue of *Good Housekeeping*[34]), but it was understood that shapely legs were also an asset. Moreover, convenience and speed of preparation took precedence over the fine taste or impressive appearance of the final product of the kitchen. Although advertisers' cartoon marriages were still made or broken by the fluffiness of the wife's cakes, it was increasingly made from a mix, and "Quick 'N Easy" was the order of the day. "Quick Stunts with Hunts" were possible using canned tomato sauce.[35] White sauce, the mainstay of prewar home economists and cooking schools, became a relic of the past, replaced by condensed cream-of-mushroom soup in various guises. "Creamiest Dreamiest Creamed Dishes . . . Cream Sauces Too . . . This *Easy* Way!" said Campbell's. Its "Baked Chicken Puff," made by mixing cream-of-mushroom soup with some cooked chicken, canned green beans, cheese and eggs, was a complete meal in itself "and so quick, so easy!"[36]

Poverty was deemed to have virtually disappeared from the land, and with it went concern over the nutrition of the poor. Unlike its earlier editions in the 1920s and 1930s, the 1954 edition of Lydia Roberts's standard text on child nutrition did not even mention poverty as a cause of malnutrition. Malnutrition itself was now regarded as a clinical disorder which struck at random on the class scale, to be cured by trained dietitians using clinical methods.[37]

It is difficult to pinpoint exactly when the reaction against all of this began. The revised look at malnutrition dates at least from the rediscovery of poverty in the early 1960s, and particularly from Michael Harrington's influential book *The Other America,* which used evidence of persisting hunger and malnutrition to arouse concern over the plight of the millions of Americans living in poverty.[38] As a result of this and other *exposés,* federal programs to give the poor surplus farm products were instituted, followed by a food-stamp program which expanded the choice of free foods for the poor. There was also revived interest in school lunch programs to combat malnutrition, and federal aid was extended to subsidize them. When the late 1970s and early 1980s brought a renewal of complacency regarding malnutrition, as well as a turn against government programs to aid the poor, there were charges that hunger and malnutrition were again on the rise. One research group which advocated expanding nutrition programs issued eleven major reports from 1983 to mid-1986 in an attempt to document this. Its portrait of the diets of the poor in rural America has a familiar ring: not enough fresh vegetables, fruit, milk, beef, or chicken and therefore deficiencies in protein, vitamins A and C, iron, and calcium. This was reflected in stunted growth, learning disabilities, and significantly higher infant mortality rates for rural over urban America: 16.29 deaths per thousand versus 11.13. Despite dire warnings such as these, the Reagan Administration tried persistently to cut back on many of the nutrition programs. But the programs which had been created to meet the 1960s concerns over malnutrition could not easily be killed, and in fiscal 1986 the federal government still spent $18.3 billion on nutrition programs.[39]

In the mid-1960s as well, renewed concerns over health began to sweep the middle classes, inaugurating what seems to be the century's second Golden Age of Food Quackery. In part, the upsurge of concern over health originated in the neo-romantic youth rebellion and "counter-culture" of the late 1960s, which extolled all that was individual and natural and denigrated the mass-produced and artificial. This was abetted by media stories, akin to the "muckraking" exposés of Dr. Wiley's time, which reported that researchers had discovered that certain commonly used food additives caused cancer or other horrific ailments. Vitamin vendors and others who sensed the lucrative possibilities of the new concerns quickly set to work exploiting them. As James Harvey Young has written, "an integrated myth emerged of considerable persuasiveness: improper diet caused all disease; food wasn't what it used to be because of worn-out soil; chemical fertilizers poisoned the land and hence the food grown on it; pesticides heaped on more poison; food processing destroyed nutrients; you might not realize you were sick, but you really were, suffering from subclinical deficiencies."[40]

While food processors were initially able to neutralize this thrust by replacing or deleting the offensive additives and repackaging their products as "All-Natural," "Nature's Own," "Country Pride," and so on, concern over additives fed a resurgence of concern over nutrition and health, particularly as the "baby boomers" matured into a generation of extraordinarily self-absorbed people with pronounced narcissistic tendencies.

The parallels with the 1920s are striking. Again, apparent breakthroughs in nutritional science have combined with social changes to arouse renewed concern over food intake. From the mid-1970s on, the almost daily reports that linked diet to a host of afflictions have helped expand the "natural" foods thrust far beyond its original countercultural adherents, creating an atmosphere not unlike that which encouraged the middle class of the years 1905–25 to change its eating habits. Now, as in those years, concern has spread far beyond dangerous additives to encompass the nature of foods themselves.

Most upsetting has been evidence which seemed to indicate that many of the most commonly used foods in the American diet were lethal. Fear of cholesterol turned consumers against dairy products and eggs. By 1983, consumption of the former had dropped by 20 percent from 1950 levels and that of eggs had plummeted by a third. Consumption of whole milk, the miracle food of the 1920s, dropped by over half![41] Porterhouse steak and roast beef, which historically symbolized masculine success and contentment, now connoted heart attacks and stroke to the health-conscious and in the 1970s beef consumption began a steady decline as consumers turned to poultry and fish in the belief that they were less dangerous.[42] Those who use salt, perhaps man's oldest taste-enhancer, are now regarded with the same mixture of horror and pity as greets smokers and the only familiar star in the firmament seems to be the persistence of the American sweet tooth.[43]

On the other hand, as in the 1920s, previously denigrated foods are now promoted as "protective" foods: it has been years since middle-class people believed that carrots improved eyesight, but now they are told they prevent cancer. They have long since stopped forcing cod liver oil down their children's throats to head off rickets, but have now begun to take it themselves because fish oils may reduce heart disease. Tofu not only brings good health, it is also good for the environment. And so on.

Books advocating special diets which claim to prevent cancer, heart disease, and other killers top the best-seller lists, their authors ubiquitous guests on television talk shows. Either the heights of promotional genius were scaled or the *reductio ad absurdum* was plumbed with the appearance of a book entitled *Eat to Win,* which managed to capitalize on both the nutrition and the concurrent physical fitness craze by promising success in athletics to those who followed its dietary nostrums. Food processors have responded nimbly, churning out foods in low-calorie, low-sodium, low-cholesterol, low-fat, caffeine-free, high-fructose, high-protein, high-calcium, and high-fiber forms.

Various forms of vitamin-mania have been made possible by the ability to mass-produce vitamins in affordable mega-doses. Abetted by new scientific and pseudo-scientific discoveries, this has brought a resurgence of the 1920s hopes that vitamins were miracle cures for afflictions ranging from cancer to the common cold. A 1986 survey indicated more shoppers cited vitamin/mineral content as a factor in determining what foods to buy than any other consideration.[44]

A growing obsession with slimness echoed that of the 1920s. "Babe" Paley, the late point-person of the New York social scene summed up much of the philosophy of the emerging "Yuppie" generation best when, in the early 1970s, she declared, "You can't be too rich or too thin." However, to a much greater extent than in the earlier era, excess weight is now regarded as a health as well as an aesthetic problem. In the 1920s, "dieting" had been regarded as a primarily female pursuit. Now, excess weight conjures up visions of heart disease, diabetes, and other ailments, and slimness has come to connote good health as well as attractiveness. For the first time, then, men have become an important segment of the market for "diet" or, as they are now called, "calorie-reduced" foods. Nimble advertisers have even persuaded "macho-men" that drinking "Lite" beer or eating "Lean Cuisine" does not call their masculinity into question.[45]

With the upper and middle classes of both sexes now weight-conscious, and concern over obesity drifting down to the working class as well, the market for foods purporting to help weight-loss has expanded enormously. By 1984, almost 20 percent of the $290 billion spent on retail foods in the United States went for special "light" and "diet" foods.[46] When one considers that this does not include expenditures for fruits, vegetables, cottage cheese, and hundreds of other items purchased by weight-conscious people, the implications of this figure for the number of weight-conscious Americans is quite staggering.

But "natural foods" and frozen "Lean Cuisine" are not the whole story. In the mid-1960s, William Paley, the head of CBS and "Babe's" husband, had architect Eero Saarinen design a particularly elegant restaurant for the ground floor of the new head office building of CBS, where he and his friends could dine on fine French food. For the upper and middle class, food was again becoming the important denoter of status it had been at the turn of the century. Again, French food took the lead. Jacqueline Kennedy added luster to the glittering Kennedy image by importing a French chef to supervise the White House kitchen. Although not a fan of classic French cuisine, even folksy Lyndon Johnson felt constrained to keep French cooking as the public cooking of the White House for fear of being labeled an unsophisticated yokel by the Eastern Establishment he feared, courted, and despised.

French cooking now arose from the ashes in middle-class America. By then, "classic" cuisine was in retreat among French trend-setters themselves, and a renewed appreciation for bourgeois and provincial cooking, of a kind which could be imported into American restaurants and home kitchens, was on the ascendant. By the late 1960s, and early 1970s, then, from Bangor to San Diego, cities whose finer restaurants had been endless variations on the steak, lobster, and roast beef theme began to sprout French restaurants called "L'Auberge," or, failing that, "continental" ones of the type Calvin Trillin has labeled the "La Casa de la Maison House, Continental Cuisine" genre.

Middle-class home cooking received an energetic push back in the French direction when Julia Child, a foreign service officer's wife, parlayed the knowledge of French food gained during her husband's posting in France into an immensely successful French cookbook for middle-class Americans and what must have been the world's most popular television cooking series. By 1974 the first volume of the book had sold over 1.25 million copies, a total exceeded only by a few long-standing standard American cookbooks such as Irma Rombauer's *The Joy of Cooking.*[47] Thenceforth, mere beef in red wine sauce, bereft of *lardons* and small white onions, could no longer be fobbed off as *Boeuf bourguignon* in America, and no upper-middle-class kitchen was complete without an authentic copper bowl for whisking egg whites. Even those uninitiated into the finer points of the controversy over what constitutes an authentic *cassoulet* replaced tea sandwiches with quiche on ladies' luncheon plates, and Jell-O molds went the way of *Tyrannosaurus rex.*

With self-assured but competitive New Yorkers in the lead, the plunge into foreign cuisines became quite frenetic. This was first apparent in the restaurant industry. *Northern* Italian, Shanghai, Szechuan, Hunan, and ever-more obscure forms of Chinese food came to the fore, followed closely by Greek, Indian, Middle Eastern, Indochinese, and even Afghan and Ethiopian cuisines.[48]

Before long, middle-class home cooking, barely adjusted to the renewed French influence, was invaded by other foreign foods and terms. Suddenly, the canned-mushroom-soup and bottled-mayonnaise concoctions on the women's pages of newspapers and in women's magazines were giving way to the peasant dishes of the Third World. Pita bread joined Wonder Bread on supermarket shelves and American women were initiated into the mysteries of *polenta* and *baba ghanush*. Now even Mexican food, historically the object of fear and revulsion outside the Southwest, has shot up in status among the *cognoscenti*. What purport to be versions thereof have even become the theme of mass-market fast-food chains. Perhaps this is the last major foreign lode to be mined, at least for the moment, for it has been followed by a "rediscovery" of the American culinary tradition. Now well-heeled lawyers and bankers pay outrageous prices for the very catfish and hush puppies Riverbottom people had rejected as "nigger food."

There remain limits to how far culinary horizons can expand. Particularly when it hits the mass market through chain restaurants and frozen foods, much foreign food is unrecognizable as such, certainly to people from the purported countries of origin. Innards, extremities, and many other parts of animals' carcasses are still taboo, along with much of the seafood consumed in the rest of the world. Garlic, hot peppers, and spices are rigorously restricted in mass-market items, while bland, cheesy-looking substances which make the previous generations's Velveeta seem like Roquefort have replaced tangy cheeses.[49]

While the gap between image and reality is by no means as great as in the 1920s, when pashas' palaces served ham and cheese sandwiches, it has come from essentially the same source: the tension between the customer's desire to be titillated by something distinctive and the wish for the reassuringly familiar item on the plate. In these circumstances, historic Anglo-American food tastes remain remarkably resilient. Indeed, with the spread of soft drinks, snack foods, and fast-food chains throughout much of the world, with the Chinese government not only manufacturing Coca-Cola but also trying to encourage the consumption of Wonder-Bread-style bread in sandwiches, it seems that American food tastes and habits are having a greater impact on many foreign countries than foreign foods are having in America.

The apparent expansion of American culinary horizons has been much remarked upon, and although it is little more than skin deep it has distracted from other, more significant changes in American eating habits. As in the 1910s and 1920s, changes in the roles of females in the work force have had profound effects on food habits. In the 1920s, the increased proportion of single girls in white-collar occupations had profoundly affected the pattern of who ate what and where. Now, a surge in the number of working wives, mainly middle and lower-middle class, and the consequent rise of the two-income family has helped transform both restaurant and home cookery. While the single girls of the 1920s fueled a boom in cafeterias, lunch counters, and sandwich shops, the married women workers of the post-1960 era, and their families, have created a market for fast-food and other chain restaurants to relieve them from the burden of family meal preparation. With added income and less time for cooking, they also constitute a ready market for prepared foods, purchased at "take-home" outlets, supermarket "deli-counters," or even, as Charlotte Perkins Gilman had fantasized (although she certainly did not have pizza in mind) delivered by automobile piping hot to the home. The microwave oven and new forms of processing, preserving, and packaging enable food processors and retail grocery outlets to sell more food that necessitate only defrosting, boiling, or the most cursory last-minute preparation at home. Indeed, one of the common predictions of the turn-of-the-century home economists seems well on the way to being borne out: that food preparation would follow the other traditional household arts outside the home. However, the home economists had envisioned this as part of a process which would still leave mother as supreme guardian of the fires of home and family life, and never dreamed that it would happen as a consequence of women themselves leaving the home.

Delayed marriages, postponed child-bearing, and smaller families have reinforced the trend, begun in the 1920s, toward relegating the family dinner to a relic of the past. Single men and women living on their own and flush teen-agers swell the market for fast-food restaurants as well as for snack foods which could be eaten (sometimes literally) on the run. It even seems that the concept of the meal itself is being challenged by a new form of eating, aptly labeled "grazing."

In the process, the restaurant industry has undergone the same kind of restructuring that transformed the food-processing industry earlier in the century, as a few giants have emerged to dominate the chain and franchised restaurant sector. This has furthered the process of nationalizing and homogenizing American food tastes and habits which has been going on for at least two hundred years. In the 1920s critics complained that restaurant-goers in the farthest reaches of the country faced similar meals. Now, the meals are not just similar, they are identical, for the success of the new systems is based on the customer's certainty that wherever he or she goes, the product will indeed be exactly the same.

The trend toward homogeneity has not been limited to chain restaurants. The giant food processors, themselves the objects of a dizzying series of takeovers and mergers in the 1970s and 1980s, now play more important roles in supplying prepared, mainly frozen, foods to restaurants. Like the canned spaghetti which was such a hit with the cafeterias of the

1920s, their frozen Chicken Kiev and Shrimp à la Whoever save expensive labor costs and allow for large mark-ups. With most restaurant cooking requiring only a knowledge of defrosting, reheating, deep frying, and assembly, the pattern apparent in the 1920s was repeated and reinforced: the restaurant industry boomed, but the demand for well-trained, talented cooks did not begin to keep pace. Now unskilled or semi-skilled adult labor could be replaced by untrained, part-time, even cheaper teen-age labor.

Americans at today's table are therefore beset by apparent contradictions. On the one hand, there has been a marked movement toward homogeneity, toward the creation of a national diet. On other hand, one of the characteristics of this diet is a bewildering array of food choices, including many which purport to be foods of different cultures. Concerns for convenience and nutrition seem to outweigh economy as the main motives for food choices, but the recession of the early 1970s which, combined with rising prices for beef and other grain-fed commodities, encouraged middle-class consumers to adjust their eating habits, serves as a reminder that price still does matter.

As for nutrition, there seems little agreement on anything except that it must be important. As in the 1920s, many of the experts are firm in their pronouncements but vague in their proof. McCollum, the great guru of the Newer Nutrition, may have been right about vitamin D and rickets, but was not so right about white bread and was completely wrong regarding acidosis. The nutrition-conscious eater has no way of knowing whether today's experts, still engaged in the same scramble for research funds that consumed Atwater and his generation, are any more reliable guides than McCollum. As one expert on consumer attitudes toward nutrition recently said: "At one time or another, all of us must have felt that for every Ph.D there is an equal and opposite Ph.D."[50] With some justification, other wags have pointed out that a person who followed all of the experts' warnings against eating certain foods would surely die of malnutrition (whatever that really is).

Consumer surveys indicate that consumers' nutritional concerns are as variable as experts' advice. From 1983 to 1986, for example, the proportion of shoppers questioned who expressed concern over chemical additives in their foods declined by almost 60 percent, those concerned about preservatives fell by close to 70 percent and those looking for "natural" foods dropped by 250 percent. On the other hand, those concerned about fats and calories almost doubled and those avoiding cholesterol rose by more than 150 percent.[51]

Perhaps as a result of confusing signals being emitted by the "experts," few middle-class Americans seem to stick to one set pattern of eating.

Buffetted from food scare to food scare, enticed by the convenience (and, let it be said, the taste of) fast foods, unable to resist snack foods and "grazing," yet still relishing the occasional Julia Child-like triumph in the kitchen, *Homo Americanus* and family present a confused picture. As *Fortune* magazine noted, "The same working mother who repairs to McDonald's three times a week may settle down on the weekend for a bout of gourmet cooking. Diet sodas with pizza, health food for lunch, and junk food for dinner—the trends in the market for food are precisely as consistent as the eating habits of Americans."[52]

Beneath the turbulent surface, however, there are still calm, steady currents originating from bygone eras, for, although confused and confusing, contemporary attitudes toward food are still solidly grounded in the ideas which helped transform the American diet some one hundred years earlier: that taste is not a true guide to what should be eaten; that one should not simply eat what one enjoys; that the important components of food cannot be seen or tasted, but are discernible only in scientific laboratories; and that experimental science has produced rules of nutrition which will prevent illness and encourage longevity. All of these have been necessary underpinnings for the nutrition-consciousness of the 1970s and 1980s. We will never know, of course, what Atwater, Atkinson, Richards, Fletcher, Chittenden, and the other purveyors of these ideas would have thought of the outcome of their dietary bequest to the nation. We can be quite certain, however, that they would have recognized their own contribution to laying down its roots.

Over the years since Atwater, Atkinson, and Richards began their crusade, the American diet has indeed been radically transformed. As this book has tried to demonstrate, the years from about 1880 to 1930 were crucial in shaping the nature and direction of this process. During this time, material, social, and ideological forces converged to shape new ways of eating and new attitudes toward food. The material environment of America—its changing geography, expanding transportation networks, burgeoning financial and manufacturing institutions, and growing cities—both provided the stimulus and set the bounds for dietary change. Social changes connected with this, factors such as the rise of the urban working and middle classes, the servant shortage, the growth of bureaucracy, professionalism, and the changing female labor force, created an atmosphere receptive to certain kinds of ideas regarding food. The intellectual climate of the times, particularly the reverence for experimental science, made the middle class particularly receptive to the ideas of the New and Newer Nutritions.

However, as the rest of the twentieth century also demonstrated, the right social and intellectual climate was not, in itself, enough. In order for new nutritional ideas to be adopted by mainstream Americans and for national food habits to change, it was necessary for the changes to be actively fostered by the most powerful institutions in society, namely, government and the giant food corporations. The former, working through formal and informal educational systems, and the latter, with their influence over and advertising in the mass media, have been the only forces with the necessary resources to spread the message on a mass basis.

As we have seen, even with these substantial resources, it has not been easy to deliberately change food habits. The federal government had only limited success during World War I. The effectiveness of formal nutrition education in the schools is open to question. The giant corporations contributed to the widespread familiarity with some of the basic concepts of the New and Newer Nutritions but on a selective and skewed basis, often spreading as much misinformation as information. Their impact on consumer behavior is difficult to gauge, for, to a great extent, corporate food promotion and advertising followed rather than spurred changing food habits. Nevertheless, it is impossible to conceive of dietary change taking place in America without the active participation of these two forces. In the end, though, the propagation of the new ideas by powerful forces was not, in itself, enough. As Herbert Hoover discovered during the war— when workers ignored the Food Administration and ate more, rather than less, beef—food habits do not change merely in response to appeals to the mind, or even the heart. To be accepted, new ideas about food must also fit in with peoples' social and economic aspirations.

Notes

Introduction

1. Waverley Root and Richard de Rochemont, *Eating in America* (New York: William Morrow, 1976), 10.

2. These they cooked and seasoned in the manner that had won favor in seventeenth- and eighteenth-century England. As Root said, the term "as American as apple pie" could not be more inaccurate, for the dish (and the apple) is an import from England. *Ibid.*, 61–65.

3. The Dutch also had an early influence, but their cooking was so similar to the British that it was absorbed leaving hardly a trace. *Ibid.*, 302–9. One can also make an argument for Scandinavian inputs, as well as those of others, but at that stage the arguments get increasingly arcane.

4. Jean-Claude Bonnet, "Le réseau culinaire dans l'Encyclopédie", *Annales. Economies, Sociétés, Civilisations,* Vol. 31 (1976), 891–914.

5. Evan Jones, *American Food: The Gastronomic Story,* 2nd ed. (New York: Vintage Books, 1981), 123.

6. Susan Williams, *Savory Suppers and Fashionable Feasts: Dining in Victorian America* (New York: Pantheon, 1985), 113.

7. Juliet Corson, *The Cooking Manual* (New York: Dodd, Mead, 1879), 83.

8. Cited in *The Ladies' Home Magazine,* Vol. 16, no. 6 (Dec. 1860), 372. Pears and berries were popular during their seasons, but little interest was shown in other fruits. Lemons, oranges, bananas, and pineapples were imported to America, but only the well-to-do could afford them.

9. For example, Edgar W. Martin, *The Standard of Living in 1860* (Chicago:

Univ. of Chicago Press, 1942), 54–55. Waverley Root disagreed with this common assessment of the monotony of the pre-Civil War diet, pointing to the wealth of recipes for vegetables in cookbooks. However, aside from the problem involved in using proscriptive literature to prove the point (Martin used production and, where available, consumption statistics), he did concede that after 1860 there seems to have been a move away from variety on this score, something he ascribed to urbanization and industrialization, and said Americans remained suspicious of fruits and vegetables until about World War I. Root, *Eating in America,* 139–43.

10. "Herbs, Their Domestic Uses, Properties, Culture," *Godey's Lady's Book and Magazine,* No. 86, [1873], 178.

11. *The Ladies' Magazine,* Vol. 6, [1833], 437.

12. Root, *Eating,* 107. Indeed, it remained a relative rarity in England until quite recently. It was normally unavailable in the greengrocers in the sizable Midlands town in which I lived in the late 1970s and had to be purchased at a shop which specialized in imports from the Continent.

13. Sidney Mintz, *Sweetness and Power* (New York: Viking, 1985), 188. Mintz also cites the statement of the revolutionary leader John Adams that "molasses was an essential ingredient in American independence" (*Ibid.,* p. 256) in support of this but Adams was more likely thinking of its importance in making rum than in the delightful taste it adds to Indian pudding.

14. Elizabeth Ayrton, *The Cookery of England* (Harmondsworth: Penguin, 1974), 429–30; cited, 120.

15. Mary Cabell Tyree, *Housekeeping in Old Virginia* (Louisville: John Morton, 1879).

16. Beecher and Beecher Stowe, *American Woman's Home,* 190.

17. Although many North Americans have the impression that sweetness is a common component of Chinese cooking, this is not so. Only the Cantonese-speakers (a minority of only 200 million or so) sweeten main courses to any significant degree, and they do so with a relatively light hand.

18. Anthony Trollope, *North America* (London: Chapman and Hall, 1862), Vol. I: 181.

19. Thomas Hamilton, *Men and Manners in America* (Edinburgh: William Blackwood, 1833), 24.

20. This was not simply the result of "a desire to have more than is paid for," on the American plan, he thought, for he had witnessed the same phenomenon in places on the European plan, and concluded that it was "simply a bad and ugly habit." P. Blouet [pseud. Max O'Rell], "Reminiscences of American Hotels," *The North American Review,* Vol. 152, No. 1 (Jan. 1892), 89.

21. Gen. Rush C. Hawkins and W. J. Fanning, "The American Hotel of Today," *ibid.,* Vol. 157, No. 8 (Aug. 1893), 198; "A Curious Find at the Hotel Brevoort," *The Chef,* Vol. 1, No. 1 (Feb. 1910), 19.

22. Frances Trollope, *Domestic Manners of the Americans* (1832) (New York: Dodd, Mead, 1927), 50–52.

23. Catharine Beecher and Harriet Beecher Stowe, *The American Woman's Home* (New York: J. B. Ford, 1869), 168.

24. Corson, *The Cooking Manual,* 8.

25. Hamilton, *Man and Manners in America,* 43.

26. Michael Chevalier, *Society, Manners and Politics in the United States* (Boston, 1839), 284.

27. Arthur M. Schlesinger, Jr., *Paths to the Present* (Boston: Houghton Mifflin, 1964), 226.

28. Robert Lacour-Gayet, *Everyday Life in the United States before the Civil War, 1830–1860*, trans. Mary Ilford (New York: Ungar, 1969), 45.

29. Hamilton, *Man and Manners in America*, 43.

Chapter 1.

1. Arthur M. Schlesinger, Jr., *Learning How to Behave* (New York: Macmillan, 1946), 28.

2. Jefferson Williamson, *The American Hotel* (New York: Knopf, 1930), 214.

3. Joseph Conlin, "Beans, Bacon, and Galantine Truffles: The Food of the Western Miners," *Arizona and the West*, Vol. 23, No. 1 (Spring 1981), 48.

4. Williamson, *The American Hotel*, 214.

5. Beecher and Beecher Stowe, *American Woman's Home*, 190, 179.

6. Colson, *Cooking Manual*, 3.

7. Mary E. Sherwood, *Etiquette. The American Code of Manners.* (New York: Routledge, 1884), 11.

8. [Abby B. Longstreet], *Social Etiquette of New York* (New York, 1878), 12; cited in Schlesinger, *Learning How to Behave*, 29.

9. Joseph Conlin, "Consider the Oyster," *American Heritage*, (Feb.–March, 1980), 65–66.

10. Menu reproduced in Charles Anhofer, *The Epicurean* (Chicago: Hotel Monthly Press, 1920), 1106.

11. Ibid., 1107. Delmonico's major bow in the direction of the New World was to use first-class American ingredients when possible.

12. Jean-Paul Aron, "Sur les consommations avariées à Paris dans le deuxième moitié du xixe siècle, *Annales E. S. C.*, 30 e année, No. 2–3 (mars–juin 1975); *Le mangeur du XIXe siècle*, (Paris: Robert Laffont, 1973), 296–99.

13. Thomas Duncan, *How to be Plump* (Chicago: Duncan Bros., 1878), 18–19.

14. Lois Banner, *American Beauty* (Chicago: Univ. of Chicago Press, 1983), 112–31.

15. Chris Chase, *The Great American Waistline* (New York: Coward, McCann, 1981), 12.

16. Karl Schriftgiesser, *Oscar of the Waldorf* (New York: Dutton, 1943), 38.

17. Veronique Nahoum, "La belle femme, ou le stade du miroire en histoire," *Communications*, No. 31 (1979), 26–30.

18. David Potter, *People of Plenty* (Chicago: Univ. of Chicago Press, 1955).

19. Thorstein Veblen, *Theory of the Leisure Class* (New York: Macmillan, 1899, 1912). While Veblen pays little attention to the role of food habits in this process, a recent French work places great emphasis on their importance in the process of creating class distinctions. Pierre Bourdieu, *La Distinction—Critique social du jugement* (Paris: Editions de Minuit, 1982), 20; (English edition: trans. Richard Nice, Distinction: *A Social Critique of the Judgement of Taste* (Cambridge: Harvard Univ. Press, 1984).

20. Sarah J. Hale, *Mrs. Hale's New Cook Book* (Philadelphia: Peterson & Bros., 1857), 499, 497.

21. Catharine Beecher, *Treatise on Domestic Economy for the Use of Young Ladies at Home and School* (Boston: T. H. Webb, 1843), 44–52; cited in Katherine Kish Sklar, *Catharine Beecher, A Study in Domesticity* (New York: Norton, 1976), 306.

22. Ward McAllister, *Society as I Have Found It* (New York: Cassell, 1890), 234–35, 157.

23. *Ibid.*, 100–1.

24. Mary E. Sherwood, *The Art of Entertaining* (New York: Dodd, Mead, 1892), 143.

25. See the menus in the Menu Collection, Schlesinger Library, Radcliffe College, Cambridge, Massachusetts, and those in the Menu Collection, Rare Books Division, New York Public Library, Box 1.

26. Helen Duprey Bullock Papers, Schlesinger Library, Radcliffe College, Folder 15.

27. The Occidental Hotel in Leadville, Colorado, probably was more deserving of the title, for it actually hired away one of Delmonico's chief chefs. Conlin, "Beans, Bacon," 49–51.

28. Aron, *Le mangeur*, 207.

29. See, for example, the breakfast menus of Saratoga's American and Grand Union hotels in The Menu Collection, NYPL, Box 1.

30. Grand Union Hotel, Children and Nurses' Dining Room Menu, [1883], Menu Collection, NYPL, Box 1.

31. Sherwood, *Etiquette*, 365.

32. *Ibid.*, 363.

33. Samuel Eliot Morison, *One Boy's Boston* (Boston: Houghton Mifflin, 1962), 49.

34. Cited in Schlesinger, *Learning How to Behave*, 42.

35. The fashionable hour for dinner in New York in the 1880s was 7:00 p.m., somewhat earlier than in the rest of the country. Sherwood, *Etiquette*, 371.

36. Morison, *One Boy's Boston*, 52.

37. Although they were great favorites in Philadelphia, where the elite tended to eat late, high teas were never too popular with males because of the absence of alcoholic beverages. Sherwood, *Etiquette*, 370.

38. Urbain-Dubois, *Cuisine artistique* (Paris: Dentu, 1882), x.

39. Williamson, *The American Hotel*, 215.

40. Williams, *Savory Suppers*, 152.

41. Cited, with attribution to a number of works, in Schlesinger, *Learning How to Behave*, 41.

42. Morison, *One Boy's Boston*, 49, 52.

43. The "ideal" number of servants for the "ultra-fashionable," according to a turn-of-the-century book on the topic, was ten or eleven: chef, cook, kitchen maid, kitchen scullery, one or two laundresses, parlor maid and three or four "men." Charles W. Nichols, *The Ultra-Fashionable Peerage of America* (New York: George Harjes, 1904), 74.

44. Gwendolyn Wright, *Building the Dream: A Social History of Housing in America* (New York: Pantheon, 1981), 111. Depending on how one defines it, about 15 percent of Americans could be called urban middle class in 1880. For

detailed analyses of the statistics on domestic servants see David M. Katzman, *Seven Days a Week: Women and Service in Industrializing America* (New York: Oxford Univ. Press, 1978).

45. Catherine Owen (Helen Nitsch), *Ten Dollars Enough* (Boston: Houghton Mifflin, 1886) 8.

46. Those who aspired to "fancy cooking" would have to buy additional equipment, such as ice cream freezers and charlotte russe molds. Maria Parloa, *Miss Parloa's New Cook Book and Marketing Guide* (Boston: Estes and Lauriat, 1880), 66–67.

47. Parloa, *New Cook Book*, 410; Massachusetts, Bureau of Statistics of Labor, *Twenty-eighth Annual Report* (March, 1898), 12–21; Daniel Walkowitz, *Worker City, Company Town* (Urbana: Univ. of Illinois Press, 1978), 105.

48. Catherine Owen (Helen Nitsch), *Culture and Cooking* (New York: Cassell, Peter Galpin & Co., 1881) 70.

49. Parloa, *New Cook Book*, 405.

50. Williams, *Savory Suppers*, 67.

51. *Ladies' Home Journal*, Oct. 1886, 6.

52. A Boston Housekeeper, *An American Family Cook Book* (New York: Felt, 1865), xii.

53. *Godey's Lady's Book and Magazine*, Vol. 90 (1875), 471; Vol. 95 (1877), 21.

54. Tarbox, *What to Eat for Breakfast*, 47.

55. For example, see Juliet Corson, *Cooking Manual*, 4–5.

56. For example, the menus of the annual reunions of Boston's Brahmin OMJ Society from 1878 to 1884 followed the latest trends in that the nomenclature became progressively more French over the six years (even though the dishes remained mainly American and English in their straightforwardness). Yet although a wide variety of meats, seafood, and game was served, there was not one menu on which pork appeared. Hotel and Restaurant Menu Collection, Schlesinger Library.

57. *Godey's Lady's Book and Magazine*, Vol. 95 (1877), 395.

58. Parloa, *New Cook Book*, 403–11.

59. *Good Housekeeping*, Vol. 10, No. 10 (March 15, 1890), 229.

60. Mary J. Lincoln, *Mrs. Lincoln's Cook Book* (Boston: Roberts, 1883), 36.

61. *The American Code of Manners*, cited in Schlesinger, *Paths to the Present*, 226.

62. Although constipation tends to be more common in females than males, Victorian taboos inhibited women from complaining about it.

63. Evidence that middle-class bodies and waistlines were getting larger came in the 1880s, when dealers in ready-to-wear clothing, whose major market lay in the middle class, adopted a larger scale of sizes. Schlesinger, *Paths to the Present*, 229.

Chapter 2.

1. P. H. Lindhert and Jeffrey G. Williamson, "Three Centuries of American Inequality," in P. Usedling, ed., *Research in Economic History*, Vol. 1 (Greenwich: JAI Press, 1976), 69–123.

2. Robert W. Fogel, Stanley Engerman, and James Trussell, "Exploring the Uses of Data on Height," *Social Science History*, Vol. 6, No. 4 (Fall 1982), 416–17. A recent study of birth weights in industrializing Montreal provides further evidence

that industrialization and urbanization meant poorer nutrition for the nineteenth-century North American working class. Peter Ward and Patricia C. Ward, "Infant Birth Weight and Nutrition in Industrializing Montreal," *American Historical Review,* Vol. 89, No. 2 (April 1984), 324–45.

3. Catherine Owen, *Culture and Cooking,* 95.

4. John Modell, *Family Budget Study: Massachussets, 1874,* Dataset ICPSR 9032, (Ann Arbor, Mich.: Inter-University Consortium for Political and Social Research, 1983).

5. Families of four to six with total annual incomes of over $800 consumed over twice as much beef per capita as those earning under $400.

The data, which includes some statistics on five European nations as well, is compiled in computer readable form in U.S. Department of Labor, *Cost of Living of Industrial Workers in the United States and Europe, 1888–1890,* Dataset ICPSR 7711, (Ann Arbor, Mich.: Inter-University Consortium for Political and Social Research, 1984). The dubious utility of the numerical means calculated from the data, as opposed to their rank order, results in part from the large number of missing cases in most categories, and the fact that many seem to have been entered as zeros as well as the usual "99999." This means that, in excluding the responses of "0" in order to exclude non-respondents, some respondents who actually did not consume any of a given item over the year were likely excluded as well, thus elevating the values of the means.

6. Later, the president of the American Federation of Labor, Samuel Gompers, echoed this theme, quoting Blaine's warnings in AFL's own anti-oriental campaign. Samuel Gompers, *Meat vs. Rice. Some Reasons for Chinese Exclusion,* U.S. Senate, 57th Cong., 1st sess., Doc. No. 137 (Washington: GPO, 1902), 24.

7. The best-off (those living on over $800) drank only about 20 percent more than those with incomes below $400.

8. Although the number of respondents who estimated beef consumption in the latter two is really too low to be significant, the fact that many more gave estimates for fresh pork consumption would seem to indicate that this was one of the cases where a significant number of the responses of "0" may well have meant no fresh beef at all.

9. Illinois Bureau of Labor Statistics, *Biennial Report,* No. 3 (1884), 370–71, in Irving Yellowitz, ed., *The Position of the Worker in American Society, 1865–1896* (Englewood Cliffs, N.J.: Prentice-Hall, 1969), 74–76.

10. U.S., Commissioner of Labor, *Sixth Annual report: Costs of Production* (Washington: GPO, 1891), 693 ff., cited in Smuts, *Women and Work*), 11.

11. Daniel Walkowitz, *Worker City, Company Town,* (Urbana: University of Illinois Press, 1978,) 103–4. Wages in other industries followed similar patterns. Statistics for all industrial occupations in Massachussets in 1881 show unskilled male labor being paid about $7.50 to $10.00 a week, with women and children receiving down to $3.00. The average weekly wages of most skilled workers, on the other hand, was well over $16.00 and ranged up to almost $28.00 for "heaters" in the metal industry. The lowest paid of the semi-skilled, in the low-paying cotton and wool industries, averaged over $11.50 a week. State of Massachusetts, Bureau of Labor Statistics, *Twenty-Eighth Annual Report,* March, 1898, (Boston: State Printers, 1898), 12–21.

12. Trachtenberg, *Incorporation,* 95.

13. He calculates that $228.00 was needed to keep a family consisting of hus-

band and wife in the bare necessities with proportionally more for those with children. He estimates that, in addition to the 20 percent below this line, 40 percent of the families dependent on the iron industry and about two-thirds of those in the cotton mills lived at or just above this line. Walkowitz, *Worker City*, 103–4.

14. "Cost of Living of Industrial Workers," Dataset ICPSR 7711.

15. As we shall see in Chapter 4, labor leaders such as Eugene V. Debs who opposed efforts to persuade workers to economize on food accused reformers of trying to reduce the American worker's diet to the low level of his European counterparts. Their assessment of the relative merits of the diets on both sides of the ocean was supported by the dietary surveys of the time, which consistently showed American workers eating more than the British and Europeans.

16. Frederick L. Olmsted, *A Journey in the Back Country* (New York: 1860), 396; *The Seaboard Slave States*, 698, cited in Richard Cummings, *The American and His Food*, 86–87.

17. Throughout the century, the infant death rate varied between 222 and 237 per thousand for females and an astounding, in modern terms, 266 and 278 for males. This helped reduce the mean life expectancy at birth for blacks during the century to 33.7 years. Jack Eblen, "New Estimates of the Vital Rates of the United States Black Population during the Nineteenth Century," *Demography*, Vol. 11, No. 2 (May 1974), 301–19.

18. Paul Buck, "The Poor Whites of the Ante-bellum South," *American Historical Review*, Vol. 31, No. 3 (Oct. 1925), 46.

19. Elizabeth W. Etheridge, *The Butterfly Caste: A Social History of Pellagra in the South* (Westport: Greenwood, 1971), 9.

20. Jacqueline Jones, *Labor of Love, Labor of Sorrow: Black Women, Work, and the Family from Slavery to the Present* (New York: Basic Books, 1985), 106, 83.

21. *Ibid.*, 88–89.

22. Theodore C. Blewgen, *Norwegian Migration to America* (Northfield: Norwegian-American Historical Association, 1940), 195.

23. In the eastern states, rural infant mortality rates seem to have been somewhat lower than those of the cities, and those of farmers were considerably lower than those of the foreign-born workers at the bottom of the working class socioeconomic pole. Michael R. Haines, "Mortality in Nineteenth Century America: Estimates from New York and Pennsylvania Census Data. 1865 and 1900," *Demography*, Vol. 14, No. 3 (Aug. 1977), 311–30.

24. John Ise, *Sod and Stubble* (New York, 1940), cited in Robert W. Smuts, *Women and Work in America* (New York: Schocken, 1971), 8.

25. Katzman, *Seven Days* 59–61.

26. James Cowan to Major Herbert Cowan, Jan. 28, 1888, Letters from Emigrants to America Collection, London School of Economics, London, U.K.

Chapter 3.

1. Williams, *Savory Suppers*, 113.

2. Eric Lampard, *The Rise of the Dairy Industry in Wisconsin* (Madison: State Historical Society of Wisconsin, 1963), 196.

3. Williams, *Savory Suppers*, 114.

4. In the nine years from 1872 to 1881, for example, the price of rump steak in Massachusetts dropped by about one-third. Massachusetts, Bureau of Labor Statistics, *Twenty-eighth Annual Report* March 1898, (Boston: State Printers, 1898), 23.

5. *Ibid.,* 23–25. The impact of these declines on the lower classes was tempered by falling or stable wage rates and income for many workers and farmers.

6. Alfred S. Eichler, *The Emergence of Oligopoly: Sugar Refining as a Case Study* (Baltimore: Johns Hopkins, 1969), 36.

7. *Ibid.,* 68–69.

8. Mary J. Lincoln, *The Boston Cook Book* rev. (Boston: Little, Brown, 1900), 458.

9. Sidney Mintz, *Sweetness and Power: The Place of Sugar in Modern History* (New York: Viking, 1985).

10. Cummings, *American and His Food,* 114, 236.

11. Alonzo E. Taylor, "Consumption, Merchandising, and Advertising of Foods," *Harvard Business Review* April, 1924, 281–95.

12. Maurice Aymard, "Pour l'histoire de l'alimentation: quelques remarques de méthode," *Annales. E. S. C.* 30e année, No. 2–3 (mars-juin, 1975).

13. Gerald Carson, *Corn Flake Crusade* (New York: Rinehart & Co., 1957), 162–75.

14. *Ibid.,* 196–99.

15. Ralph M. Hower, *The History of an Advertising Agency* (Cambridge: Harvard Univ. Press: 1939), 634–42, cited in Naomi Aronson, "Working Up an Appetite," in Jane R. Kaplan, ed., *A Woman's Conflict* (Englewood Cliffs: Prentice-Hall, 1980), 216.

16. William G. Panschar, *Baking in America: Economic Development,* Vol. 1 (Evanston: Northwestern Univ. Press, 1956), 82–83.

17. Robert C. Alberts, *The Good Provider: H. J. Heinz and his 57 Varieties* (Boston: Houghton Mifflin, 1973), Ch. 9.

18. *Ibid.,* 47, 149.

19. Edward C. Hampe, Jr., and Merle Wittenberg, *The Lifeline of America* (New York: McGraw-Hill, 1964), 119–23.

20. *Ibid.,* 121–23.

21. Moreover, the usual combination of expensive new techniques for mass production and a growing number of mergers was already laying the groundwork for the rise of a few giant wholesale bakers. Their packaged breads, sold on grocers' shelves, were already driving the craftsmen who ran small bakeries out of business. Panschar, *Baking in America,* 83–87.

22. *New York World,* July 18, 1910.

23. C. McCurdy, "American Law and the Marketing Structure of the Large Corporation, 1875–1890," *Journal of Economic History,* Vol. 38, No. 3 (1978), 644, cited in Eric B. Ross, "Patterns of Diet and Forces of Production: An Economic and Ecological History of the Ascendancy of Beef in the United States Diet," in Eric Ross, ed., *Beyond the Myths of Culture* (New York: Academic Press, 1980), 202.

24. Bertram B. Fowler, *Mean, Meat, and Miracles* (New York: Julian Messner, 1952), 108–9.

25. Actually, their number varied somewhat, depending on competition, mergers, and so on. They began as the Big Four, became the Big Five and then the Big

Six and then finally the Big Five again. Although they hardly deserved the muckraking label, "The Greatest Trust in the World," in 1905 the four largest of them slaughtered from 45 to 50 percent of the country's beef cattle. Alfred Chandler, Jr., *Strategy and Structure* (Cambridge: M.I.T. Press, 1962), 25–26; Gabriel Kolko, *The Triumph of Conservatism* (New York: The Free Press, 1963), 53; Ross, "Patterns of Diet," 202–3.

26. Kolko, *Conservatism*, 101–6.

27. *Harper's Magazine Advertiser*, Vol. 64 (Dec. 1906), n.p.

28. Alberts, *Good Provider*, 49–50, 172–6. The legislation was also supported by a number of other food processing interests, including the brewers', butter makers', and confectioners' associations. The main organized opposition came from patent medicine and whiskey producers. Kolko, *Conservatism*, 108–9.

29. Alberts, *Good Provider*, 166.

30. Maurice Natenberg, *The Legacy of Dr. Wiley* (Chicago: Regent House, 1957), 40.

31. Honoré Willsie, "Canning and the Cost of Living," *Harper's Weekly* Nov. 1, 1913, 8–9.

32. *Harper's Magazine Advertiser*, Vol. 64 (Dec. 1906), n.p.

33. *Ibid.*

34. *Ibid.*, Vol. 60 (Feb. 1905), n.p.

35. H. A. Ross, *The Marketing of Milk in the Chicago Dairy District*, University of Illinois Agricultural Experiment Station, Bulletin No. 269 (June 1925), 464; "Outline of Mrs. White's Career in Social Work," Eva White Papers, Schlesinger Library, Box 1, Folder 1; Irene Till, *Milk, the Politics of an Industry* (New York: McGraw-Hill, 1938), 451–52.

Chapter 4.

1. *The Ladies' Home Magazine*, Vol. 15, No. 3 (March 1860), 183.

2. *Ibid.*, Vol. 16, No. 6 (Dec. 1860), 372.

3. Wilbur O. Atwater, "The Pecuniary Economy of Food," *Century Magazine*, Vol. 35, No. 3 (Jan. 1888), 437–46.

4. Atwater, "The Chemistry of Foods and Nutrition," *Ibid.*, Vol. 34, No. 1 (May 1887), 59–74.

5. Wilbur O. Atwater, "The Chemistry and Economy of Food," *Proceedings* of the 3rd Annual Session, National Convention of Chiefs and Commissioners of Bureaus of Labor (Boston, 1885), 215–22; "Chemistry of Foods", 72–73; "Pecuniary Economy of Food," 445.

6. Wilbur O. Atwater to Edward Atkinson, Oct. 11, 1890, Edward Atkinson Papers, Massachusetts Historical Society, Boston, Mass. (hereafter cited as *AP*).

7. Atkinson, "Comparative Nutrition," Rumford Kitchen Leaflet No. 4 in, *The Rumford Kitchen Leaflets,* ed. Ellen H. Richards (Boston: Rockwell and Churchill, 1899), 6.

8. "The Aladdin Oven," *Popular Science Monthly*, Nov. 1889. Later versions used more lamps and had asbestos linings. Edward Atkinson, *Science of Nutrition*, 4th ed. (Boston: the author, 1892), 3–7.

9. Mary Hinman Abel, *Practical, Sanitary, and Economic Cooking Adapted to*

Persons of Moderate and Small Means (Rochester: American Public Health Association, 1890).

10. Mary Hinman Abel, *"The Story of the New England Kitchen, Part II,"* in Ellen Richards, ed., *The Rumford Kitchen Leaflets* (Boston: Rockwell and Churchill, 1899), 154; Atkinson, *Science of Nutrition,* 65.

11. In the early 1880's, for example, Helen Campbell, a pioneer in the movement to teach home economics to the poor, had written: "That cooking schools and knowledge of cheap and savory preparation of food must soon have their effect on the percentage of drunkards no one can question." Cited in Mrs. James T. Fields, *How to Help the Poor* (Boston: Houghton Mifflin, 1884), 112.

12. Richards to Atkinson, April 10, 1896, *AP;* Edward James and Janet Wilson James, eds., *Biographical Dictionary of Notable American Women* (Cambridge: Harvard Univ. Press, 1971), 145.

13. Abel, "Story of the New England Kitchen, Part II, *Rumford Kitchen Leaflets,* 134.

14. It is curious that they idolized Rumford, for when the cheap soup he prescribed for the inmates of the Munich workhouse was adopted by other poorhouses in Europe its introduction was often followed by decimating outbreaks of scurvy and soaring death rates. Although they cannot be faulted for not recognizing that the concoction of herring and pulses was deficient in vitamins, some quick calculations using the tools of the "New Nutrition" would have told them that the recommended servings of the much-vaunted soup provided only a starvation ration of 1,000 calories a day per person. J. C. Drummond, *The Englishman's Food* (London: Jonathan Cape, 1939, rev., 1957), 257–58, 330.

15. Ellen H. Richards, "Scientific Cooking: Studies in the New England Kitchen, *Forum,* Vol. 15 (May, 1893), 355–59.

16. Maria Parloa, "The New England Kitchen," *Century Magazine,* Vol. 21, No. 12 (Dec. 1891), 315; Richards to Atkinson, Dec. 19, 1889, *AP.*

17. Richard to Atkinson, Nov. 11, 1889, *AP.*

18. Richards, "The Wholesale Preparation of Food," in Atkinson, *The Science of Nutrition,* 64.

19. A normal loaf cost six to eight cents in the bakeries. Richards to Atkinson, March 8, 1890, *AP.*

20. Atkinson, Richards, and Abel, "The Right Application of Heat to the Conversion of Food Material," *Proceedings of the 39th Meeting of the American Association for the Advancement of Science,* Aug. 1890 (Salem: AAAS, 1891), 419–21.

21. Abel, "Story of the New England Kitchen, Part II," 136–37; Parloa, "New England Kitchen," 317.

22. Abel, "Story of the New England Kitchen, Part II," 138; Richards to Atkinson, Oct. 1, 1891, *AP.*

23. Abel, "Story of the New England Kitchen, Part II," 138; James and James, *Notable American Women,* 145; Richards, "Public Kitchens in Relation to School Lunches and Restaurants," Rumford Kitchen Leaflet No. 17, in Richards, ed., *Rumford Kitchen Leaflets.* Previously, janitors had sold sandwiches and other cold foods to children who did not bring packed lunches but the nutritionists were unanimous about the need for hot lunches. Cold food was wasteful, they thought, for the body consumed much of the food's energy in raising it to the proper temperature for digestion. Indeed, Atkinson's first foray into the technology of

food reform involved inventing a workman's lunch pail in which lunches could be slow-cooked during the morning to be hot and ready to eat at lunchtime.

24. Mary H. Moran and Julia Pulsifer, "Boston's Public School Lunches," reprinted article (Boston: Women's Educational and Industrial Union); "The New England Kitchen and School Lunch, typescript in Mary H. Abel Papers, Schlesinger Library, Radcliffe College.

25. Abel, "New England Kitchen, Part II," 139.

26. Abram Hewit to Atkinson, Sept. 19, 1890, Oct. 1, 1890, *AP*.

27. Thomas Egleston to Atkinson, March 9, 1891; Andrew Carnegie to Atkinson, March 21, 1891, *AP*. Carnegie was already acquainted with Atkinson and had engaged him in a lively correspondence regarding the tariff. See various letters in the later 1880's in *ibid.*

28. Egleston to Atkinson, Nov. 20, 1891, Nov. 27, 1891, Jan. 23, 1892, *AP*.

29. Abel, "New England Kitchen, Part II," 142.

30. Egleston to Atkinson, Feb. 26, 1892, May 26, 1893, *AP*.

31. *New York Observer,* Sept. 21, 1893; Hull House, *Year Book,* 1925, in Jane Addams Papers, Settlement House Collection, Sophia Smith Collection, Smith College.

32. Abel, "New England Kitchen, Part II," 148; Philadelphia College Settlement House, Seventh Report (Sept. 1895 to Oct. 1896), 24, in Settlement House Collection, Sophia Smith Collection, Smith College.

33. Richards to Atkinson, March 23, 1893, *AP;* James and James, *Notable American Women,* 145; Richards, ed., *The Rumford Kitchen Leaflets.* Their use of the state pavilion was faciliated by Carroll Wright, then Massachusetts Commissioner of Labor, later the head of the U.S. Bureau of Labor Statistics, who was a keen sympathizer with their scientific approach to the industrial crisis.

34. Richards to Atkinson, April 1, 1893; Booker T. Washington to Atkinson, May 20, 1895, Oct. 31, 1895, *AP*.

35. College Settlements Association, Fourth Annual Report (1892–93), 23, Seventh Annual Report (1895–96), 24, Eighth Annual Report (1896–97), 30, Ninth Annual Report (1897–98).

36. Hull House, *Year Book* (1925).

37. Atkinson to Havemeyer, Feb. 19, 1894, March 4, 1894, *AP*.

38. *Ibid.*

39. Richards to Atkinson, Nov. 22, 1894, *AP*.

40. See Atkinson, *Science of Nutrition,* 4th Edition, 1–10, 52–57; Atkinson to his Customers, April 22, 1890, Richards to Atkinson, April 12, 1892, *AP*.

41. Egleston to Atkinson, Feb. 26, 1892, *AP*.

42. Ellen H. Richards, *The Cost of Food: A Study in Dietaries* (New York: John Wiley, 1902), 51.

43. Egleston to Atkinson, Dec. 22, 1894, Atkinson to Egleston, Nov. 6, 1895, Egleston to Atkinson, Nov. 9, 1895, March 12, 1896, *AP*.

44. Egleston to Atkinson, Feb. 26, 1892, *AP*.

45. Atkinson, *Suggestions for the Establishment of Food Laboratories in Connection with the Agricultural Experiment Stations,* U.S. Department of Agriculture, Office of Experiment Stations, Bulletin No. 17 (1893); Egleston to Atkinson, May 26, 1893, Atkinson to Havemeyer, Feb. 19, 1894, *AP*.

46. George Rosen, "Ellen Richards (1842–1911)," *American Journal of Public*

Health, Vol. 64, No. 8 (1974). See the contributions by Abel and Richards to Atwater's *Chemistry and Economy of Food*, and Abel, *Sugar as Food*, U.S. Department of Agriculture, Office of Experiment Stations, Farmer's Bulletin 93 (1899), and *Beans, Peas, and Other Legumes as Food*, Farmer's Bulletin 121 (1900).

47. Richards to Atkinson, Nov. 26, 1897, *AP*.

48. Robert Clarke, *Ellen Swallow, The Woman Who Founded Ecology*, (Chicago: Follett, 1973), 129.

49. Moran and Pulsifer, "Boston's School Lunches"; "The New England Kitchen and School Lunch," unsigned memorandum, [1944?], Abel Papers; Unsigned, untitled memorandum on WEIU lunch programs, [1955?] WEIU Papers, Schlesinger Library, Radcliffe College.

50. Indeed, as at least one of his detractors pointed out, the Ricardian Iron Law of Wages, which he often cited, would dictate that cheaper food be invariably followed by lower wages. Reply to Atkinson by R. M. Chamberlin, in Atkinson, *The Margin of Profits*, 56–57, cited in Harold Williamson, *Edward Atkinson* (Cambridge: Harvard Univ. Press, 1934), 272.

51. Eugene V. Debs, editorial, *Locomotive Fireman's Magazine* (June, 1892), cited in Williamson, *Edward Atkinson*, 272.

52. For example, Atwater, "Pecuniary Economy of Food," 437; Atkinson, *Science of Nutrition*, 47.

53. Abel, "New England Kitchen, Part II," 151.

54. Abel, "King Palate," Rumford Leaflet No. 3, in Richards, ed., *Rumford Leaflets*, 36.

55. George F. Kunz, "Tribute to Ellen H. Richards," Association of Collegiate Alumnae, [1912], 299, copy in Ellen H. Richards Papers, Smith College.

56. Sample menus in the WEIU Papers and in Richards, "An Account of the New England Kitchen and the Rumford Food Laboratory," reprint of paper presented to the Massachusetts Medical Society, June 1892, and "Count Rumford and the New England Kitchen," *The New England Kitchen Magazine*, Vol. 1, No. 1 (April 1894), 14.

57. They remained defensive about this move, which apparently drew middle- and upper-class criticism. "Although nothing has been so severely criticized as the use of pork in some of the dishes," they reported, "the results have justified it. It enters into the food of the common people nearly the world over. They are accustomed to it, and the flavor it gives is appetizing. However the question may stand for the wealthy, it is doubtful if the poor man in this country can get on comfortably without pork." "Count Rumford and the New England Kitchen," 8.

58. Atwater, "How Food Nourishes the Body," *Century Magazine*, Vol. 34, No. 2 (June 1887), 237; "Pecuniary Economy of Food," 438–43.

59. Atkinson, *Science of Nutrition*, 16; Howard Lewis, "Fifty Years of Study of the Role of Protein in Nutrition," in Adela Beeuwkes et al., eds., *Essays in the History of Nutrition and Dietetics* (Chicago: American Dietetic Association, 1967), 70–73.

60. Atwater, *Chemistry and Economy of Food*, 212–13.

61. Atwater, "The Potential Energy of Food," *Century Magazine*, Vol. 34, No. 3 (July 1887), 405.

62. Richard Cummings, *American and His Food*, (Chicago: Univ. of Chicago Press, 1939), 130.

63. Richards to Atkinson, Nov. 1897, *AP*.

64. *Ibid.*

65. Cited in Caroline L. Hunt, *The Life of Ellen H. Richards* (Boston: Whitcomb and Barrows, 1918), 233–34.

Chapter 5.

1. Mrs. John [Mary E.] Sherwood, *Manners and Social Usages* (New York: Harper and Bros., 1887), 273.

2. Sherwood, *Manners and Social Usages,* rev. (New York: Harper, 1907), 131–32.

3. Robert and Helen Lynd, *Middletown* (New York: Harcourt, Brace, 1929), 154.

4. See Laura Shapiro, *Perfection Salad* (New York: Farrar, Straus and Giroux, 1986), particularly Chap. 4, for an amusing account of this process.

5. Ella Lyman Cabot, Household Account Books, 1895–1901, Ella Lyman Cabot Papers, Schlesinger Library, Radcliffe College, Box 12.

6. Mary Hinman Abel, "Labor Problems in the Household," Fifth Lake Placid Conference on Home Economics, *Proceedings* (1903), 30.

7. *Ibid.,* 42.

8. *Ibid.,* 46.

9. Mary Hinman Abel, "Labor Problems in the Household," Fifth Lake Placid Conference on Home Economics *Proceedings* (1903), 29.

10. Helen Campbell, "Household Economics as a University Movement," *Review of Reviews,* Vol. 13 (March 1896), 299.

11. "Domestic Reform League," and "The School for Housekeeping," unsigned, [1902?], ms., in Women's Educational and Industrial Union Papers, Schlesinger Library, Radcliffe College, Box 1, Folders 5 and 9.

12. School for Housekeeping, Comments of the Press, [1899], *ibid.,* Box 1, Folder 9.

13. Sarah Tyson Rorer, *Book News,* Vol. 12 (March, 1894), 280, cited in Emma Weigley, *Sara Tyson Rorer* (Philadelphia: American Philosophical Society, 1977), 79.

14. Abel, "Labor Problems in the Household," 33.

15. *Ibid.,* 40.

16. Susan Strasser, "Mistress and Maid, Employer and Employee: Domestic Service Reform in the United States, 1897–1920," *Marxist Perspectives,* Vol. 1, No. 4 (1978), 60–63.

17. Edward Bellamy, "A Vital Domestic Problem. Household Service Reform," *Good Housekeeping* (hereafter *GH*), Vol. 10, No. 4 (Dec. 21, 1889), 74–77.

18. "Household Industrial Problems," Report of a Committee, Tenth Lake Placid Conference on Home Economics, *Proceedings* (1908), 161.

19. Ellen B. Dietrick, "Some Forms of Cooperation," *GH,* Vol. 11, No. 7, (Aug. 2, 1890), 150.

20. Catherine Selden, "The Tyranny of the Kitchen," *North American Review,* Vol. 157, No. 4 (Oct. 1893), 431–40.

21. Dolores Hayden, *The Grand Domestic Revolution* (Cambridge: MIT Press, 1981), 218.

22. Selden, "Tyranny," 438.

23. Editorial, *GH,* Vol. 10, No. 5 (Jan. 4, 1890), 117–18.

24. Ellen Richards, "The Wholesale Preparation of Food," in Atkinson, *The Science of Nutrition* (Springfield: Clark, Bryan, 1893), 64.

25. *GH,* Vol. 10, No. 1 (Jan. 4, 1890), 118.

26. *Boston Congregationalist,* [Jan. 1890?], cited in *GH,* Vol. 10, No. 7 (Feb. 1, 1890), 167.

27. Dietrick, "Some Forms of Cooperation," 150.

28. Fannie Fuller, "Practical Cooperation," *GH,* Vol. 11, No. 6 (July 19, 1890), 126.

29. Dietrick, "Some Forms of Cooperation," 149. It should be noted, however, that Peirce's goals were wider-ranging than liberation from servants, and included liberating housewives from housework in order to bring them out of the home and into full-time jobs. Susan Strasser, *Never Done: A History of American Housework* (New York: Pantheon, 1982), 199–201.

30. Mrs. Arthur C. Neville, "The Essentials of Cooperation," Ninth Lake Placid Conference on Home Economics, *Proceedings* (1907), 131–32.

31. Iva Peters, *Agencies for the Sale of Cooked Food Without Profit* (Washington: USGPO, 1919), 46–47.

32. Caroline Hunt, "Household Industrial Problems," 133.

33. Selden, "Tyranny," 440.

34. Charlotte Perkins Gilman, *Women and Economics* (Boston: Small, Maynard, 1898), 243–44, 230–31, 236–39.

35. As was noted with regard to the New England Kitchen, these were very important considerations at the time, for it was thought that it was healthier and more efficient for the body to consume hot rather than cold food.

36. Campbell, "Household Economics," 299.

37. Hunt, "Household Industrial Problems," 163.

38. Women's Educational and Industrial Union, "The Cost of Homemade and Prepared Foods," [1900], WEIU Papers, Box 1; Women's Education and Industrial Union and Boston Branch, Association of Collegiate Alumnae, *Comparison of the Cost of Home-Made and Prepared Food,* Massachusetts Labor Bulletin No. 19, Aug. 1901.

39. WEIU, "Trained and Supplementary Workers in Domestic Service," 1–2.

40. Hayden, *Domestic Revolution,* 218–19.

41. Charlotte Perkins Gilman, *What Diantha Did* (London: Unwin, 1912), 208.

42. Bellamy, "Vital Domestic Problem," 77.

Chapter 6.

1. Ellen Richards, "The Public Kitchens in Relation to School Lunches and Restaurants," Rumford Kitchen Leaflet No. 19, in Richards, ed., *The Rumford Kitchen Leaflets* (Boston: Rockwell and Churchill, 1899), 165.

2. Ellen H. Richards, *The Cost of Living as Modified by Sanitary Science,* (New York: John Wiley, 1900), 2.

3. Henrietta I. Goodrich, "Standards of Living: An Introduction," Fourth Lake Placid Conference on Home Economics, *Proceedings* (1902), 36.

4. The interest in human nutrition research was also shared by Atwater's immediate successor as Director of the Office, Walter Allen, a German-trained chemist

who held the position from 1889, when Atwater returned to Middletown, to 1893, when True assumed the position he would hold, with title changes, for the next thirty-five years. Charles E. Rosenberg, "The Adams Act: Politics and the Cause of Scientific Research," *Agricultural History*, Vol. 38, No. 1 (1964), 3.

5. Edward Atkinson to Ellen Richards, July 3, 1893. J. Sterling Morton to Adkinson, May 23, 1893, Edward Atkinson Papers, Massachusetts Historical Society; Edward Atkinson, *Suggestions for the Establishment of Food Laboratories,* U.S. Department of Agriculture, Office of Experiment Stations, Bulletin No. 17 (Washington: GPO, 1893), 19.

6. "The People's Food—A Great National Inquiry," *Review of Reviews,* Vol. 13, No. 6 (June 1896), 683.

7. Wilbur O. Atwater and Edward D. Rosa, "Description of a New Respiration Calorimeter and Experiments on the Conservation of Energy in the Human Body," USDA, Office of Experiment Stations Bulletin No. 63 (Washington: GPO, 1899).

8. True to Atwater, Feb. 14, Feb. 23, 1895, March 2, 1896; Atwater to True, April 9, 1896, U.S. Department of Agriculture, Files of the Office of Experiment Stations, Record Group 164, Series 51, File 1, National Archives, Washington, D.C. (hereafter OES Papers), Correspondence of Alfred C. True, 1893–1929 (hereafter True Correspondence); Governor cited in "The People's Food," 681.

9. True to Atwater, April 11, 1896; Atwater to True, April 14, 1896; True to Atwater, April 17, 1896; Atwater to True, March 22, 1897; True to Atwater, March 23, 1897, True Correspondence, OES Papers.

10. Atwater to Carroll Wright, Oct. 21, 1896, True Correspondence, OES Papers.

11. He hoped to establish what was the "normal" human basal metabolism rate by determining the basal metabolism rate of human beings under all conceivable conditions. John T. Edsall and David Bearman, "Historical Records of Scientific Activity: A Survey of Sources for the History of Biochemistry and Molecular Biology," *Proceedings of the American Philosophical Society,* Vol. 123, No. 5 (Oct. 15, 1979), 288.

12. Wilbur O. Atwater, "Memorandum Regarding Investigations in the Comparative Nutrition of Mankind," [Feb. 1902], True Correspondence, OES Papers.

13. Charles F. Langworthy, "Food and Diet in the United States," USDA, *Yearbook of the Department of Agriculture, 1907* (Washington: GPO, 1907), 361–78.

14. Caroline Hunt, *The Life of Ellen H. Richards* (Boston: Whitcomb and Barrows, 1918), 235.

15. Mary J. Lincoln, "The Pioneers of Scientific Cookery," *Good Housekeeping,* Vol. 51 (Oct. 1910), 470–74.

16. Juliet L. Bane, *The Story of Isabel Bevier* (Peoria: Charles Bennet, 1955), 17.

17. Janet M. Hill, "The Boston Cooking School," *The Boston Cooking School Magazine,* Vol. 1, No. 1 (June 1896), 4.

18. In her office she displayed photos of Atwater, True, and Richards, labeled "My Bountiful Benefactors." Bane, *Bevier,* 22.

19. Bailey Burritt to Albert Milbank, Aug. 30, 1916, New York Association for Improving the Condition of the Poor, Records, in Community Service Society Records, Manuscript Division, Columbia University Libraries, New York. (hereafter CSS Papers), File 325–26.

20. Ben Andrews to True, Jan. 2, 1913, True Correspondence, OES Papers.

21. First, Second, and Third Lake Placid Conferences on Home Economics, *Proceedings* (1901), 3.

22. Isabel Bevier, *Nutrition Investigations in Pittsburgh, 1894–1896,* OES Bulletin No. 52 (Washington: GPO, 1898).

23. Atwater to True, May 14, 1900, True Correspondence, OES Papers. On the extensive lobbying efforts by Atwater and True among home economists and university administrators see the letter files for 1899, 1900, and 1901.

24. She was an apostle of the new "Vienna method," which had been introduced into the United States at the Philadelphia Exposition of 1876. Lincoln, "Pioneers of Scientific Cookery," 471.

25. Bane, *Bevier,* 53.

26. Amy Daniels, "The Inductive Method in Cookery," Fifth Lake Placid Conference on Home Economics, *Proceedings* (1903), 55–57.

27. U.S. Department of Agriculture, *Year Book, 1897,* cited in Isabel Bevier and Susanna Usher, *The Home Economics Movement* (Boston: Whitecomb and Barrows, 1906), 37.

28. Helen Campbell, "Household Economics as a University Movement," *Review of Reviews,* Vol. 13 (March, 1896), 296.

29. Whether Ely himself repeated them at Illinois is not clear. In typically obtuse style, Campbell wrote that Illinois had "secured a repetition of eight of the lectures given at the University of Wisconsin." Campbell, "Household Economics," 296–97.

30. The outline, which indicates they ranged over ancient history, evolutionary theory, chemistry, architecture, physiology, upholstery, and indeed much of human knowledge, is reprinted in Campbell, "Household Economics."

31. Henry C. Sherman to A. C. True, August 12, 1910, True Correspondence, OES Papers; Bane, *Bevier,* 34.

32. He told Congress that the land grant colleges were "the single most effective agencies in the development of home economics." Bevier and Usher, *Home Economics Movement,* 23–43.

33. Rosenberg, "Adams Act," 5, 11.

34. Isabel Bevier, "The U.S. Government and the Housewife," *American Kitchen Magazine,* Vol. 11, No. 3 (Dec. 1899), 77–79.

35. Bane, *Bevier,* 34.

36. The Boston school system was a leader along this path. Its first cookery courses were initially financed by Pauline Agassiz Shaw, who later funded the New England Kitchen. At first, in the 1880s, she underwrote the lessons in an industrial school and then helped persuade the school board to take over the program and expand it into the grammar schools. North Bennet Street Industrial School, Report, 1887–88, North Bennet Street Industrial School, Records, Schlesinger Library, Series I, Box 1, Folder 2.

37. Previously, graduation from some form of cookery course was the most that was required of urban domestic science teachers.

38. Richards herself, for example, set up the Boston program and her students initially taught it. North Bennet Street Industrial School, Report, 1887–88.

39. Atwater, "Memorandum for Dr. True," [May 1898], True Correspondence, OES Papers.

40. Louise E. Hogan, *History and Present Status of Instruction in Cooking in the Public Schools of New York City.* USDA, OES Bulletin No. 56 (Washington: GPO, 1899), 10–23.

41. Mother's Club of Cambridge, Minutes of Meetings, [1886], Schlesinger Library, Radcliffe College.

42. Helen Campbell, "Household Economics," *Review of Reviews,* Vol. 13, (March 1896), 296–97.

43. *Ibid.,* 297. Seven years later, the NHEA became an official arm of the General Federation.

44. Mary Pattison, *Principles of Domestic Engineering* (New York: Trow Press, 1915), 1. Significantly, scientific home economics encountered a wall of indifference, if not hostility, in most of the South, for its hard-pressed economy still continued to provide an adequate supply of cheap black servant labor for kitchen and dining room. Moreover, there was stiff resistance among whites to learning new methods of cookery because of the strong association between blacks and cooking as an occupation. Ivy F. Harner, "Household Economics in the Institutes of the South," Fourth Lake Placid Conference, *Proceedings,* (1902), 14–15.

45. However, delicatessens, which were sprouting in lower-middle class and working-class areas did not meet their approval, for their spicy meats and condiments were regarded as uneconomical and conducive to intemperance.

46. Pattison, *Principles of Domestic Engineering,* 17.

47. Martha B. and Robert W. Bruere, *Increasing Home Efficiency,* (New York: Macmillan, 1912), 104.

48. *Ibid.,* 105–6.

49. Richards, *The Cost of Food: A Study of Dietaries* (New York: Wiley, 1902), 101.

50. Fannie Merritt Farmer, *The Boston Cooking School Cook Book* (Boston: Little, Brown, 1896), vii, v.

51. "Menus for February," *American Kitchen Magazine,* Vol. 10, No. 5 (Feb. 1899). The suggested menus and dishes in home economics texts, which often used the New Nutrition to teach the virtues of simple, economical cooking, were even simpler: for example, the Boston school system's high school text, Josephine Morris *Household Science and Arts* (New York: American Book Co., 1912).

52. Farmer, *Boston Cooking School,* 512. Her rival, Mary J. Lincoln clung to the big breakfast as well. Even her *Home Science Cook Book,* intended to suggest "short cuts for those who believe in simplifying life," still recommended breakfasts based on what it saw as the usual breakfast in "well-to-do American households," that is fruit, cereal, eggs, fish or meat and potatoes, and warm bread, or griddle cakes, or doughnuts. Mary J. Lincoln, *The Boston Cook Book,* Revised ed. (Boston: Little, Brown), 1900; Mary J. Lincoln and Anna Barrows, *The Home Science Cook Book* (Boston: Whitcomb and Barrows, 1911), 1.

53. Weigley, *Rorer,* 132–39.

Chapter 7.

1. William C. Birge, *True Food Values and their Low Costs* (New York: Sully and Kleinteich, [1910?]), 46.

2. Some foods had to be chewed more. He found, for example, that one-fifth of an ounce of shallot "required seven hundred and twenty-two mastications before disappearing through involuntary swallowing." Horace Fletcher, *The New Glutton or Epicure* (New York: Frederick Stokes, 1906), 127.

3. *Ibid.*

4. "Experiments in Feeding," *Harper's Weekly*, Feb. 13, 1904, 229.

5. He himself had a weakness for sweets, and while not pressing these or any other particular foods on others, he would recommend that like him, people should ingest most of their calories in the form of carbohydrates.

6. Report of Michael Foster, April 26, 1902, in Fletcher, *New Glutton or Epicure*, 18–20.

7. *Ibid.*, 11–12.

8. Michael Foster to Henry P. Bowditch, Jan. 25, 1902, Manuscripts and Rare Books Division, Countway Library, Harvard Univ. Medical School, Boston, Mass.

9. Michael Foster, "Experiments upon Human Nutrition," April 26, 1902, in Fletcher, *New Glutton or Epicure*, 18–24. He also thought that he could spend most of the time using the new equipment to pursue his other interests. Foster to Bowditch, Oct. 6, 1902, Countway Library.

10. In 1903, when a close associate of Foster's and Bowditch, the British physiologist Arthur Gangee, was contracted by the Carnegie Institution to prepare a report on the current state of research into human nutrition, he avoided Fletcher for fear of annoying the Institution's trustees. Within a year Foster was growing wary as well. He wrote Bowditch that he had a letter from Fletcher "which has taken an appreciable portion of my alloted days to read . . . but have not learned much from it. . . . The men here who went 'chewing'——first all reported that they felt in most surpassing health——and then they *all*——(all except Higgins) broke down." Arthur Gangee to Bowditch, March 2, 1903; Foster to Bowditch, July 7, Jan. 29, 1904, Countway Library of Medicine.

11. Isaac F. Marcosson, "Perfect Feeding of the Human Body," *World's Work*, Vol. 7 (Feb. 1904), 4460.

12. Louis Berman, *Food and Character* (Boston: Houghton Mifflin, 1932), 239.

13. Russell H. Chittenden, "Physiological Economy in Nutrition," *Popular Science Monthly*, Vol. 63 (1903), 123–31.

14. "The Quick Lunch of the Army," *Harper's Weekly*, July 7, 1902, 740.

15. Horace Fletcher to William James, Nov. 7, 1905. William James Papers, Houghton Library, Harvard University.

16. "Experiments in Feeding," 229.

17. C. F. Langworthy, "Progress in Nutrition Investigations, 1905–6," Eighth Lake Placid Conference, *Proceedings* (1906), 68.

18. Horace Fletcher, "Modern Theories of Diet," Tenth Lake Placid Conference on Home Economics, *Proceedings* (1908), 174.

19. Chittenden, "Physiological Economy," 123, 131.

20. Woods Hutchinson, "The Dangers of Undereating," *Cosmopolitan*, Vol. 47 (1909), 388.

21. Francis G. Benedict to Henry Bowditch, Oct. 18, 1909, Countway Library of Medicine.

22. John H. Kellogg, "Recent Dietetic Experiments," Ninth Lake Placid Conference on Home Economics, *Proceedings*, (1907), 122.

23. Horace Fletcher, "Fletcher Experiments," Ninth Lake Placid Conference on Home Economics, *Proceedings* (1907), 112.

24. Henry James to Horace Fletcher, May 3, 1907, Dec. 4, 1907. Henry James Papers, Houghton Library, Harvard University.

25. Henry James to Fletcher, Sept. 21, 1905, *Ibid.*

26. Henry James to Fletcher, July 22, 1908, *Ibid.*

27. Harvard *Crimson,* Nov. &, 1905; Fletcher to William James, Nov. 7, 1905, Sept. 27, 1908, William James Papers.

28. Whorton, *Crusaders,* 201.

29. Ronald Numbers, *Prophetess of Health: a Study of Ellen G. White* (New York: 1976); Whorton, *Crusaders,* 201–4.

30. Dale Brown, *American Cooking* (New York: Time-Life), 1968, quoted, with no page number, in Root and de Rochemenot, *Eating in America,* 228.

31. Kellogg, "Recent Dietetic Experiments," 118–23. His pseudoscientific medical journal was perhaps aptly named *Modern Medicine.* The one oriented towards a lay audience was called *Good Health.*

32. Gerald Carson, *Corn Flakes Crusade,* Chap. 8–14.

33. Bowditch to Charles S. Minot, March 24, 1906, Countway Library.

34. However, like so many ill people, he concluded "if he can do me good I don't care what people say of him." *Ibid.*

35. John H. Kellogg to Fletcher, Nov. 26, 1902, in Fletcher, *New Glutton,* 50–1.

36. Whorton, *Crusaders,* 205; Carson *Corn Flakes Crusade,* 232–33.

37. John H. Kellogg, "Recent Dietetic Experiments," Ninth Lake Placid Conference on Home Economics, *Proceedings,* (1907), 123.

38. Fletcher to William James, Sept. 27, 1908, William James Papers; Horace Fletcher, "Modern Theories of Diet," Tenth Lake Placid Conference on Home Economics, *Proceedings* (1908), 170–1.

39. *Ladies' Home Journal,* Nov. 20, 1902, 20.

40. Emma Weigley, *Sara Tyson Rorer,* 140.

41. For example, J. B. Huber, "Do we Eat Too Much?" *Scientific American* Vol. 97 (Sept. 1909), 167, 257–8.

42. Henry C. Sherman, *The Chemistry of Food and Nutrition* (New York: Macmillan, 1911).

43. Henry C. Sherman, *Food Products* (New York: Macmillan, 1914), 215–16.

44. Horace Fletcher to Irving Fisher, July 29, 1914, Horace Fletcher Papers, Houghton Library, Harvard Univ. cited in Green, *Fit,* 303.

45. C. F. Langworthy, *Food Customs and Diet in American Homes,* USDA, Office of Experiment Stations, Bulletin No. 110 (Washington: GPO, 1911), 17.

46. Berman, *Food and Character,* (Boston: Houghton Mifflin, 1932), 244.

47. John T. Edsall and David Bearman, "Historical Records of Scientific Activity: A Survey of Sources for the History of Biochemistry and Molecular Biology," *Proceedings of the American Philosophical Society,* Vol. 123, No. 5 (Oct. 15, 1979), 288–89; Aaron J. Ihde and Stanely Becker, "Conflict of Concepts in Early Vitamin Studies," *Journal of the History of Biology,* Vol. 4, No. 1 (1971), 1–33.

48. Caroline Hunt, *Ellen Richards,* 140–47. Mary Hinman Abel, who remained active in the home economics movement into the 1920's, lived to a ripe old age, dying in 1938 at age 88.

49. Henry James to Fletcher, Sept. 22, 1908, Henry James Papers.

50. Henry James to William James, Feb. 13, 1902; Fletcher to William James, "Washington's Birthday," 1909, William James Papers; Henry James to Fletcher, June 22, 1909, Henry James Papers.

51. Bernarr McFadden, *Strength from Eating* (New York: Physical Culture Publishing, 1901), 27.

52. Francis Crowninshield, *Manners for the Metropolis* (New York: Appleton, 1909), 40.

53. P. R. Kelley, "Diet in Students' Boarding House, University of Minnesota", *Cooking Club Magazine,* Vol. 12 (1910), No. 11, 10–11.

54. Gustav Mann, Oral History Interview, 1952, Bancroft Library, University of California, Berkeley, 36.

55. Menus in Menu Collection, Rare Books and Manuscripts Division, New York Public Library, New York.

56. Bailey Burritt to Dr. Armstrong, July 13, 1916, CSS Papers, Box 51, File 325–33.

57. Parloa, *New Cook Book,* xxx.

58. When the increase in the number of families in the nation is taken into account, potential employers had only half as many servants available in 1920 as in 1900. Katzman, *Seven Days a Week,* 58.

59. Alice G. Kirk, *Practical Food Economy* (Boston: Little, Brown, 1917), 3.

Chapter 8.

1. Kittredge, "Housekeeping Centers," 189.

2. Bailey Burritt to Ranulph [*sic*] Kingsley, July 7, 1917, New York Association for Improving the Condition of the Poor, Records, in Community Service Society, Records, Division of Archives and Manuscripts, Columbia University Libraries, New York. (hereafter CSS Papers), Box 50, File 325–2a.

3. Frank Manny, "Food Facts," CSS Papers, Box 51, File 325-3.

4. Frank Manny, "Nutritional Guidance," Feb. 29, 1916, *ibid.,* Box 50, 325-2a.

5. The NYAICP even funded Henry C. Sherman's attempts to revise Atwater's standards. Henry C. Sherman, "Memorandum of Proposed Projects," [1916]; Dr. Armstrong to Bailey Burritt, April 16, 1916, CSS Papers, Box 51, File 325-3.

6. Max Rubner, who inherited Voit's mantle as the world's leading nutritional scientist, lent great weight to this idea. Max Rubner, "The Nutrition of the People," Fifteenth International Congress of Hygiene and Demography, *Transactions* (Washington: GPO, 1913), Vol. 1, 394–95.

7. New York Society for Improving the Condition of the Poor, "Inventory of New Exhibit," CSS Papers, Box 52, File 325-3.

8. Weigley, *Rorer,* 139.

9. "The Abuse of Alcohol from a Sanitary Standpoint," *American Kitchen Magazine,* Vol. 5, No. 1 (April 1896), 32–35.

10. Jacob Riis, *Children of the Poor* (New York: 1893), 197.

11. Alice Norton, "Domestic Science as a Social Factor," Sixth Lake Placid Conference on Home Economics, *Proceedings* (1904), 16.

12. "The Abuse of Alcohol," *ibid.,* 33.

13. Jane Addams, "Immigration: A Field Neglected by the Scholar," *The Commons,* Jan. 1905, 16.

14. CSS Papers, Box 53, Folder 345.

15. Committee of Fifty, *Saloon Substitutes,* cited in Frank H. Streightoff, *The Standard of Living among the Industrial People of America,* (Boston: Houghton Mifflin, 1911), 91.

16. William Healy, *The Individual Delinquent* (Boston: Little, Brown, 1915), 280.

17. In 1899, a total of 311,715 non-Canadian immigrants were admitted to the United States. Within five years, that annual rate had more than tripled, and in the ten years from 1901 to 1910 close to 9 million immigrants arrived, the large majority of whom were Italians, Jews, Poles, or non-German-speaking denizens of the Hapsburg Empire. Jeremiah W. Jenks and W. Jett Lauck, *The Immigration Problem* (New York: Funk and Wagnalls, 1926), 667.

18. Peter R. Shergold, *Working Class Life: The "American Standard" in Comparative Perspective, 1899–1913,* (Pittsburgh: Univ. of Pittsburgh Press, 1982), 225.

19. Werner Sombart, *Why Is There No Socialism in America?,* (1906), trans. Patricia M. Hocking and P. T. Husbands, (White Plains: M. E. Sharpe, 1976), 106.

20. The latter was a sign of a poorer diet, at least by the lights of the people involved, for bread consumption normally declines as meat consumption rises.

21. U.S. Congress, Senate, 62nd Cong., 1st sess., *Cost of Living in Principal Industrial Towns of the United States,* Senate Doc. No. 38 (Washington: GPO, 1911), 41–57.

22. Margaret Byington, *Homestead. The Households of a Mill Town* (New York: Charities Publication Committee, 1910), 63–4.

23. Peter Roberts, *Anthracite Coal Communities* (New York: Macmillan, 1904), 106.

24. Byington makes this point mainly with regard to Slavs, but it is a generalization that would apply to many other immigrant groups as well. Byington, *Homestead,* 70.

25. *Ibid.,* 77.

26. Louise B. More, *Wage-Earners' Budgets* (New York: Henry Holt, 1907), 205.

27. The Simmons College faculty featured a specialist in teaching home economists how to teach cooking to immigrants who would troop from settlement house to settlement house, her class in tow, giving live demonstrations of how it should be done. Boston Post, clipping, [1911] in Eva White Papers, Box 3, Folder 31(a).

28. Winifred S. Gibbs, *Economical Cooking* (New York: New York Book Co., 1912).

29. Robert Woods, "Notes on the Italians in Boston," *Charities,* Vol. 12 (1904), 81.

30. Winifred S. Gibbs, "Dietetics in Italian Tenements," *Public Health Nurse Quarterly,* Vol. 6 (1914), No. 1, 43.

31. Breckinridge, *New Homes for Old,* 56.

32. Gerd Korman, *Industrialization, Immigrants, and Americanizers* (Madison: State Historical Society of Wisconsin, 1967), 103.

33. Newspaper clippings, [1916–17?], in Eva White Papers, Box 3, Folder

32v(a), 14-e, Schlesinger Library. When finally under way, however, it seemed to be aimed primarily at training them as domestic servants. Katherine Brooks, "Practical Training for Girls to be Continued by National Civic Federation," [1916], *ibid.*, 16-D.

34. Jane Addams, *Twenty Years at Hull House* (New York: New American Library, 1961), 253.

35. Erik Amfithreatrof, *The Children of Columbus* (Boston: Little, Brown, 1973), 240.

36. Manny, "Nutritional Guidance."

37. Kittredge, "Housekeeping Centers," 190.

38. Isabel F. Hyams, "The Louisa May Alcott Club," Second Lake Placid Conference in Home Economics *Proceedings* (1900), 19.

39. Boston *Post*, Feb. 24, 1917.

40. Josephine Morris, *Household Science and Arts* (New York: American Book Co.), 1912.

41. Indeed, in many immigrant households the kitchen doubled as a bedroom at night. A sampling of 15,000 prewar immigrant families by the U.S. Immigration Commission showed that this was not uncommon; 771 or over 5 percent of them had people sleeping in the kitchen as well. Breckenridge, *New Homes,* 62.

42. Boston *Post*, Oct. 8, 1911.

43. Women's Municipal League, undated flyer in Eva White Papers, Box 3, Folder 31(a).

44. Winifred S. Gibbs, "Dietetics in Italian Tenements," *Public Health Nurse Quarterly,* Vol. 6 (1914), No. 1, 46.

45. Velma Phillips and Laura Howell, "Racial and Other Differences in Dietary Customs," *Journal of Home Economics,* Sept. 1920, 397.

46. In one study of immigrant diets a number reported that no, they had not Americanized their diet because they did not like the American diet of sweet cakes. Sophinisba P. Breckinridge, *New Homes for Old* (New York: Harper and Brothers, 1921), 131.

47. *Ibid.,* 131–32.

48. David Brownstone, *Island of Hope, Island of Tears* (New York: Rawson Publishers, 1979), 17.

49. Christine Ellis, interview in Staughton and Mary Lynd, eds., *Rank and File* (Boston: Beacon Press, 1973), 15.

50. John C. Kennedy, et al., *Wages and Family Budgets in the Chicago Stockyards District,* (Chicago: Univ. of Chicago Press, 1914), 50.

51. *Ibid.,* 126.

52. Breckinridge, *New Homes,* 58–9, 130.

53. Florence Nesbitt, *Household Management* (New York: Russell Sage Foundation, 1918), 109.

54. Peter H. Bryce, "A Year's Change in Food Habits," *American Journal of Public Health,* Vol. 9, No. 2 (Jan. 1919), 109.

Chapter 9.

1. See, for example, Robert C. Chapin, *The Standard of Living Among Workingmen's Families in New York City* (New York, Charities Publication Committee,

1907); Louise B. More, *Wage-Earners' Budgets* (New York: Holt, 1907); and Scott Nearing, *Financing the Wage-earner's Family* (New York: B. W. Huebch, 1913).

2. "KFB" to Charles Hecht, Dec. 9, 1916, CSS Papers, Box 51, File 325-3.

3. *New York Times*, Feb. 3, 20, 23, 24, March 1, March 19, 21, 22, 23, 25, 1917; Bruno Lasker, "The Food Riots," *The Survey*, Vol. 37, (March 3, 1917), 638.

4. Boston *Post*, Feb. 24, 1917; *NYT*, Feb. 24, 1917.

5. *NYT*, Feb. 22, 1917.

6. *NYT*, Feb. 23, 1917; "Rushing into Dictatorship," *The Nation*, Vol. 104, No. 2696 (March 1, 1917), 213; Boston *Post*, Feb. 23, 1917.

7. "Minutes of Conference on Distributive Cooperation," July 19, 1913," CSS Records, Box 51, File 325-3.

8. *NYT*, Jan. 7, Feb. 24, 1917.

9. *NYT*, Feb. 24, 1917.

10. Burritt to Walter Long, April 23, 1913, Burritt to Prof. James Ford, May 15, 1913, CSS Papers, Box 52, File 325-3; "A Review and Program of the Department of Social Welfare of the NYAICP, Nov. 7, 1923," CSS Papers, Box 53, Folder 325–26.

11. *NYT*, Feb. 23, 25, 1917; Lasker, "Food Riots," 638.

12. *NYT*, Feb. 26, March 1, March 6, 1917.

13 "People's Kitchen Statement," *NYT* July 19, 1915.

14. "Supplementary Memorandum Regarding Public Kitchen," [Jan.–Feb. 1915]; Burritt to Dr. Armstrong, Feb. 27, 1915, CSS Papers, Box 55, File 345.

15. Burritt to Armstrong, Jan. 5, 1915, *ibid.*

16. Armstrong to Burritt, Aug. 18, 1915, *ibid.*

17. EFB to John Elliot, Feb. 23, 1915, Dr. Armstrong to Mr. Brown, March 24, 1915, Burritt to Cornelius Bliss, Aug. 8, 1915, Armstrong to Burritt, Aug. 8, 1915, *ibid.*

18. "Summary 2nd Annual Report of Committee on Public Kitchens," Feb. 20, 1917, *ibid.*

19. James P. Holland to Edward Brown, Jan. 21, 1916; Brown to Holland, Jan. 22, 1916, *ibid.*

20. Burritt to Mrs. James Burden, Feb. 25, Nov. 17, 1920, March 17, 1921; Burritt to Cornelius Bliss, Dec. 20, 1920, *ibid.*

21. By these standards, depending on their occupation, those who were "poorly nourished" did not consume at least 100 to 150 grams of protein per day, 50 to 70 grams of fat and 350 to 600 grams of carbohydrate per 70-kilogram male. To meet his minimum requirements for proteins and carbohydrates, a 70-kilogram male at hard work would have to consume about 7,000 calories a day!

22. Frank Underhill, "Report on Nutrition Investigation, New York, 1907, Buffalo, 1908," in Chapin, *The Standard of Living*, 319–25.

23. He also concluded that seventy-six percent of the families he studied whose incomes were between $400 and $600 were "under fed" as well as 32 percent of those earning between $600 and $799. Chapin, *The Standard of Living*, 127.

24. Frank Streightoff, *The Standard of Living among the Industrial People of America* (Boston: Houghton Mifflin, 1911), 98.

25. Byington, *Homestead*, 70–74.

26. The NYAICP continued to use Atwater's requirements as the basis for its relief and other nutritional programs as late as 1916. Bailey Burritt to Henry C. Sherman, March 9, 1916, CSS Papers, Box 52, File 325-3.

27. Also, when food prices began to rise after 1907, the standard seemed in need of constant upward revision. Frank Manny, "Summary of Estimates Concerning Defective Nutrition," Nov. 26, 1917, CSS Papers, Box 50, File 325-a.

28. Most relied on measurements taken twenty years earlier by Bowditch in two private schools in New York and Chicago, supplemented by data provided by Luther Holt, a Park Avenue pediatrician (of whom more will be heard anon) on the earlier years. Only those, such as the U.S. Children's Bureau, whose later charts integrated some of the data collected by the anthropologist Franz Boas on the measurements of the native-born children of immigrants began to compensate for this class and ethnic bias. See Lydia Roberts, "A Review of Some Recent Literature on Malnutrition in Children," *Journal of Home Economics,* Vol. 11 (Jan. 1919), 5–12, for a summary of the various approaches to actually diagnosing malnutrition.

29. In 1920 the chief statistician for Metropolitan Life recalled that as early as 1905 he had come to realize that, when it came to ascertaining the nutritional status of Italian-Americans, "so-called standard tables were inadequate." This belief was reinforced by anthropometric investigations he did for the army in 1917–18 which led him to conclude that "military standards of height were totally inadequate" for native-born Americans of Italian ancestry and that the standard tables "were no standard at all when applied to widely different racial elements." Frederick Hoffman to Bailey Burrit, Dec. 8, 1920, CSS Papers, Box 50, File 325-2a.

30. Frank Manny, "Summary of Estimates."

31. One such mother, an Italian in very comfortable circumstances, was initially disturbed enough to agree to start serving her daughter eggs and milk every morning for breakfast. However, likely after realizing that it was the diagnosis, not the feeding, which was faulty, she reneged, telling nutritionists: "Louisa eats what the family eats." Florence Nesbitt, *Household Management* (New York: Russell Sage Foundation, 1918), 108–9.

32. John Gilbert, *The Growth and Development of Italian Children in New York City* (New York: New York Association for Improving the Condition of the Poor, 1922).

33. Using this method the estimated number of New York City schoolchildren suffering from defective nutrition in 1917 was 130,000. Manny, "Summary of Estimates."

34. Alan Brown and G. Albert Davis, "The Prevalence of Malnutrition in the Public School System of Ontario," *Canadian Journal of Public Health,* Vol. 12, No. 2 (1921), 66–72.

35. William R. P. Emerson, "Scales, a Tape-measure, and Conservation; Malnutrition among Schoolchildren," *New Republic,* Vol. 15 (June 29, 1918), 257.

36. Frances Perkins, "Some Facts Concerning Undernourished Children," *Survey,* Vol. 25, No. 1 (Jan. 1910), 68–72.

37. Josephine Baker to Walter Bensel, July 9, 1913, CSS Papers, Box 50, File 325-2c.

38. Frank Manny, "Summary of Estimates," Nov. 26, 1917, CSS Papers, Box 50, File 225a.

39. Frank Manny, "Defective Nutrition and the Standard of Living," Nov. 19, 1917, CSS Papers, Box 50, File 325-2a.

40. Among 1916 inductees into the Army, Jews were slightly shorter than Italians, Slavic immigrants were about as short as Italians but Magyars were shortest of all. Frederick L. Hoffman, *Army Anthropometry and Medical Rejection Statistics,* (Newark, N.J.: Prudential Press, 1918), 29.

41. An analysis of physical examinations of World War I inductees concluded that poor eyesight was "so markedly prevalent among Polish Jews as to be one of their racial characteristics." U.S. Surgeon-General's Office, *Defects Found in Drafted Men* (Washington: GPO, 1920), 285.

42. In New York City the Dumferline Scale showed slum-dwelling children of the native-born (a high proportion of whom were likely black), to be the most undernourished, but they were followed closely by Jews. Italians fared somewhat better, and the native-born children of Germans and Irish topped the scale. Manny, "Defective Nutrition."

43. Manny, "Summary of Estimates;" Manny, "Memoranda Concerning Nutrition Study," Dec. 24, 1917, CSS Papers, Box 51, File 325-2-F.

44. F. Eugenia Whitehead, "Nutrition Education for Children in the U.S. since 1900—Part I," in Adelia Beeuwkes, et. al., *Essays in the History of Dietetics* (Chicago: American Dietetic Association, 1967), 39–40.

45. Indeed, it kept the NEK itself going for a while, and survived the NEK by over ten years, until 1907, when the Women's Educational and Industrial Union took over its direction. Mary H. Moran and Julia Pulsifer, "Boston's Public School Lunches," [1907], reprinted by WEIU, copy in WEIU Papers, Schlesinger Library, Radcliffe College.

46. Mable H. Kittredge, "Housekeeping Centers in Settlements and Public Schools," *The Survey,* May 3, 1913, 189.

47. C. F. Langworthy, "Home Economics Work in the United States for Men and Boys," *Journal of Home Economics,* Vol. 5 (1913), 139.

48. Elizabeth Milbank Anderson to R. Fulton Cutting, March 15, 1913, CSS Papers, Box 53, File 325-6.

49. New York School Lunch Committee, Memorandum in Support of 1915 Budget Estimates of the Board of Education for Equipment of School Kitchens," Sept. 14, 1914, CSS Papers, Box 50, File 325-2c.

50. Burritt to Theodore Roosevelt, April 16, 1913, CSS Papers, Box 49, Folder 325-2.

51. "A Review of the Program of the Department of Social Welfare of the NYAICP, Nov. 17, 1923," CSS Papers, Box 53, Folder 325-6.

52. Langworthy, "Home Economics Work," 139.

53. "A Review of the Program of the Department of Social Welfare."

54. *NYT,* Dec. 2, 1917.

55. *NYT,* March 24, 1918.

56. In early 1917, they had contemplated denouncing the Department of Health's wide definition of malnutrition and in December, the head of the AICP nutrition section had told its director that the Dumferline categories were too subjective to be of much use. Haven Emerson to Burritt, April 16, 1917; Frank Manny to Bailey Burritt, April 17, 1917, CSS Papers, Box 50, File 325-a; Manny, "Memoranda."

57. He expressed similar concerns to Luther Holt, adding that "there are as yet no figures that are very meaningful." Burritt to Josephine Baker, May 23, 1918;

Burritt to Luther Holt, May 23, 1918, CSS Papers, Box 50, File 325-2a. Holt, who stood by height/weight ratios as the only important criterion, condemned the Dumferline scale and called Baker's figures "at variance with what is true." Luther Holt, "Standards for Growth and Nutrition of School Children," *Archives of Pediatrics,* Vol. 35 (1918), 339.

58. Report of Special Committee on School Luncheons, New York City Board of Education, [March, 1919?], CSS Papers, Box 49, Folder 325-2.

59. Burritt to R. Fulton Cuttin, Dec. 12, 1919, CSS Papers, Box 50, File 325-2a.

60. John Gelbhert to Burritt, Jan. 23, 1920, *ibid.*

61. Albert Milbank to William Matthews, Dec. 19, 1918, CSS Papers, Box 52, Folder 325-6.

62. Baker had always urged that nutrition education be an integral part of school lunch programs. *NYT,* March 24, 1918.

63. Deprived of the last vestiges of a role in the process, the social workers began playing down the importance of school lunches in the battle against malnutrition. They were merely "an accessory to" nutrition classes, school medical services, and home visits by social workers, said the head of the social welfare department of the NYAICP. John Gelbhert, "A Review and Program of the Department of Social Welfare of the NYAICP," Nov. 17, 1923, CSS Papers, Box 53, File 325-6.

64. For example, although many of the children in the special open-air school in Boston's Franklin Park were Jews, who abided by most of the orthodox dietary laws, a social worker involved in the school lunch program noted approvingly that "these laws have been set aside, that every known law of health may be followed for the child's improvement." She did concede that perhaps exceptions might be made for the children of rabbis and "on their ceremonial holidays." M. Eleanor Stewart, "Experiment of Anemic Children in the Winchell School, March 1 to June 22, 1910," Eva White Papers, Schlesinger Library, Radcliffe College, Box 1, Folder 17.

65. See, for example the New York City school lunch menus in the CSS Papers, Box 50, File 325-2.

66. Leonard Covello, *The Heart is the Teacher* (New York: McGraw-Hill, 1958), cited in Cordasco, *The Italians,* 265.

67. John Fante, "Odyssey of a Wop," *American Mercury,* Vol. 30, No. 12 (Sept. 1933), 89–97.

68. Frances Perkins had noted this in 1910, when she wrote that "perhaps we shall come to realize that malnutrition exists in all classes of society and is often due as much to unwise feeding as underfeeding. Perkins, "Some Facts," 71.

69. His Boston classes, for which he claimed immense successes, were run from his clinic at the prestigious Massachusetts General Hospital, and while subsequent New York classes achieved only mixed success, this was not apparent until 1921. Jean L. Hunt, et. al., *Health Education and the Nutrition Class* (New York: Dutton, 1921), 27.

70. Camelia W. Uzell, "A Demonstration in Health Education," *The Survey,* Vol. 40 (June 1, 1918), 258.

71. Emerson, "Scales," 257.

72. Studies of malnutrition among the poor had shown that poverty was the cause in only 5 percent of the cases, he said, and "a study of the diets of the poor in

New York and Boston shows an excess of protein and that they are entirely adequate in all other materials for growth." Neither was malnutrition a question of cookery. "The children will do well enough on the food the household usually provides," he said. *Ibid.,* 258.

73. "The first appeal is made to the universal human wish to be as good as the next one," wrote one enthusiast. Uzzell, "A Demonstration," 258.

74. "Health first and education later," should be the slogan, he said, for if the war continued the older of his subjects might be declared unfit for national service. Emerson, "Scales," 259.

75. Emerson, "Is Your Child Underweight?," *Woman's Home Companion,* Vol. 46 (Aug. 1919), 13–14; "Climb to the Normal Weight Line", *ibid.,* Vol. 46 (Sept. 1919), 30–2; "Does Your Child Get Tired?," *ibid.,* Vol. 46 (Dec. 1919), 36–9; Eugenia Whitehead, "Nutrition Education," 40.

76. Whitehead, "Nutrition Education," 40.

77. Lydia J. Roberts, *Nutrition Work with Children* (Chicago: Univ. of Chicago Press, 1927).

Chapter 10.

1. See, for example, *Laides' Home Journal,* 7 (April 1890), 25; Alice Kessler-Harris, *Women Have Always Worked: A Historical Overview* (Old Westbury, N.Y., 1981), 73, 76.

2. C. H. F. Routh, *Infant Feeding and Its Influence on Life; or, The Causes and Prevention of Infant Mortality* (London, 1863), 351–52.

3. Eustace Smith, *On the Wasting Diseases of Infants and Children* (London 1868), 35; *Harper's Bazaar,* June 19, 1869, p. 399.

4. See remarks by Joseph E. Winters at a meeting of the New York Academy of Medicine, reported in *Medical Record,* 30 (Dec. 4, 1886), 638; *Harper's Magazine Advertiser,* 81 (July 1890), 137.

5. [Mellin's Food Company], *The Care and Feeding of Infants* (Boston, 1895), 69; *LHJ,* 17 (March 1900), 20; *LHJ,* 10 (Sept. 1893), 24; Woolrich & Company, *Infant Mortality: Prime Cause and Remedy* (Palmer, Mass. 1882), 7–9. Woolrich & Company produced Ridge's Food. Advertisements for dried milk preparations that stressed that their product was safer than impure milk conveniently ignored the fact that, especially for the poor, impure water was also a dangerous substance.

6. *LHJ,* 10 (Sept. 1893), 30; [Mellin's Food Company], *The Care and Feeding of Infants* (Boston, 1900); *ibid.,* (Boston, 1904); *ibid.,* (Boston, 1913); *ibid, Advice to Mothers on the Care and Feeding of Infants* (Boston, 1898); and *ibid., The Home Modification of Cow's Milk* (Boston, 1900). Mellin's Food Company was particularly successful in impressing physicians, but other companies also realized, in the early stages of the industry, that courting family doctors could pay off handsomely. See, for example Woolrich & Company, *Infant Mortality.* For a discussion of the development of this relationship, see Rima D. Apple, "'To Be Used Only under the Direction of a Physician': Commercial Infant Feeding and Medical Practice, 1870–1940," *Bulletin of the History of Medicine,* 54 (Fall 1980), 402–17.

7. James O. Jordan and Frank E. Mott, "Condensed Milk and Its Value for General Use and for Infant Feeding," *American Journal of Public Hygiene,* 6 (1910),

400; Arthur V. Meigs, *Milk Analysis and Infant Feeding* (Philadelphia, 1885), 83–84.

8. See advertisements for "'Cleanfont,' the Modern Nursing Bottle" and "'Mizpah' 'Valve Nipples,'" in *LHJ*, 11 (Nov. 1894), 25, 32.

9. Lacta-Preparata advertisement, *Harper's Magazine Advertiser*, 81 (July 1890), 148; Meigs, *Milk Analysis*, 83–86; J. Lewis Smith, "The Feeding of Infants Deprived of Breast Milk," *Medical Record*, 30 (Dec. 4, 1886), 638; L. Emmett Holt, "Where Does the Medical Profession Stand Today on the Question of Infant Feeding?" *Archives of Pediatrics*, 14 (Sept. 1897), 818.

10. American Pediatric Society, "Collective Investigation of Infantile Scurvy in North America," *Archives of Pediatrics*, 15 (July 1898), 498, 500; I. L. Polozker, "What Should Be Taught Concerning Proprietary Foods and Condensed Milk," *Pediatrics*, 21 (Sept. 1909), 581–82; "Condensed Milk as a Food for Infants," *ibid.*, 23 (Dec. 1911), 699–701.

11. Polozker, "What Should Be Taught," 584; Clifford G. Grulee, *Infant Feeding* (Philadelphia: Saunders, 1916), 135.

12. Edwards A. Park and Howard H. Mason, "Luther Emmett Holt (1855–1924)," in *Pediatric Profiles*, ed. Borden S. Veeder (St. Louis: Mosby, 1957), 44.

13. Thomas Morgan Rotch, "An Historical Sketch of the Development of Percentage Feeding," *New York Medical Journal*, 85 (March 23, 1907), 532; Thomas Morgan Rotch, "The Value of Milk Laboratories for the Advancement of Our Knowledge of Artificial Feeding," *Archives of Pediatrics*, 10 (Feb. 1893), 97.

14. Rotch, "The Artificial Feeding of Infants," *Archives of Pediatrics*, 4 (Aug. 1887), 458–80; Rotch, *The American Methods in the Modification of Milk in the Feeding of Infants* (London: British Medical Journal, 1902), 29.

15. Rotch, "Historical Sketch," 536; Appendix to an offprint of Rotch, "Value of Milk Laboratories," Thomas Morgan Rotch Papers, Countway Library of Medi-Harvard University, Boston, Mass.

16. Rotch, *American Methods*, 2; Rotch, "Artificial Feeding of Infants," 469–70; for an outline of the situation by 1913, see Julius Friedenwald and John Ruhrah, *Diet in Health and Disease*, rev. (Philadelphia: Saunders, 1913), 254–55.

17. Rotch, "Some Considerations regarding Substitute Feeding during the First Year," *Archives of Pediatrics*, 21 (Aug. 1904), 561–75; Rotch, *Pediatrics: The Hygienic and Medical Treatment of Children* (Philadelphia: Lippincott, 1896), 230–83; Rotch, "The Essential Principles of Infant Feeding and the Modern Methods of Applying Them," *Journal of the American Medical Association*, 41 (Aug. 8, 1903), 349; Rotch, "The Cardinal Principles for the Successful Feeding of Infants," *Interstate Medical Journal*, 17 (May 1910), 305–15; Rotch, "Opening Address of the President before the New England Pediatric Society," *Boston Medical and Surgical Journal*, 158 (March 19, 1908), 36–38; Park and Mason, "Luther Emmett Holt," 45, 47; Rotch, *American Methods*, 25.

18. Park and Mason, "Luther Emmett Holt," 45; [Mellin's Food Company], *The Mellin's Food Method of Percentage Feeding*, (Boston, 1908).

19. H. J. Gerstenberger, discussion of J. Madison Taylor, "The Curative Powers in Human Milk," in American Academy of Medicine, *Prevention of Infant Mortality: Being the Papers and Discussions of a Conference Held at New Haven, Conn., November 11, 12, 1909*, 73; Hastings H. Hart and Ira S. Wile, discussion of J. P.

Crozer Griffith, "The Influence of Diet on Infant Mortality," in *ibid.*, 52–53; Anna Rochester, *Infant Mortality: Results of a Field Study in Baltimore, Md., Based on Births in One Year* (Washington: GPO, 1923), 55.

20. Rotch, *American Methods*, 46; William H. Park and L. Emmett Holt, "Report upon the Results of Different Kinds of Pure and Impure Milk in Infant Feeding in Tenement Houses and Institutions of New York City," *Archives of Pediatrics*, 20 (1903), 881–909. Thomas Morgan Rotch seemed blithely unconcerned about the question of the price of clean milk in general, calling it a question "very much more dwelt upon by the rich than by the poor." Rotch, "The Pasteurization of Milk for Public Sale," *American Journal of Public Hygiene*, 3 (May 1907), 142.

21. L. Emmett Holt, "Infant Mortality and Its Reduction, Especially in New York City," *Journal of the American Medical Association*, 54 (Feb. 26, 1910), 685; Ira S. Wile, "Educational Responsibilities of a Milk Depot," in American Academy of Medicine, *Prevention of Infant Mortality*, 139; William H. Davis, "Statistical Comparison of the Mortality of Breast-Fed and Bottle-Fed Infants," in *Transactions of the Fifteenth International Congress on Hygiene and Demography, Washington, September 23–28, 1912* (Washington: GPO, 1913), Vol. 6, 184–90; Taylor, "Curative Powers in Human Milk," 66.

22. Smith, "Feeding of Infants," 637; American Pediatric Society, "Collective Investigation of Infantile Scurvy," 502. Before the mid-1880s many doctors advised heating milk, not to purify it but because the most popular physiological theories of the day held that warm liquids were more digestible than cold ones. See, for example, Marion Harland [Mary Virginia Terhune], *Common Sense in the Nursery* (New York, 1885), 115–16.

23. American Pediatric Society, "Infantile Scurvy," 502–3; Holt, "Where Does the Medical Profession Stand?" 819. Sterilization was still the favored process in Germany, whence much of the lead in the field had originally come. *Ibid.*

24. Manfred J. Waserman, "Henry L. Coit and the Certified Milk Movement in the Development of Modern Pediatrics," *Bulletin of the History of Medicine*, 46 (July to Aug. 1972), 359–90; Henry Dwight Chapin, *The Theory and Practice of Infant Feeding with Notes on Development* (New York: Wood, 1902), 105–14.

25. Pasteurized Milk Laboratories, *Directions for Manufacturing Home Pasteurizer—Systems Nathan Straus*. Predictably, Rotch opposed compulsory pasteurization because he felt that milk should be heated to different levels for different infants. He also argued that different localities required different systems for ensuring the cleanliness of milk. See Rotch, "Pasteurization of Milk," 138–43.

26. Robert W. Bruere, "A Plan for the Reduction of Infant Mortality," in American Academy of Medicine, *Prevention of Infant Mortality*, 128; Charles E. North, "Milk and Its Relation to Public Health," in *A Half Century of Public Health: Jubilee Historical Volume of the American Public Health Association*, ed. Mazyck P. Ravenel (New York: American Public Health Ass'n, 1921), 279; U.S. Department of Labor, Children's Bureau, *Baby-Saving Campaigns: A Preliminary Report on What American Cities Are Doing to Prevent Infant Mortality* (Washington: GPO, 1913), 20–21. In Boston the reformers thought they must first convince the masses of the value of "pure milk." Thus, in 1910 settlement houses sold certified milk at below the price of "dipped" milk, with the reformers absorbing the losses. More typically, however, the milk stations were chary of charging less than the

prevailing rate for fear of alienating the "dairy interests." See *ibid.,* 23; and "Outline of Mrs. White's Career in Social Work," typescript, Folder 1, Box 1, Eva White Papers, Schlesinger Library.

27. *Boston Post,* Oct. 11, 1911; Henry Street Settlement, *Report, 1893 to 1913* (New York, 1913), 18; Children's Bureau, *Baby-Saving Campaigns,* 23, 25; American Association for Study and Prevention of Infant Mortality, *Transactions of the First Annual Meeting: Johns Hopkins University, Baltimore, November 9 to 11, 1910,* 316.

28. Friedenwald and Ruhrah, *Diet in Health and Disease,* 271–91; Elizabeth Peabody House, Station No. 2, Final Report, Dec. 1911, Folder 17, Box 1, Eva White Papers.

29. American Association for Study and Prevention of Infant Morality, untitled leaflet, Sept. 1, 1910, Rotch Papers; Children's Bureau, *Baby-Saving Campaigns,* 22; Chas. H. Verrill, "Infant Mortality and Its Relation to the Employment of Mothers in Fall River, Mass.," *Transactions of the Fifteenth International Congress on Hygiene and Demography,* III, pt. 1, pp. 334–36.

30. In 1863, for example, C. H. F. Routh, England's great pediatrician and pioneer in the study of infant feeding, wrote that 24 percent of babies either died or "did not thrive" on breast milk. Routh, *Infant Feeding,* 32–3.

31. Thomas S. Southworth, "The Possibilities of Maternal Nursing in the Prevention of Infant Mortality," in American Association for Study and Prevention of Infant Mortality, *Transactions of the First Annual Meeting,* 252–53; Herman Schwarz, "Nursing Statistics Derived from the Study of the Infancy of 1,500 Children, and a Contribution to the Cause of the Summer Infant Mortality," in *ibid.,* 208; Rotch, "Notes on Infant Feeding," *Archives of Pediatrics,* 6 (July to Aug. 1889), 476; Rotch, "The Management of Human Breast Milk in Cases of Difficult Digestion," *ibid.,* 7 (Nov. 1890), 841–54; Davis, "Statistical Comparison," 184.

32. Wilbur C. Phillips, "Infants' Milk Depots and Infant Mortality," in American Association for Study and Prevention of Infant Mortality, *Transactions of the First Annual Meeting,* 79; S. Josephine Baker, "The Reduction of Infant Mortality in New York City," in *Transactions of the Fifteenth International Congress on Hygiene and Demography,* III, pt. 1, pp. 145–47, 149.

33. Park and Holt, "Report upon the Results of Different Kinds of Pure and Impure Milk," 887.

34. In Montclair, for example, over 26 percent of the children of fathers in the highest income bracket had been weaned completely by the end of the third month. In contrast, only 12.7 percent of those whose fathers were in the lowest bracket had been weaned by that age. Margaretta A. Williamson, *Infant Mortality: Montclair, N.J.: A Study of Infant Mortality in a Suburban Community* (Washington: GPO, 1915), 23. In England as well, while many prominent reformers ascribed high levels of infant mortality among the poor to artificial feeding, a 1910 government study indicated that about 80 percent of working-class mothers breast-fed their infants. Carol Dyhouse, "Working-Class Mothers and Infant Mortality," *Journal of Social History,* 12 (Winter 1978), 255. A 1910 investigation of Fort William, Ontario, indicated that similar class differences existed in Canada. There, the Medical Officer of Health discovered that it was in the prosperous part of the city that most mothers had abandoned breast feeding. Robert Wodehouse, "Vital Statistics Pertaining to Infant Mortality," *Public Health Journal,* 11 (Aug. 1911),

363, cited in Rosemary Gagan, "Disease, Mortality and Public Health in Hamilton, Ontario, 1900–1914" (M.A. thesis, McMaster University, 1981), 125.

35. Williamson, *Infant Mortality: Montclair,* 22–3.

36. *Ibid.,* 23. In New Bedford, Mass. and Manchester, N.H., for example mortality rates were 201.9 and 242.9 per 1,000 live births respectively in the lowest income bracket and ranged in a quite orderly progression down to 59.9 and 58.3 per 1,000 in the highest. Even in Saginaw, Michigan, whose immigrants were mainly British, Canadian, and German, with child-rearing habits quite similar to those of the native born, infant mortality correlated with income. Nila F. Allen, *Infant Mortality: Results of a Field Study in Saginaw, Mich., Based on Births in One Year* (Washington: GPO, 1919), 30–1.

37. Park and Holt, "Pure and Impure Milk," 887.

38. A physician addressing a 1909 conference on infant mortality typified these people when he said:

Poorer mothers do not refrain from or cease nursing because of social duties, nor is unwillingness the dominant cause of their failure. Unsatisfactory maternal nursing among them depends upon underfeeding of the mother, poor obstetric attention at birth, being turned out from a maternity hospital almost too weak to walk steadily and returning to a home lacking in hygiene, but filled with work, overwork, worry, general diseases such as tuberculosis, infections, ignorance of the necessity of breast-feeding, promises of proprietary food advertisements. Finally, physicians themselves, all too frequently, advise discontinuance of breast milk, without an effort to secure adequate quantity or quality, by correcting underlying faulty conditions.

Nevertheless, he still thought the crux of the problem to be not poverty but mothers' ignorance, conveniently separating the two. Wile, "Educational Responsibilities of a Milk Depot, 146.

39. Rowland G. Freeman, Pasteurization of Milk," *Journal of the American Medical Association,* 54 (Jan. 29, 1910), 372; Waserman, "Henry L. Coit," 375–76; North, "Milk and Its Relation to Public Health," 274–77; Irene Till, "Milk—The Politics of an Industry," in Walton Hamilton et. al., *Price and Price Policies* (New York, 1938), 450–51; H. A. Ross, *The Marketing of Milk in the Chicago Dairy District* (Urbana, Ill: Univ. of Illinois 1925), 464.

40. The pendulum continued to swing away from the theories of Justus von Liebig, Rotch, and Holt until at least 1962, when without knowledge of the irony involved, *Pediatrics,* coauthored by Holt's son and the lineal descendant of Holt's famous *The Diseases of Infancy and Childhood* (1897), rejected the entire theoretical basis of Holt's generation of infant feeders. "In modifying milk for infant feeding it is neither possible nor necessary to overcome all the differences between cow's milk and breast milk; in fact, the most successful artificial feedings have differed widely from breast milk in composition." L. Emmett Holt, Jr., Rustin McIntosh, and Henry L. Barnett, *Pediatrics* (New York: Appleton-Century-Crofts, 1962), 218.

41. Apple, "Commercial Infant Feeding," 408–13.

42. Naomi Aronson, "Working Up and Appetite: The Food Industry Supplies Demand" in J. R. Kaplan, ed., *A Woman's Conflict: The Special Relationship Between Women and Food* (Englewood Cliffs: Prentice-Hall, 1980), 223.

43. Robert Morse Woodbury, "Economic Factors in Infant Mortality," *Journal of the American Statistical Association,* 19 (June 1924), 137–55. Although Akron, Ohio, for example, had a compulsory pasteurization law and regular inspection of its milk supply by public-health officials, infant mortality rates in its poorer wards in 1914 were just about as high as those in similar wards in other cities without pasteurization, ranging up to 112.9 per 1,000 live births in the area with highest mortality. Theresa S. Haley, *Infant Mortality: Results of a Field Study in Akron, Ohio, Based on Births in One Year* (Washington: GPO, 1920), 16.

44. C.-E.A. Winslow and Dorothy F. Holland, "The Influence of Certain Public Health Procedures upon Infant Mortality," *Human Biology,* 9 (May 1937), 133–74.

45. See, for example, Edward Meeker, "The Improving Health of the United States, 1850–1915," *Explorations in Economic History,* 9 (Summer 1972), 353–73; Robert Higgs, "Mortality in Rural America, 1870–1920: Estimates and Conjectures," *ibid.,* 10 (Winter 1973), 177–95; Michael R. Haines, "Mortality in Nineteenth Century America: Estimates from New York and Pennsylvania Consensus Data," 1865 and 1900," *Demography,* 14 (Aug. 1977), 311–31; John P. Fulton, "Mortality Decline in the State of Rhode Island, 1860–1970: A Comparison with England and Wales" (Ph.D. diss., Brown University, 1978), 123–38; Gretchen A. Condran and Eileen Crimmins-Gardner, "Public Health Measures and Mortality in U.S. Cities in the Late Nineteenth Century," *Human Ecology,* 6 (March 1978), 27–54. Although the authors disagree on many specifics, and Fulton does attempt to show that cleaner milk played a role of some importance, evidence in these studies would seem to downplay the importance of either medical intervention or public health and sanitation in reducing mortality, leading to the conclusion that rising standards of living, and especially of nutrition, played a major role.

46. *Journal of the American Medical Association,* 247 (Feb. 19, 1982), 1027. The link between low birth weight, low economic status, and high rates of infant mortality in the United States is demonstrated in the same number. See J. David Erickson and Tor Bjerkedal, "Fetal and Infant Mortality in Norway and the United States," *ibid.,* 9870–91.

47. Henry Dwight Chapin, "Child-Study in the Hospital—A Record of Six Hundred Cases," *Forum,* 17 (March 1894), 125–28.

48. Michael C. Latham, "Nutrition and Infection in National Development," in *Food: Politics, Economics, Nutrition, and Research,* ed. Philip H. Abelson (Washington: American Ass'n for Advancement of Science, 1975), 69.

Chapter 11.

1. Albert S. Crockett, "Hearty Eaters," *Saturday Evening Post,* Vol. 202, No. 16, Oct. 26, 1929, 105.

2. He saw considerable significance in the title that he chose for his post as head of the Food Administration: not Director, or Chief, but Administrator. Mark Sullivan, *Our Times: The United States, 1900–1925,* Vol. 5 (New York: Scribners, 1933), 413.

3. "Eat Less and Save Millions of Lives" was the title of one of Hoover's admonitions to the nation. Herbert Hoover to the American People, Sept. 21, 1918, in

United States Food Administration, Records, National Archives, Washington, D.C. (hereafter FA Records), Record Group 4, 12 HA D2, Box 492, File 228.

4. Even before the new knowledge of vitamins revolutionized attitudes towards vegetables, the FA was encouraging their cultivation in War Gardens as cheap, filling foods, using slogans such as "We Can Can Vegetables and the Kaiser Too." Charles Pack, *The War Garden Victorious* (Philadelphia, 1919), 15, cited in Cummings, *The American and His Food,* 139.

5. The advertiser's conviction that product names were all-important led FA administrators struggling to overcome American aversions to eating whale and porpoise to try to have them labeled "sea beef" or "sea steak." Maxcy R. Dickson, *The Food Front in World War I* (Washington: American Council on Public Affairs, 1944), 63.

6. The President's wife was the first to sign, in a public ceremony, after Hoover privately assured Wilson that "the card is not so binding as to cause anyone any great embarrassment in its execution." Herbert Hoover to Woodrow Wilson, June 23, 1917, Herbert Hoover Papers, Hoover Institution Archives, Stanford Univ., Palo Alto, Calif. (hereafter Hoover Papers) Box 6.

7. See Files of Women's Publications and Women's Pages Section, FA Records, 5HA-A4, Box 325, File 398.

8. Dickson, *Food Front,* 62.

9. Unsigned memo to Ray Wilbur, Sept. 11, 1917; Wilbur to Abby Marlatt, Oct. 6, 1917, FA Records, 5HA-4, Box 325, File 398.

10. Or, as in the face of a feared potato glut in the spring of 1918, just one year after the riots over potato shortages, employ surplus foodstuffs.

11. Minutes, Conference of Educational Directors, Feb. 28 to March 1, 1918, Hoover Papers, Stanford Univ., Palo Alto, Calif., Box 41.

12. Hoover to Women in the Graduating Classes of the Colleges and Universities, FA Records, 5HA-A8, Box 327, File 59.

13. Ida Tarbell, Introduction, "Ten Lessons in Food Conservation," ms. in *ibid.,* 5HA-A8, Box 327, File 59.

14. Albeit on rather shaky grounds: they were said to provide "mineral matter," particularly lime, for strong bones, iron, whose benefits were unknown, and water, as well as the two newly-discovered "vitamines," A and B. USFA, *Food Saving and Sharing,* (Garden City: Doubleday, 1918).

15. USFA, *Food and the War,* (Boston: Houghton Mifflin, 1918).

16. She also billed herself as "Domestic Science Expert, Universal Film Company." Ida C. Bailey Allen, *Mrs. Allen's Book of Meat Substitutes* (Boston: Small, Meynard, 1918).

17. Thetta Quay Franks, *Daily Menus for War Service* (New York: Putnam's, 1918).

18. Unfortunately, the results are of little value. The homes were not selected in any scientific way. Most of the surveyors were college girls majoring in home economics and a very high proportion of those surveyed seem to have been their instructors, parents, relatives, and friends of the family. The sample was therefore weighted heavily towards well-off farmers and the middle class. The few workers surveyed were almost all skilled workers and the only blacks were those associated with Tuskegee College, which was one of the cooperating institutions. There were practically no immigrants and the sample was skewed geographically by the hap-

hazard location of the cooperating institutions. Thus, for example, only one farm family from California participated. Moreover, the schedules were much too detailed even for this upscale sample, requiring participants to calculate weights, measures, and costs to a very fine degree. Most were therefore filled out inadequately or improperly. U.S. Bureau of Human Nutrition and Home Economics, Records, Food and Nutrition Division, Schedules Relating to a National Dietary Study of Families, 1917–19, Boxes 1–4, National Archives, Washington, D.C.

19. Memo, "Bi-weekly Staff Meeting," Office of Home Economics, March 28, 1918, Bureau of Human Nutrition, Records, Box 594.

20. Richard O. Cummings, "Publicity, Posters, Campaigns, and Propagandistic Methods of the United States Food Administration, 1917–1920, "A Preliminary Survey of Materials in the National Archives," U.S. Department of Agriculture, Jan. 1942, 4.

21. Menu, "Special. Meatless Tuesday, Dec. 19, 1917," Chicago, Milwaukee and St. Paul Railway, FA Records, 12HM-A3, Box 325.

22. Lilian Dynevor Rice, "Recipes that Serve Your Country," *Women's World,* Feb. 1918, 20.

23. Pamphlet, FA Records, 12HM-A1, Box 492, File 329.

24. Richard O. Cummings, "Publicity," 3, 16.

25. Hoover to Woodrow Wilson, May 31, 1917, Hoover Papers, Box 6. Some months later, Ray Wilbur recommended to Hoover that he not give in to suggestions that the nation's bakers be allowed to produce only whole wheat bread because there was no conclusive evidence of the superiority of whole over refined wheat. "Many people suffer from constipation and whole wheat bread relieves them," he wrote, but this did not justify forcing it on the majority, who did not like it. Ray Wilbur, draft memorandum, Aug. 31, 1917, FA Records, 5HA-A4, Box 325.

26. Julian Street, "What's the Matter with American Food?" *Saturday Evening Post,* Vol. 203, No. 38 (March 21, 1931), 10.

27. Unsigned, [Langworthy?], undated [April, 1919?], memo, Bureau of Human Nutrition Records, RG 176, Subject Correspondence of the Chief of the Bureau (Alfred True) 1917–30, Box 595.

28. Cummings, "Publicity," 5.

29. Ray Wilbur to J. W. Hollowell, Dec. 6, 1917, FA Records, 5HA-A4, Box 325. A few days later he labeled Kansas City the "furthest behind" of any place he had been because of "misrepresentation" by Senator Read (a detractor of Hoover) the meat packers, and Germans. Ray Wilbur, Report on Kansas City, Dec. 27, 1917, FA Records, 5HA-A4, Box 325.

30. Cummings, "Publicity," 8.

31. EAR to Jane Addams, Sept. 21, 1917, FA Records, 12HM-A3, Box 584.

32. Obviously impressed by the New Nutrition, he hoped that "the stress of war" would help them overcome their bad habit of eating too much wasteful and harmful food such as sugar. "We need to learn food values and eat not simply because eating is pleasant, but because through proper food we may build strong healthy bodies," he said. Dickson, *Food Front,* 75.

33. FA Records, 12HN-A3, Box 589.

34. Jane Addams File, FA Records, 5HA-A1, Box 288.

35. See correspondence in this regard in FA Records, 12HM-A3, Box 584.

36. F. G. Woodward, Memorandum, Sept. 6, 1917, FA Records, 12HM-A3, Box 584.

37. Jno. [sic] M. Parker to R. E. Mermerlstern [sic], Oct. 22, 1917, FA Records, 12HM-A3, Box 584. "It is hardly fair," said the Massachusetts agent of the FA, "to ask wage earners with families to cut down on rations when they have all they can do to keep their homes going." However, he added, "much can be done in showing how far a dollar can go." Newspaper clipping, [Boston *Post?*], [Jan. 1918], Eva White Papers, Schlesinger Library, Box 2, Folder 32v (a), 103.

38. Frank Gudas to United States Food Administration, Sept. 19, 1917, FA Records, 12HM-A3, Box 584.

39. Dennison House, Minutes of Board of Directors Meeting, Oct. 15, 1917, Dennison House Records, Schlesinger Library, Radcliffe College, Box 3, Folder 9.

40. Unsigned carbon copy of letter from Vernacular Press Section to Ben Allen, Oct. 6, 1917, FA Records, 12HM-A3, Box 584.

41. Mermelstein to Max Rhoade, Oct. 5, 1917, FA Records, 12HM-A3, Box 584. This is a rather Roman Catholic concept of Yom (not "your") Kippur, the Day of Atonement, and there are no other "holy days" upon which Jews are required to fast.

42. "Transcript of Conference of Educational Directors," Hoover Papers, Box 41.

43. *New York Times,* June 10, 12, 15, 18, 1917.

44. Mrs. W. J. Jennings to Herbert Hoover, July 14, 1917, FA Records, 5HA-A8, Box 327.

45. Ida Tarbell to W. H. Kistler, Aug. 8, 1917, *ibid.*

46. Dickson, *Food Front,* 102.

47. *Ibid.,* 93.

48. *Ibid.,* 101.

49. C. F. Langworthy, "Memorandum Regarding the Present Use of Meat in the United States," Dec. 8, 1921, Bureau of Human Nutrition and Home Economics Records, Box 594.

50. This was reflected in a widening price spread between the two kinds of pork. E. L. Rhoades, *Merchandising Packinghouse Products* (Chicago: Univ. of Chicago Press, 1929), 115.

51. Transcript of Conference of Educational Directors, Washington, Feb. 28 to March 1, 1918, Hoover Papers, Box 41.

52. U.S. Secretary of War. Commissary General of Sustenance, *Manual for Army Cooks* (Washington: GPO, 1896), 186–91. The presence of this section is puzzling, for it predates the Spanish-American War and the subsequent occupations of various parts of the Caribbean and Central America and yet was almost fifty years after the invasion and occupation of Mexico. However, a good part of the Army was stationed in the Southwest, and the instruction that *metates* could "be purchased at any Mexican store" (190) shows that at least one of the authors had been stationed in that area.

53. U.S. War Department, Office of the Quartermaster-General, *Manual for Army Cooks, 1916* (Washington: GPO, 1917). Among the answers given to the obvious question regarding food conservation: Why should civilians be forced to substitute other grains for white flour in order for the Army to eat only wheat bread?, the Army answered "The human element: Soldiers cannot adjust to new

diets very well, for they cannot substitute other things for new items on their menus such as different breads they do not like. They will simply eat less bread with a consequent loss of vitality and failure to replenish the tissues expended under the severe physical hardships of the campaign." Lt. Col. Frank Geere, *Wheat Bread for Soldiers in the Field* (pamphlet), (Boston: Association of Collegiate Alumnae, 1918).

54. Mary I. Barber, ed., *History of the American Dietetic Association* (Philadelphia: Lippincott, 1959), 198–205.

55. The Jewish comedian Buddy Hackett has remarked that it was not until he joined the Army and ate non-Jewish food that he realized that the pain in his chest which had been with him all of his life could go away. So spicy and garlicky was its Rumanian variant that Zero Mostel used to claim that "Rumanian-Jewish food killed more Jews than Hitler."

56. See Harvey A. Levenstein, "The American Response to Italian Food," *Food and Foodways*, Vol. 1, No. 1 (1985), and Harvey A. Levenstein and Joseph Conlin, "Les habitudes alimentaires des immigrants italiens en Amérique du Nord," *Culture Technique*, No. 16 (1986).

57. Christine Frederick *Selling Mrs. Consumer*, 130.

Chapter 12.

1. Elmer McCollum, *The Newer Knowledge of Nutrition* (New York: Macmillan, 1918): E. Neige Todhunter, "Some Aspects of the History of Dietetics," *World Review of Nutrition and Dietics*, Vol. 18, (1973) 1–46; Aaron J. Ihde and Stanley L. Becker, "Conflict of Concepts in Early Vitamin Studies," *Journal of the History of Biology*, Vol. 4, No. 1 (Spring 1971), 1–33; U.S. Congress, Senate, Select Committee on Nutrition and Human Needs, *The Role of the Federal Government in Human Nutrition Research*, 94th Cong., 2d sess., 1976, 10–13.

2. Henry C. Sherman, *Food Products* (New York: Macmillan, 1914), 79–81; Lafayette B. Mendel, *Changes in the Food Supply and their Relation to Nutrition* (New Haven: Yale Univ. Press, 1916), 49–50. Sherman, much involved with home economists who demanded precise rules and scientific-sounding formulae, eventually came up with a neat but vague rule. Cereals and spreads should be used plentifully and in addition an equal amount of the food budget was to be spent on each of three categories: 1) meat and fish; 2) fruit and vegetables; and 3) milk. Baily Burrit to Dr. Ira S. Wile, April 25, 1918, CSS Papers, Box 50, File 325-3.

3. McCollum, *Newer Knowledge*, 82.

4. USFA, *Food and the War* (Boston: Houghton Mifflin, 1918).

5. Elizabeth Etheridge, *The Butterfly Caste* (Westport: Greenwood, 1971), Chap. 7, 8, 9.

6. Food economy was mentioned only in the context of "True Economy in Health." Lucy Gillett, *Food for Health's Sake* (New York: Funk and Wagnall's, 1924), v, 42, 31.

7. Frederick Palmer, "How Long Do You Want to Live?," *Collier's* Oct. 14, 1922.

8. Winifred D. Wandersea, *Women's Work and Family Values, 1920–1940* (Cambridge: Harvard Univ. Press, 1981), 3.

9. In early 1918, its pamphlet, "Milk, the Indispensable Food for Children," went through its first printing of twenty thousand copies within a matter of weeks and a second printing was rushed through in response to the unheard of demand from mothers for information on milk's importance. Dorothy R. Mendenhall, *Milk, the Indispensable Food for Children* (Washington: GPO, 1918); Memorandum for Miss Lathrop [author's signature undecipherable] April 4, 1918, U.S. Children's Bureau, Records, Record Group 102, U.S. Bureau of the Census. National Archives, Washington, D.C., Box 85.

10. "Food Mergers—What Has Happened, and Why," *Business Week,* Nov. 14, 1929, 29.

11. This excludes the liquor and beverage industry, hard hit by prohibition, and tobacco. *Historical Statistics of the United States, Colonial Times to 1970* (Washington: GPO, 1973), 684.

12. *Ibid.*

13. Alonzo Taylor, "Consumption, Merchandising, and Advertising of Foods," *Harvard Business Review,* April 1924, 281–95.

14. *Macaroni Journal,* Sept. 15, 1926.

15. H. C. Nulmoor, "Asparagus Becomes a Best Seller," *American Restaurant Magazine,* Feb. 1928, 48–49.

16. General Mills, "Outline of Career in Advertising of Marjorie Child Husted," Feb. 1950, Marjorie C. Husted [Betty Crocker] Papers, Schlesinger Library; F. J. Schlink, *Eat, Drink, and Be Wary* (New York: Covici, Fried, 1935), 18–19.

17. Second only to toiletery and drug manufacturers. Cummings, *American and His Food,* 156.

18. *Good Housekeeping,* March 1919; *The Delineator,* Vol. 96, No. 3 (March 1920), 56; *Ibid.,* Vol. 96, No. 4 (April 1920), 50.

19. *The American Magazine,* April 1922, 37.

20. *The Literary Digest,* June 10, 1922; The *American Magazine,* Jan. 1922, 35. By the end of the decade, Fleischmann's success in the health food market and its extensive distribution network had made it a prime candidate for takeover. It was bought by J. P. Morgan and Co. and merged into Standard Brands, Inc. "Food Mergers—What Has Happened, and Why," *The Business Week,* Sept. 14, 1929, 29.

21. *GH,* Sept. 1928, 129. This was an attempt to take advantage of the discovery that iodine, which it added to its salt, helped prevent the development of goiters.

22. *GH,* April 1928, 166.

28. James H. Young, *The Medical Messiahs* (Princeton: Princeton Univ. Press, 1967), 335.

24. *GH,* April 1928, 199.

25. Schlink, *Eat, Drink, and Be Wary,* 107.

26. Irene Till, *Milk, The Politics of an Industry* (New York: McGraw-Hill, 1938), 45–52.

27. "Food Mergers," *The Business Week,* Sept. 14, 1928, 29.

28. Till, *Milk,* 451–52.

29. *GH,* Sept. 1928, 257.

30. *GH,* Sept. 1928, 168.

31. The mother understood, then, that there "couldn't be a simpler way to build up health" than by adding Cocomalt to the child's milk to make it more palatable and nutritious. *GH,* Sept. 1928, 194.

32. *Ladies Home Journal,* Sept. 1928, 109.

33. It remained close to or over that level until 1942, when it began a slow decline. "Apparent Civilian Per Capita Consumption of Foods: 1849 to 1970," in U.S. Bureau of the Census, *Historical Statistics of the United States, Colonial Times to 1970* (Washington: GPO, 1975), 331. In 1953, the U.S. Department of Agriculture had substantially lower estimates of consumption than *Historical Statistics* later published, but the overall trend was similar, showing a 4 percent rise in per capita consumption of all dairy products from 1909 to 1930 and a 3 percent rise in that of milk. U.S. Department of Agriculture, *Consumption of Foods in the United States,* 1909–52, Agricultural Handbook No. 62 (Washington: GPO, 1953), 137–38, 144, cited in Panschar, *Baking in America,* 104. Although pasteurization likely played a role as well by giving milk a clean bill of health, its overall effect on consumption was likely minor for where milk did have an unhealthy connotation, it was mainly, as the last chapter indicated, as a warm weather baby-killer.

34. McCollum, Orent-Keiles and Day, *The Newer Knowledge of Nutrition* (New York: Macmillan, 1929), 598.

35. McCollum and Nina Simmonds, *Food, Nutrition, and Health,* (New York, Macmillan, 1928).

36. General Mills, "Outline of the Career of Marjorie Hulsted"; Schlink, *Eat, Drink, and Be Wary,* 14–19.

37. Schlink, *Eat, Drink, and Be Wary,* 212, 222; Helen Pundt, *AHEA, A History of Excellence* (Washington: American Home Economics Association), 51, 56.

38. Editorial, *Journal of Home Economics,* Vol. 19, No. 4, (April 1927), 46.

39. Rena Jenkins, Home Economics Survey, July 12, 1926, in Julia Jaffrey to Louise Stanley, July 14, 1926, U.S. Bureau of Human Nutrition and Home Economics, Records. RG 176, National Archives, Washington, D.C., Box 595.

40. Lydia J. Roberts, "The Dietitian and Normal Nutrition," *Journal of the American Dietetic Association,* Vol. 5, No. 1 (June 1919), 11.

41. The course also dealt with proper table manners. Whereas one section of the book mentions that many were so poor that lunches consisted only of a tortilla with nothing on it, the girls were still instructed to set tables with white table cloths and silencers ("or, if the table be of pleasing appearance, doilies may be used.") Pearl I. Ellis, *Americanization Through Homemaking* (Los Angeles: Wetzel, 1929), 26, 31, 19.

42. In a 1920 advertisement extolling the quality of Del Monte canned goods she noted that "the war taught us that properly canned fruits and vegetables are absolutely essential in a food crisis; reconstruction is teaching us that these same foods are a strong ally during a shortage of domestic help." *The Delineator,* Vol. 96, No. 2 (Feb. 1920), 99. Conveniently ignored, of course, were her prewar admonitions against the waste of money which expenditure on fruit, particularly canned fruit, represented.

43. *Macaroni Journal,* May 15, 1923.

44. John T. Edsall and David Bearman, "Historical Records of Scientific Activity: A Survey of Sources for the History of Biochemistry and Molecular Biology," *Proceedings of the American Philosophical Society,* Vol. 123, No. 5 (Oct. 15, 1979), 287–88.

45. *Ibid.,* 286–88.

46. Gove Hambidge, "The Grocery Revolution," *Ladies' Home Journal*, Nov. 1928, 121.

47. Clarence Lieb, "Our Changing Ideas about Diet," *Woman's Home Companion*, Vol. 55, No. 6 (June 1928), 11.

48. "The cook will no longer be called upon to denature the articles which he cooks; the miller will no longer be required to remove the wholesome parts of the grain; the manufacturer will not be required to predigest the foods which pass through his hands," he wrote in 1919. Harvey Wiley, "Food Reconstruction," *GH*, Vol. 68, No. 2 (Feb. 1919).

49. *GH*, July 1928, 108, Sept. 1928, 131.

50. *Macaroni Journal*, Oct. 15, 1926.

51. Mary E. Spencer, *Food and Nutrition* (n.p: National Catholic Welfare Conference, n.d.).

Chapter 13.

1. Alice Kessler-Harris, *Out to Work* (New York: Oxford Univ. Press, 1982), 217–30; Sophinisba P. Breckinridge, "The Activities of Women Outside the Home," in President's Committee on Recent Social Trends, *Recent Social Trends in America* (N.Y.: McGraw-Hill, 1933), Vol. 2, 721.

2. Breckinridge, "The Activities of Women Outside the Home," 721.

3. The change was also accompanied by a change in the servants' complexion, as black women replaced immigrant white women in northern cities. Maurine W. Greenwald, *Women, War, and Work* (Westport: Greenwood, 1980), 23.

4. Ruth Cowan, in her article, "A Case Study of Technological Change: The Washing Machine and the Working Wife," in Mary S. Hartman and Lois Banner, eds. *Clio's Consciousness Raised* (New York: Harper and Row, 1974), 245–52, and in her book, *More Work from Mother* (New York: Basic, 1983), links higher standards of cleanliness, made possible by improved household technology, to the continuing pressure to keep women tied to the household, but this would not seem to be the case with food, at least from about 1915 to 1930.

5. Winifred D. Wandersee, *Women's Work and Family Values, 1920–1940* (Cambridge: Harvard Univ. Press, 1981), 3.

6. Robert S. and Helen Lynd, *Middletown: A Study in American Culture* (New York: Harcourt and Brace, 1929), 154.

7. William Ogburn, "The Family and Its Functions," *Recent Social Trends*, Vol. 2, 667.

8. Gove Hambidge, "The Grocery Revolution," *Ladies' Home Journal*, Nov. 1928, 99.

9. E. G. Montgomery, "Points Brought Out in the Canned Food Survey," U.S. Department of Commerce, 1926, cited in Christine Frederick, *Selling Mrs. Consumer*, 162.

10. Lynds, *Middletown*, 153–54.

11. Frederick, *Selling*, 120.

12. "Time-Saving Meals," *Good Housekeeping*, April 1919.

13. "'Home Cooking' Made This Man Famous," *The American Restaurant*, Dec. 1926, 80.

14. Admittedly, some presidents, notably Herbert Hoover, were not exactly sylph-like, but even he was not particularly heavy in 1928, when he swept to victory.

15. B. Johnston, *Eat and Grow Fat* (New York: Sherwood, 1917); Johnston, *Eat and Grow Slender* (New York: Sherwood, 1917). Among the reasons given for gaining weight was that thin people tend to be more nervous than fat people and should therefore put on weight to calm down. Also, "hard brain work uses up a great amount of force, and this is largely supplied by the consumption of fats, starch, and sugar. A well known English lawyer always takes a meal of some easily digested fatty food before making a great intellectual effort." [20.]

16. *GH*, Vol. 68, No. 3 (March 1919), 118.

17. Lulu Hunt Peters, "Watch Your Weight!" *American Magazine*, Vol. 93, No. 3 (March 1922), 56–57.

18. Ruth Wadsworth, "The Old Order Changeth," *Women's Home Companion*, May 1923.

19. "Food and Health," *Literary Digest*, Vol. 76 (Mar. 24, 1923), 76.

20. Helen M. Welles and Belle de Graf, *Food and How to Cook It* (Philadelphia: National, 1928), xiii.

21. Mary D. Chambers, *One-Piece Dinners* (Boston: Little, Brown, 1924), 1, 45.

22. Christine Frederick, "Improving Our Restaurants," *The American Restaurant*, Jan. 1928, 68.

23. William Allen White, "The Supremacy of Beefsteak," in "When Americans Dine," *The Nation*, Vol. 117, No. 3051 (Dec. 26, 1923), 731.

24. Frederick, "Improving Our Restaurants," 68.

25. Wells and de Graf, *Food*, 127.

26. *Ibid.*, 218–19.

27. The book still went through four printings from 1925 to 1929, but one suspects that captive student audiences might have played a role in this. Claire de Pratz, *French Home Cooking* (New York: Dutton, 1936).

28. Xavier Raskin, *The French Chef in the American Kitchen* (Chicago: Rand-McNally, 1922).

29. Mary T. Luck and Sybil Woodruff, *The Food of Twelve Families of the Professional Class* University of California Cost of Living Studies III (Berkeley: Univ. of California Press, 1931), 277.

30. Hawley, *Economics of Food Consumption*, 112, 250–51.

31. Menu, "Dinner Given by the Mayor of Boston for Charles Lindbergh, Oct. 18, 1927," Menu Collection, Manuscripts Division, New York Public Library, Box 1.

32. *Ibid.*, Box 1.

33. Wells and de Graf, *Food*, 64.

34. Christine Frederick, "Improving Our Restaurants," *The American Restaurant*, Jan. 1928, 68.

35. J. O. Dahl, "The Trend Towards Simplified Cooking as Seen by Hotel and Food Executives," *Hotel Management and Food Profits*, March 1931, 100.

36. "What Is an 'American Dinner'?" *The Nation*, Vol. 117, No. 3041 (Oct. 17, 1923), 428.

37. "When We Americans Dine: A Symposium on the Great American Dinner," *The Nation,* Vol. 117, No. 3051 (Dec. 26, 1923), 731–34.

Chapter 14.

1. This emphasis on the irrational, non-economic basis of food choices dominated the work of the wartime Committee on Food Habits of the National Research Council, which Mead headed. See National Research Council, *The Problem of Changing Food Habits,* Report of the Committee on Food Habits, NRC Bulletin No. 108 (1943), and in particular her essay "The Problem of Changing Food Habits," 20–31.

2. Mary Douglas, "Deciphering a Meal," *Daedalus,* Vol. 101 (1972), 61–82; Marvin Harris, *Cannibals and Kings: The Origins of Culture* (New York: Random House, 1977).

3. Marvin Harris, "How Beef Became King," *Psychology Today,* Vol. 12, No. 5 (Oct. 1978), 88–94; Eric B. Ross, "Patterns of Diet and Forces of Production: An Economic and Ecological History of the Ascendancy of Beef in the United States Diet," in Eric B. Ross, ed. *Beyond the Myths of Culture* (New York: Academic Press, 1980), 181–225. Harris summarized his views on the material basis of food habits in a paper criticizing Mary Douglas and the "idealists" which he presented to a conference of anthropologists in Florida in 1983 but the copy of the paper which I have is labeled "not for publication."

4. Douglas, "Deciphering," 62; Harris, unpublished.

5. Paul Douglas, *Real Wages in the United States, 1890–1926* (Boston: Houghton Mifflin, 1930), 582.

6. M. Ada Beney, *Cost of Living in the United States, 1914–1936* (New York: National Industrial Conference Board, 1938), 43–47; U.S. Bureau of the Census, *Historical Statistics of the United States* (Washington: GPO, 1975), 213.

7. The largest survey of the decade, a 1924 study of over 12,000 families in 42 states by the Bureau of Labor Statistics, showed that on average over 38 percent of their expenditures still went on food. Hawley, *Economics of Food Consumption,* 250–51. The figures are not out of line with those of Paul Douglas, who calculated that the proportion of the workers' budgets devoted to food dropped from an average of 43.1 percent in 1901 to 38.2 percent in 1918. Douglas, *Real Wages,* 495.

8. *Historical Statistics,* 213.

9. J. C. Kennedy, et. al., *Wages and Family Budgets in the Chicago Stockyard District* (Chicago: Univ. of Chicago Press, 1914), 72.

10. As a result, their diets were adjudged, by 1930 standards, to be much healthier than those of 1914, with more than adequate supplies of calories, proteins, calcium, phosphorus, iron, and "likely" (because there was still great uncertainty regarding requirements) vitamins A and C. Lucy H. Gillett and Penelope B. Rice, *Influence of Education on the Food Habits of Some New York City Families* (New York: New York Association for Improving the Condition of the Poor, 1931), 15–19. I have not discussed the 1928 families who were "influenced" by nutritional social workers since they were clearly atypical.

11. Lynds, *Middletown,* 157–58.

12. In March, 1923, 1500 girls from Muncie's 9,200 homes were taking home

economics courses and a goodly proportion must have been working class. Many of the 7500 or so copies of women's magazines sold in Muncie that month must have circulated among working class women, *ibid.*

13. Gillett and Rice, *Influence,* 15–17.

14. White wheaten flour was not "enriched" with vitamins and minerals until the 1940s.

15. Gillett and Rice, *Influence,* 34.

16. Of course these things are impossible to calculate with any precision, but Norman Clark does make a good argument that, contrary to previously accepted wisdom, Prohibition did result in a significant drop-off in working-class alcohol consumption. Norman H. Clark, *Deliver Us from Evil: An Interpretation of American Prohibition* (New York: Norton, 1976), Chap. 8.

17. Irving Bernstein, *The Lean Years* (Baltimore: Penguin, 1970), 53–54.

18. Lynds, *Middletown,* 61–63.

19. Jacqueline Jones, *Labor of Love,* 184.

20. *Ibid.,* 182–90; Alice Kessler-Harris, *Out to Work* (New York: Oxford Univ. Press, 1982), 237–38.

21. Etheridge, *Butterfly Caste,* 185.

22. Hazel K. Stiebeling, *Economic and Social Problems and Conditions of the Southern Appalachians,* U.S. Department of Agriculture Miscellaneous Publication No. 205 (Washington: GPO, 1935), 153.

23. Lydia Roberts, *The Nutrition and Care of Children in a Mountain County of Kentucky,* U.S. Department of Labor, Children's Bureau, Publication No. 110 (Washington: GPO, 1922), 4.

24. Stiebeling, *Economic and Social Problems,* 153–54.

25. Mexican-Americans in towns and cities had more adequate diets. White flour was also their staple, but they ate small but adequate quantities of meat, eggs, and cheese, as well as a lot of tomatoes and potatoes. Jet C. Winters, *A Report on the Health and Nutrition of Mexicans Living in Texas,* University of Texas Bulletin No. 3127, (July 15, 1931), (Austin: Univ. of Texas, 1931).

26. Jessie A. Stene and Lydia J. Roberts, "A Nutrition Study of an Indian Reservation," *Journal of the American Dietetic Association,* Vol. 3, No. 4 (March, 1928), 217–21.

27. Schedules of National Dietary Survey, 1917–19, U.S. Bureau of Human Nutrition, Food and Nut Division, Records, National Archives, Boxes 1–4.

28. Michael Berger, *The Devil Wagon in God's Country,* (Hamden: Archon, 1979), 154–61.

29. U.S. Department of Agriculture, Office of Cooperative Extension Work, *Cooperative Extension Work* (1929), 4, 37, 43, cited in Cummings, *American and His Food,* 175–76.

30. Dorothy Dickins, *A Study of the Food Habits of People in Two Contrasting Areas of Mississippi,* Mississippi Agricultural Experiment Station Bulletin No. 245 (Nov. 1927), 33.

31. USDA, *Cooperative Extension Work,* 43, cited in Cummings, *American and His Food,* 178.

32. South Carolina Agricultural Extension Station Bulletin 268 (Sept. 1930), cited in Julian D. Boyd, "The Nature of the American Diet," *Journal of Pediatrics,* Vol. 12, No. 2 (Feb. 1938), 247.

33. Dickins, *Food Habits,* 21.

34. Ellis Lore Kirkpatrick, *The Farmer's Standard of Living* (reprinted, New York: Arno Press, 1971), 86.

35. University of New Hampshire Extension Service, Circular 169 (June 1935), cited in Boyd, "American Diet," 247.

36. Accessibility and economics seem to have played no role, for the more remote farmers still purchased as much "refined" food in town as the others. Cummings, *American and His Food,* 168–69.

37. Margaret Coffin, *The Sources of Food Used by Maryland Farmers,* Maryland Agricultural Experiment Station Bulletin No. 346 (College Park: Univ. of Maryland, 1933), 506, cited in Cummings, *American and His Food,* 177.

Chapter 15.

1. Julian Street, "What's the Matter with Food?" *Saturday Evening Post,* Vol. 203, No. 38 (March 21, 1931), 10–11.

2. Pamphlet, "The Locke-Ober Café: A Brief History," (Boston, [1983?], 14.

3. J. O. Dahl, "An Open Letter to Chefs," *Hotel Management,* Jan. 1931, 9.

4. American Restaurant Magazine, *A Market Analysis of the Restaurant Industry* (Chicago: Paterson, 1932), 11.

5. "Locke-Ober Café," 6.

6. American Restaurant Magazine, *Market Analysis,* 23–24.

7. *Ibid.,* 11.

8. *The Restaurant Bulletin,* Vol. 1, No. 4 (Feb. 1904), 22.

9. Dinah Sturgess, "The Table d'Hote," *American Kitchen Magazine,* Vol. 10, No. 4 (Jan. 1899), 132; Richard Duffy, "New York at Table," *Putnam's,* Vol. 5, No. 5 (Feb. 1909), 569.

10. John Raklios, "How I Built a Restaurant Business," *The American Restaurant,* Dec. 1919, 19.

11. Joseph Mason, "Men and Methods," *System,* Aug. 1922, 24.

12. A typical "business lunch" at the Café Morris in Chicago in 1904 featured oysters on the shell, clam chowder, breaded whitefish or roast pork, potatoes, beans, a choice of pies or cheese and crackers, and a glass of beer, tea or coffee: all for thirty cents. "Model Business Lunch," *Restaurant Bulletin,* Feb. 1904, 22.

13. *American Restaurant,* Nov. 1919, 26–27.

14. Irving Scheyer, "Tea Room Success and Why," *ibid.,* Jan. 1919; Menu, Miss Ellis Tea Shop, Chicago, Ill., in *ibid.,* Sept. 1920.

15. "Glimpses of New York Tea Rooms," *Tea Room and Gift Shop,* Vol. 3, No. 5 (Nov. 1923), 6.

16. *Ibid.*

17. William F. Ireland, "Where the Cafeteria Was Born," *American Restaurant,* May 1920, 15–17; "The Origin of the Cafeteria—The Institution," *Journal of Home Economics,* July 1925, 392.

18. American Restaurant, *Market Analysis,* 31.

19. J. O. Dahl, "How They Are Profiting From Fashions in Food," *Hotel Management,* Oct. 1926, 59.

20. *American Restaurant,* April 1924, 52.

21. J. H. Van Leewwarden, "Drop a Coin and Get Your Pie," *American Restaurant*, July 1920, 24.

22. *Ibid.*, 24.

23. *Hotel Management and Food Profits*, March 1927, 117.

24. *Ibid.*, 101–3.

25. American Restaurant, *Market Analysis*, 53.

26. J. O. Dahl, "Do Your Customers Count Calories?," *Hotel Management and Food Profits*, Oct. 1927, 16; *Ibid.*, Feb. 1928, 63; *The American Restaurant*, Jan. 1924, 23.

27. *American Restaurant*, Jan. 1929, 52–53. Normally, restaurants aim at having food amount to about one-third of their costs.

28. American Restaurant, *Market Analysis*, 19.

29. Gustav Mann, Oral History Interview, Bancroft Library, University of California, Berkeley, 43.

30. "The 'Bark' That Leads to a Bite," *Restaurant Management*, Dec. 1928, 350.

31. *United America* Vol. 1, No. 1, Aug. 7, 1925.

32. Rian James, *Dining in New York* (New York: John Day, 1930), 206.

33. *Restaurant Management*, March, 1928, 121.

34. "Changing Over from Dining Room to Cafeteria," *Hotel Management*, Dec. 1924.

35. *American Restaurant*, Sept. 1920, 13–14.

36. "What Are They Serving?" *ibid.*, Feb. 1924, 62.

37. J. O. Dahl, "Do Your Customers Count Calories?," 17–18.

38. *Hotel Management and Food Profits*, Nov. 1931, 213.

39. In the year or so after the register was opened in May, 1926, it accumulated 378,000 entries! Jay Roberts, "Does It Pay to Employ a Dietitian?" *ibid.*, July 1927, 7–9.

40. *American Restaurant*, Jan. 1924, 23.

41. J. O. Dahl, "How Eating Habits Are Changing," *Hotel Management*, Feb. 1925, 17–19.

42. *American Restaurant*, July 1920, 28.

43. J. O. Dahl, "The Trend Towards Simplified Cooking As Seen by Hotel and Food Executives," *Hotel Management and Food Profits*, March 1931, 100.

44. "Representative Managers View the Trend," *ibid.*, 99.

45. Dahl, "Open Letter," 9.

46. "Representative Managers," 99.

47. Dahl, "Open Letter," 9.

48. *American Restaurant*, Nov. 1929, 59–60.

Chapter 16.

1. Richard Cummings also compared the two, but saw the 1896 slogan as spelling "necessity," while Hoover's "smacked of abundance." Cummings, *The American and His Food*, 164.

2. Americans could still not forego their sweets, particularly in the face of rock bottom sugar prices for much of the 1920's. By 1930, per capita sugar consumption, which had stood at about 65 pounds in 1900, had soared to almost 110

pounds, a peak which it would not again surmount. Barger, *American Agriculture,* 149–58; Marguerite C. Burk, *Trends and Patterns in U.S. Food Consumption,* U.S. Department of Agriculture Handbook No. 214 (Washington: USDA, 1961); U.S. Bureau of the Census, *Historical Statistics of the United States* (Washington: USGPO, 1975), 330.

3. Fogel, Engerman, and Russell, "Uses of Data on Height," 416.

4. Horace Gray, "Increase in Stature of American Boys in the Last Fifty Years," *Journal of the American Medical Association,* Vol. 88 (March 29, 1927), 908.

5. "Increase in Stature of American Men," Metropolitan Life, *Statistical Bulletin,* Vol. 25, No. 11 (Nov. 1944), 1–2.

6. Gordon T. Bowles, *New Types of Old Americans at Harvard and Eastern Women's Colleges,* (Cambridge: Harvard Univ. Press, 1932), 108, 132–33, cited in Cummings, *American and His Food,* 161.

7. "Increase in Stature," 2.

8. Conrad and Irene Tauber, *The Changing Population of the United States* (New York: Wiley, 1958), 269–72, tentatively estimated that there was a steady decline, while warning of insufficient data. Ainsley Coale and Melvin Zelnick, *New Estimates of Fertility and Population in the United States* (Princeton: Princeton Univ. Press, 1963), 7–9, are more decisive about a straight and steady decline, but with little more evidence. Edward Meeker, on the other hand, estimated that "average mortality and life expectancy improved little, and likely worsened, prior to 1880," and that "a fundamental transition in the state of health occurred in the decade of the eighties," (Edward Meeker, "The Improving Health of the United States, 1850–1915," *Explorations in Economic History,* Vol. 9, No. 3 (Summer 1972), 353), and in their recent work on the topic Robert Fogel and the population study group at the University of Chicago are developing a hypothesis which sees the trend in mortality rates as roughly following that which they have discovered in final height statistics: that the 1880's and early 1890's represent a bottoming out, with steady improvements following. Robert Fogel, "Nutrition and the Decline in Mortality since 1700; Some Preliminary Findings," Lecture at McMaster University, March 8, 1985.

9. Robert Higgs, who calculates that from 1880 to 1920 rural death rates declined by 30 to 40 percent, ascribes this "vital revolution" mainly to better diet. Robert Higgs, "Mortality in Rural America, 1870–1920: Estimates and Conjectures," *Explorations in Economic History* Vol. 10, No. 2 (Winter 1975), 177–95. Even S. L. N. Roa, who portrays the nineteenth century as a period of slow improvement in mortality rates, sees a great acceleration of the process the first thirty years of this century, followed by a slowing of the process in the following three decades and a leveling off of the rate of improvement in the 1960s. S. L. N. Rao, "On Long Term Mortality Trends in the United States, 1850–1968," *Demography,* Vol. 10, No. 3 (Aug. 1973), 411–13.

10. U.S. Bureau of the Census, *Birth Statistics, 1915–1918* (Washington: GPO, 1917–1920); *Vital Statistics, 1950* (Washington: GPO,) 262–63.

11. Brian McMahon, "Infant Mortality in the United States," in Carl L. Erhardt and Joyce Berlin, eds., *Mortality and Morbidity in the United States* (Cambridge: Harvard Univ. Press, 1974), 193–95.

12. For the lower one-third, however, lower income continued to be translated into poorer nutrition. This was reflected in the stark gaps which persisted between

white and non-white infant mortality rates. The earliest figures, at the turn of the century, indicated that black infants died at about twice the rate of whites. While both rates declined after 1915, the rate for non-whites declined most rapidly during the war, a fact likely connected with improved job opportunities for blacks in urban areas and wartime prosperity in the Southern rural economy. In the 1920s, however, the trend towards closing the gap, which in 1921 stood at 72.5 per thousand for whites *versus* 108.5 for non-whites was halted and slowly reversed until by the 1970s it was again almost double that of whites. Warren S. Thompson and P. K. Whelpton, *Population Trends in the United States* (New York: McGraw-Hill, 1933), 232; U.S. Bureau of the Census, *Historical Statistics of the United States,* 44.

13. U.S. Health Service, "Diets of Low-Income Families," Public Health Reports, Jan. 24, 1936, in *Monthly Labor Review* Vol. 43, No. 3 (Sept. 1936), 601.

14. This is not to say that economic distress did not contribute to poor nutrition and poor health. The studies of low-income families showed "a consistent correlation between" illness and economic status: "the lower the income the higher the sickness rate." The U.S. Public Health service saw these sickness rates as "consistent with the situation found in the food supply, which, at income levels of less than $3 or $4 per person per week showed a marked tendency to be poorly balanced, to include less than 'safe' requirements of milk and other 'protective' foods, and to be insufficient in quantity." *Ibid.,* 602–3. But this was something which had characterized low-income groups before the Depression as well. It is not clear that the Depression actually increased levels of morbidity among the poor.

15. *Good Housekeeping,* Vol. 99, No. 2 (Aug. 1934), 18, 124.

16. *GH,* Vol. 100, No. 1 (Jan. 1935), 105.

17. *GH,* 147.

18. Federal Trade Commission, Stipulation No. 02180, July 28, 1938, copy in Congress of Industrial Organizations, Washington Headquarters, Archives of Labor History and Urban Affairs, Wayne State University, Detroit, Files of D. E. Montgomery, Box 3-6.

19. *GH,* Vol. 99, No. 2 (Aug. 1934), 106, 138.

20. *GH,* Vol. 100, No. 1 (Jan. 1935), 155.

21. *GH,* Vol. 100, No., 1 (Jan. 1935), 91.

22. *GH,* Vol. 121, No. 6 (Dec. 1943), 7.

23. Paul Radin, *The Italians of San Francisco: Their Adjustment and Acculturation* (San Francisco: 1935) (Reprinted San Francisco: R and E Research, 1970), Vol. 1, 131.

24. F. Eugenia Whitehead, "Nutrition Education for Children in the U.S. Since 1900—Part II," in Adelia Beeuwkes, et. al., *Essays in the History of Nutrition and Dietetics* (Chicago: American Dietetic Association, 1967), 44.

25. John L. and Karen Hess, *The Taste of America* (New York: Grossman, 1977), 255.

26. *GH,* Vol. 121, No. 6 (Dec. 1945), 7.

27. *GH,* Vol. 115, No. 5 (Nov. 1942), 9.

28. Lydia J. Roberts, "Beginnings of the Recommended Daily Allowances," *Journal of the American Dietetic Association* Vol. 34 (1958), 107.

29. Roberts, "Beginnings," 109–11; Margaret M. Conner, "A History of Dietary Standards," in Beeuwkes, et. al., *op. cit.,* 110–13.

30. Margaret Mead, *Food Habits Research: Problems of the 1960's,* National Academy of Sciences-National Research Council Publication 1225 (Washington: GPO, 1964), 1–3; U.S. National Research Council, "Summaries of Committee Conferences," *The Problem of Changing Food Habits* (Washington: GPO, 1943), 127–57; National Research Council, Committee on Food Habits, "Translation of Scientific Findings into Living Habits, Liason Session—May 19, 1945," mimeographed copy in Library of Congress.

31. John W. Bennett, "Food and Social Status in a Riverbottom Society," *American Sociological Review,* Vol. 8, No. 5 (1943), 561–69; Herbert Passin and John W. Bennett, "Social Process and Dietary Change," in NRC, *The Problem of Changing Food Habits,* 113–23.

32. Margaret Cussler and Mary L. De Give, *'Twixt the Cup and the Lip* (Washington: Consortium Press, 1952), 110–15, ix.

33. Jennifer Colton, "Why I Quit Working," *GH,* Sept. 1951, 178.

34. *GH,* Sept. 1956, 145.

35. *GH,* Sept. 1951, 114.

36. *Ibid.,* 11.

37. Lydia Roberts, *Nutrition Work with Children* (Chicago: Univ. of Chicago Press, 1927), 131–38; *Ibid.,* rev., 1935, 201–8; Ethel Martin, *Roberts' Nutrition Work with Children* (Chicago: Univ. of Chicago Press, 1954), chap. 4, 5.

38. Michael Harrington, *The Other America* (New York: Macmillan, 1962).

39. *New York Times,* March 26, 1986.

40. James Harvey Young, "The Agile Role of Food: Some Historical Reflections," *Nutrition and Drug Interrelations* (New York: Academic Press, 1978), 11–12.

41. Bill Rados, "Eggs and Dairy Foods: Dietary Mainstays in Decline," *FDA Consumer,* Vol. 19, No. 8 (Oct. 1985), 11–12.

42. Chris Lecos, "Fish and Fowl Lure Consumers from Red Meat," *ibid.,* 21. The turn towards poultry was also the product of rising beef prices and lower prices for poultry but consumption of fish and seafood, which has soared in recent years despite steadily rising prices, would seem to indicate that this was by no means the whole story.

43. Despite charges that sugar caused cancer and other ailments, consumption of caloric sweeteners has increased quite steadily from the mid-1950s to the mid-1980s, thanks in large part to booming sales of soft drinks. Roger Miller, "Soft Drinks and Six-Packs Quench Our National Thirst," *ibid.,* 24–25.

44. Chris Lecos, "Shopping for the Second Fifty Years," *ibid.,* Vol. 20, No. 6 (July to Aug. 1986), 30.

45. Warren J. Belasco, "'Lite' Economics: Less Food, More Profit," *Radical History Review,* No. 28–30 (1984), 254–78.

46. *NYT,* Nov. 4, 1984.

47. Calvin Tompkins, "Good Cooking," *New Yorker,* Dec. 23, 1974.

48. Even southern Italian food, previously dismissed as little more than pasta and spicy tomato sauce, developed an upper-middle class following.

49. Typically, a food processor in Toronto has done very well by marketing a

full line of supposedly "Mexican food" products to restaurants by assuring them that its powdered seasoning is "adapted to Canadian tastes." Toronto *Globe and Mail,* June 2, 1986.

50. Lecos, "Shopping," 30.

51. Those concerned about chemical additives declined from 27 to 16 percent of those questioned. Those worried about preservatives fell from 22 to 15 percent, and those who wanted "natural" foods and therefore avoided "processed" foods plummeted from 12 to 3 percent. On the other hand, 17 percent of the 1986 sample avoided fats and 11 percent were concerned about calories while those avoiding cholesterol rose from 5 to 13 percent. *Ibid.,* 30.

52. Walter Kiechel III, "Two-Income Families Will Reshape the Consumer Markets," *Fortune,* March 10, 1980, 119, cited in Belasco, "'Lite' Economics," 275.

Index

Abel, Mary Hinman, 55, 75, 80; and
American Home Economics
Association, 59; death of, 231n.48;
Lomb Prize essay, 48, 57; and
public kitchens, 48, 49, 50–51, 52;
on the servant problem, 63–64;
view of working classes, 53, 56, 58
Acidosis, 153–154, 209
Adams, John, on molasses, 214n.13
Adams Act of 1906, 78
Addams, Jane, 100, 105, 142
Additives, food, 39, 204, 209; to
restore nutrients, 158
Advertising and promotion of food,
32–36, 39, 123–124, 152–160,
197–198; Food Administration
borrowed tactics from, 138, 139;
for infants, 123–124; during
1930s, 197–198; and pure-food
scare, 40; vitamins a boon to, 149
Alabama, regional dinner menus, 171
Aladdin Oven, 48, 49, 50, 51, 52,
58; later versions of, 221n.8; price
of, 54; shortcomings of, 54
Alcohol abuse: coffee and alcohol,
99–100; and poor food, 49,

222n.11; and strong seasonings,
103. *See also* Temperance advocates
Allen, Ida C. Bailey, 139–140
Allen, Walter, 266n.4
American Child Health Association,
155
American cooking: defined by
restaurateurs, 170; regional, 171;
William Allen White on, 171–172
American Federation of Labor, 26,
144
American Home Economics
Association, 59, 75, 76, 139;
relations with food processors, 156
American Journal of Public Health, on
workers' diet, 108
American Kitchen Magazine, 78, 84
American Pediatric Society, 124–125
American Public Health Association,
48, 99–100
American Red Cross, 159–160
American Sugar Refining Company,
32
Americanization of immigrants, 157,
176
Anderson, Elizabeth Milbank, 116

261